Advances in Online Therapy

Advances in Online Therapy is the definitive presentation on online psychological intervention, which takes research and experiences of online therapy a step further by applying them to therapy in a post-pandemic world.

This book addresses most of the main approaches and schools of individual, couple and family psychotherapy that are prevalent in the therapeutic field nowadays and explores how each of them adjust to online therapy. The reader will explore the main challenges and obstacles unique for each approach and how leading experts of those approaches overcome these challenges. The book also offers a relatively unique collection of the most practiced therapeutic approaches. In addition, the reader will explore specific issues that anyone who meets clients online should be aware of, like who is suitable for online counseling and who should be excluded, how to overcome resistance to online meetings, how to create online therapeutic alliance, enhancing online presence, and more. This book develops further the ideas and areas explored in the authors' previous book, *Theory and Practice of Online Therapy*.

Advances in Online Therapy aims to help mental health professionals and graduate students responsibly explore and expand their own 'online comfort zone'.

Haim Weinberg, PhD, is a clinical psychologist, group analyst, and certified group psychotherapist in California, USA.

Arnon Rolnick, PhD, is a licensed clinical psychologist with special interest in the usage of technology in psychotherapy in Tel-Aviv, Israel.

Adam Leighton is a counsellor, group facilitator, wilderness therapy facilitator, and lecturer at Ruppin Academic Center, Israel.

Library of Technology and Mental Health

Series Editor: Jill Savege Scharff, M.D.

This series, established in 2011, features authors from various parts of the global economy discuss the effects of technology on our growth and development, our relationships, our society in general, and the relevance of communication by telephone and internet to the spread of psychoanalysis. They discuss the impact of internet addiction including pornography, the effects of screen time and social media, and the value of telepsychotherapy, telepsychoanalysis, and telesupervision, all illustrated with clinical examples, ethical considerations, and personal reflections. The series editor is Jill Savege Scharff.

Distance Psychoanalysis: The Theory and Practice of Using Communication Technology in the Clinic (2011)
by Ricardo Carlino, translated by James Nuss

Psychoanalysis Online: Mental Health, Teletherapy, and Training (2013)
edited by Jill Savege Scharff

Screen Relations (2014)
by Gillian Russell

Psychoanalysis Online 2 Impact of Technology on Development, Training and Therapy (2015)
edited by Jill Savege Scharff

Psychoanalysis, Identity and the Internet: Explorations into Cyberspace (2016)
edited by Andrea Marzi

Psychoanalysis Online 3: The Teleanalytic Setting (2017)
edited by Jill Savege Scharff

Psychoanalysis Online 4: Teleanalytic Practice, Teaching, and Clinical Research (2019)
edited by Jill Savege Scharff

Advances in Online Therapy: Emergence of a New Paradigm (2023)
by Haim Weinberg, Arnon Rolnick, and Adam Leighton

"This is by far the best resource to access the accumulated therapeutic experience of remote working which has, by now, become part of all therapists' routine practice. Every therapist, regardless of orientation, should be required carefully to study the brilliant advice from the collection of master therapists the editors assembled as these clinicians adapted their practice to online working. Packed full of immediately applicable practical wisdom, this immediate classic gives us hope that with creativity and flexibility, psychological therapists are able to modify their technique and generate remarkable improvement in their clients whatever limitations are imposed on their communication medium. Undoubtedly, the most helpful book of 2022."

Professor Peter Fonagy, OBE, FMedSci, FAcSS, FBA, PhD.
Head of the Division of Psychology and Language Sciences at UCL
Chief Executive of the Anna Freud National Centre for
Children and Families, London

"This rich and comprehensive edited collection could not be more timely as we all grapple with the opportunities and challenges presented by online therapy. The editors have done an impressive job bringing together chapters on the main approaches and schools of psychotherapy inviting the contributors to reflect on how their approach has adjusted and learnt from the shift to online therapy. This is a wonderful resource and deserves to be the go-to reference book on all psychotherapy trainings."

Professor Alessandra Lemma, *fellow of British Psychoanalytic Society*
Visiting Professor, Psychoanalysis Unit, University College London and
author of "The Digital Age on the Couch"

"Online therapy is no longer unusual. After the COVID years the average therapist now has now conducted psychotherapy in a video-based online form many times. The public has come to expect that they can access and benefit from expert therapists who live far from their own hometown. These are positive changes but making online therapy work requires acknowledging and addressing its challenges in a flexible, creative, and effective way. This comprehensive volume shows you how. In a careful, systematic way it addresses setting, engagement, and the alliance; adjustments in all the major forms of psychotherapy are explored across individuals, couples, and families. Regardless of your approach, setting, or population you will find something useful on almost every page. It should be obvious to all that online therapy is here to stay – it's time to master this tool for the benefit of the lives of those we serve. Highly recommended."

Steven C. Hayes, Ph.D. *Foundation Professor of Psychology*
University of Nevada, Reno. Originator of Acceptance and
Commitment Therapy, and author of "A Liberated Mind:
How to Pivot Toward What Matters"

"An amazingly comprehensive compendium of reflections on teletherapy from therapists working from a wider range of theoretical approaches. This span makes it a terrific textbook for students of psychology, social work and counseling who are learning not only teletreatment but the range of treatment approaches, and a helpful, and very timely resource for therapists who were forced into COVID-imposed teletherapy. There's lots of useful information here on the impact of technology, the sense of intrigue that accompanies the transition from the office to the virtual space,the maintenance of empathy, the use of the whiteboard, and above all the otherness of the self that is discovered on the screen in video."

Jill Savege Scharff, MD, FABP. *Co-founder of The International Psychotherapy Institute; Clinical Professor of Psychiatry, Georgetown University Washington DC; and editor of Psychoanalysis Online Vols 1, 2, 3 and 4*

"This well-written, comprehensive and authoritative collection of articles by experienced clinicians and researchers gives a complete and state-of-the-art overview of online therapy. Anyone considering to start providing online therapy should read this book and for therapists who already work with online therapies it provides a handbook to broaden their scope and knowledge. A highly recommended book."

Professor Pim Cuijpers, Ph.D. *Department of Clinical, Neuro and Developmental Psychology, Vrije Universiteit Amsterdam, The Netherlands and director of the World Health Organization (WHO) Collaborating Centre for Research and Dissemination of Psychological Interventions, and the author of hundreds peer reviewed articles on internet based therapy*

Advances in Online Therapy

Emergence of a New Paradigm

Edited by Haim Weinberg, Arnon Rolnick, and Adam Leighton

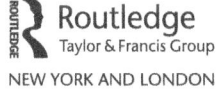

Routledge
Taylor & Francis Group
NEW YORK AND LONDON

Cover image: Getty Image

First published 2023
by Routledge
605 Third Avenue, New York, NY 10158

and by Routledge
4 Park Square, Milton Park, Abingdon, Oxon, OX14 4RN

Routledge is an imprint of the Taylor & Francis Group, an informa business

© 2023 selection and editorial matter, Haim Weinberg, Arnon
Rolnick, and Adam Leighton; individual chapters, the contributors

The right of Haim Weinberg, Arnon Rolnick, and Adam Leighton to
be identified as the authors of the editorial material, and of the authors
for their individual chapters, has been asserted in accordance with
sections 77 and 78 of the Copyright, Designs and Patents Act 1988.

All rights reserved. No part of this book may be reprinted or
reproduced or utilised in any form or by any electronic, mechanical,
or other means, now known or hereafter invented, including
photocopying and recording, or in any information storage or retrieval
system, without permission in writing from the publishers.

Trademark notice: Product or corporate names may be trademarks or
registered trademarks, and are used only for identification and
explanation without intent to infringe.

ISBN: 978-1-032-07025-4 (hbk)
ISBN: 978-1-032-07024-7 (pbk)
ISBN: 978-1-003-20502-9 (ebk)

DOI: 10.4324/9781003205029

Typeset in Baskerville
by MPS Limited, Dehradun

Contents

Contributors

Haim Weinberg, Arnon Rolnick, Adam Leighton, Introduction

Haim Weinberg, Ph.D., is a clinical psychologist, group analyst and certified group psychotherapist. He is the past president of the Israeli Association of Group Psychotherapy and of the Northern California Group Psychotherapy Society. He co-edits a series of books on the social unconscious and about online therapy.

Arnon Rolnick, Ph.D., is a licensed clinical psychologist with special interest in the usage of technology in psychotherapy. He is a certified supervisor in CBT and biofeedback and has written numerous articles on these subjects. Arnon is the head of a clinic in Tel-Aviv, Israel, which integrates various psychotherapeutic approaches.

Adam Leighton is a counsellor, group facilitator and wilderness therapy facilitator. Adam specialises in highly experiential approaches to therapy combining technology, outdoor work and ACT therapy. He established and teaches the CBT based Group Facilitation combining Outdoor Experiential Work course at the Ruppin Academic Centre.

Section I Theoretical Aspects of Online Therapy

1 Shari Geller, Cultivating Therapeutic Presence in Teletherapy.

Shari Geller, Ph.D., C. Psych., is an author, clinical psychologist, and mindful self-compassion (MSC) teacher. Shari offers training modules in therapeutic presence internationally as part of a longer-term vision of having therapeutic presence be a foundational training across psychotherapy approaches. Her publications include the books: A Practical Guide for Cultivating Therapeutic Presence, and Therapeutic Presence: A Mindful Approach to Effective Therapy co-authored with Dr. Leslie Greenberg (second edition available in October, 2022). Shari is the co-director of the Centre of MindBody Health. www.cmbh.space www.sharigeller.ca

2 Danielle Magaldi, Leora Trub, Finding Closeness while Socially Distant: Clinical Considerations for the Therapeutic Frame and Process in Teletherapy

Danielle Magaldi, Ph.D., is an Associate Professor at the City University of New York, Lehman College and a practicing psychologist. She has authored numerous chapters and articles on two under-explored research areas: the clinical implications for therapy when working with religious patients, and the impact of new technologies on our many relationships—in families, romantic attachment, adolescent development, and the therapeutic dyad. She maintains a private practice in New York City, where she works with children, adolescents, adults and couples.

Leora Trub is a practicing psychologist based in New York City, where she works with adolescents, adults and couples. She is an associate professor of psychology in the school/clinical-child PsyD program at Pace University, where she is involved in clinical training of doctoral candidates. She also runs the Digital Media and Psychology lab, which explores how technologies affect our conceptions of ourselves and our relationships with others, as well as the underlying psychological and emotional needs they meet.

3 Lou Agosta, Reflections on Empathic Presence in Online Therapeutic Relations

Lou Agosta, Ph.D., is the author of three peer-reviewed and three popular books on empathy including A Rumor of Empathy. He is a professor of medical education delivering empathy lessons at Ross Medical University at Saint Anthony Hospital, Chicago, USA. He is an empathy consultant in private practice in the Chicago area.

4 Athena Marouda – Chatjoulis, Evdokia Ntali, The Untouched – touched: Intimacy and intersubjectivity online

Athena Marouda-Chatjoulis, MSc, Ph.D, is the founder and the director of the Institute of Psychosocial Development (IPSA), Larissa, Greece. She is psychodynamic psychotherapist, group analyst, member and trainer at the Hellenic Institute for Group Analytic and Family Psychotherapy. Her research and publications are in the field of Social Psychology in the areas of interpersonal relationships, conflict resolution and decision making, and in the field of Group Analysis. She has recently retired from the position of Associate Professor in the Department of Communication and Media Studies at the University of Athens.

Evdokia Ntali is a clinical, military psychologist (PhD), collaborator of the Department of Communication and Media Studies of the National & Kapodistrian University of Athens. Her research interests focus on studying how transitional and disruptive events (personal, socio-economic) affect individual's psychic life and how new technologies mediate in these processes. She is also a trainee member of the Hellenic Society of Psychoanalytic Group Psychotherapy.

5 Vered Bar, Me and my "Otherness" or Who is the other on screen who looks exactly like me?

Vered Bar, Psy.D. Lecturer at Reichman University in master's degree programs in social psychology and organizational behavior, Senior consultant to Managers and Organizations.

Author of the book "The Split Whole - Benign Dissociation in Groups and Organizations". (Resling, 2021)

6 Hadas Mor Ofek, Zooming in Zoom: Mental-Body-Brain perspectives on Online psychotherapy sessions

Hadas Mor-Ofek, Ph.D., is a senior clinical psychologist and a supervisor. In her clinical work she integrates psychoanalytic oriented psychotherapy, cognitive-behavioral therapy and body-oriented psychotherapy. She is studying and writing about clinical implications of neuroscience. Dr. Mor-Ofek is a director of a psychotherapy training program.

Section II Individual Therapies – Specific Modalities

7 Chelsey R. Wilks, Kyrill Gurtovenko, Telehealth Delivery of Dialectical Behavior Therapy

Chelsey Wilks, Ph.D., is a clinical psychologist, assistant professor and health and data science at the University of Missouri-St. Louis. Dr. Wilks' research is in the development and evaluation of digital tools to augment and supplant therapy.

Kyrill Gurtovenko, Ph.D., is faculty in the Department of Psychiatry and Behavioral Sciences at the University of Washington and an attending psychologist at Seattle Children's Hospital. His current areas of interest and expertise include assessment and intervention for adolescent suicidality, self-injury and emotion dysregulation, Dialectical Behavior Therapy (DBT), and parenting interventions.

8 Hagara Feldman, Schema Therapy in the Online Setting – from Challenges to Opportunities

Hagara Feldman is an advanced schema therapist, supervisor and trainer; the director of "Schema Therapy Kfar Saba", which provides an ISST approved Schema Therapy accreditation program in Israel; and also, an accredited CBT supervisor. She practiced in both the public and the private sectors, in mental health and in bariatric services. She is working with various cultural groups in and outside of Israel and develops international workshops focusing on Online Schema Therapy.

9 Andrew Curreri, Molly Fitzpatrick, David Barlow, Elizabeth Eustis, Implementing the Unified Protocol via Telehealth: Adaptations and Considerations

Andrew Curreri, M.A. is a doctoral candidate in clinical psychology at Boston University, where he studies transdiagnostic approaches to understanding and treating emotional disorders. He is particularly interested in cognitive processes in emotional disorders, including repetitive negative thinking, and innovations in transdiagnostic interventions, including psychedelic-assisted psychotherapy.

Molly E. Fitzpatrick, M.A. is a Clinical Psychology Doctoral Student at William James College and holds a Clinical Fellow appointment at Harvard Medical School. Her research and clinical interests include forensic psychology, global mental health, and policy and systems-levelchange. She is currently completing her advanced practicum training on the Pediatric Inpatient Service at Cambridge Health Alliance/Harvard Medical School.

David H. Barlow, Ph.D., is Professor of Psychology and Psychiatry, Emeritus and the Founder of the Center for Anxiety and Related Disorders at Boston University. He has published over 650 articles and chapters and over 90 books and clinical manuals. He is the recipient of numerous awards, including honorary degrees from the University of Vermont and William James College, and the two highest awards in psychology, the Distinguished Scientific Award for Applications of Psychology from the American Psychological Association and James McKeen Cattell Fellow Award from the Association for Psychological Science.

Elizabeth H. Eustis, Ph.D., is a Research Assistant Professor in the Department of Psychological and Brain Sciences at Boston University. She received her Ph.D. in clinical psychology from the University of Massachusetts Boston, completed her pre-doctoral internship at The Warren Alpert Medical School of Brown University, and completed her post-doctoral fellowship at the Center for Anxiety and Related Disorders at Boston University.

10 Galit Mor, Remote Art Therapy: Engaging in a Shared Experience

Galit Mor - MAAT, BFA and a clinical Art therapy Ph.D. student at Bar-Ilan University (BIU). Her current research focuses on processing transference - counter transference through art interventions in supervision. She is an Art Therapist since 2004, an experienced supervisor, certified by the Israel Association of Art Therapists (YAHAT), and an artist. Galit practices clinical and Art -Based- supervision at her private clinic and in the public sector. As a supervisor, she is works with university students of Art Therapy, therapists, and treatment teams including educational institutes, dealing with patients, experiencing mental health issues. Galit leads workshops and teaches therapist art-based interventions, assessment methods and remote art- therapy interventions.

11 Joop Meijers, Zooming in on Experiential Dynamic Therapies

Joop Meijers, Ph.D., is a clinical Psychologist and supervisor, practicing in Jerusalem, Israel. He is specialised in Cognitive Behavior Therapy and Experiential Dynamic Therapies. In the past he was Chair of the Division of Clinical Child Psychology at the Hebrew University of Jerusalem and Chair of the Israeli Association of Cognitive-Behavior Therapy. He has written many articles and books and trained with the late Aaron Beck and Albert Ellis.

12 Brunstein Klomek Anat, Anaelle Benistri, Online-IPT- not necessarily a second best

Anat Brunstein Klomek, Ph.D., is the Dean of Baruch Ivcher School of Psychology, a clinical psychologist, Head of the Master's Program in Clinical Psychology between 2018 and 2021 at Reichman University (IDC Herzliya). Prof. Brunstein Klomek completed her post-doctoral fellowship and was an Assistant Professor in the Department of Child and Adolescent Psychiatry at Columbia University in New York. In the last years she is the academic advisor of the Israel Ministries of Health and Education as part of the national suicide prevention program.

Anaelle Benistri is a clinical psychology intern, with a B.A in psychology and education from The Hebrew University of Jerusalem and a M.A in clinical psychology from Reichman University in Israel. Her current intership is at Baruch Ivcher School of Psychology clinic in Reichman University, she provides psychotherapy to aldults, children and adolescents with a variety of psychological distress. She was co-author of a research article about the moderating role of working alliance in the association between depression and suicide ideation in messaging therapy.

13 Udi Oren, Isabelle Meignant, Online EMDR Therapy in the COVID-19 Era and Beyond

Udi Oren, Ph.D., is a licensed clinical and medical psychologist. He is an EMDR Europe accredited senior trainer, the co-founder and chairman of the Israel EMDR Association, and is the past president of the EMDR Europe Association. He is also the founder of the Israeli EMDR institute, the Israeli Center for EMDR, and of iMotion Wellness Solutions LTD.

Isabelle Meignant, M.A., is a French clinical psychologist, systémique therapist and an EMDR Europe accredited senior trainer. She is past vice-president of EMDR France, the founder and director of the school: Ecole Française de Psychothérapie EMDR, EFPE, and is the founder and president of the NGO: Action EMDR Trauma, AET. She is the author of the EMDR book for kids drawn by her sister, Cécile Meignant: Buddy the dog EMDR.

14 Yossi Ehrenreich, Arnon Rolnick, Adam Leighton, Getting a Little Closer in Every Session: The unique contribution of remote Biofeedback to psychotherapy

Yossi Ehrenreich, Ph.D., is a Senior School Psychologist (Supervisor). Licensed in Hypnosis, a certified Biofeedback and Neurofeedback practitioner and supervisor in Israel. Yossi is the chairman of the Israeli Association for Applied Psychophysiology and Biofeedback, and an adjunct lecturer at the Peres Academic Center, Rehovot. Yossi specializes in technology-based integrative psychotherapy that includes Biofeedback, Neurofeedback, and tDCS within a psychotherapy session. Yossi was the professional director at Neuroclinic: non-pharmaceutical psychiatric clinic.

15 Joseph Meyerson, Interactive Hypnosis and Hypnotic Psychotherapy Online

Joseph Meyerson, Ph.D., is a clinical and medical psychologist, hypnotic psychotherapist, supervisor, and manager at HypnoClinic, a state-approved institute for hypnosis education and training in Tel Aviv. Joseph is a Co-President of the Israeli Psychosomatic Society, Past President of the Israeli Society of Hypnosis, and Senior staff member of the Master of Arts program in Medical Psychology at Max Stern Yezreel Valley College. Joseph Meyerson has authored several papers and a book chapter on hypnotic and strategic psychotherapy, particularly on the use of dissociative-associative strategies and paramnesias in hypnotherapy.

Section III Couples & Families

16 Arnon Rolnick, Adam Leighton, Haim Weinberg, Introduction to Couple and Family Therapy

Haim Weinberg

Arnon Rolnick

Adam Leighton

17 Lorrie Brubacher, Ting Liu, Emotionally Focused Couple Therapy Online: Handholding from a Distance

Lorrie L. Brubacher is the Founding Director of the Carolina Center for EFT (Emotionally Focused Therapy). A certified trainer with the International Centre for Excellence in EFT (ICEEFT), she trains internationally, is an adjunct at University of North Carolina, Greensboro and is a therapist since 1989. Her book Stepping into Emotionally Focused Couple Therapy: Key Ingredients of Change (Routledge, 2018) is currently in 7 languages. She co-developed EFT's first interactive video training program on the EFT Attachment Injury Resolution Model and has produced many EFT couple and individual training videos.

Ting Liu, Ph.D., is a certified EFT trainer, supervisor and therapist. She is the clinical director of the Philadelphia Center for EFT and the director of the Asian Association of Emotionally focused Couple and Family Therapy. She maintains a Private Practice in Wayne, PA and provides EFT trainings internationally. Dr. Liu received her doctorate in Child Development and Family Studies with a specialization in Marriage and Family Therapy from Purdue University. She completed a postdoctoral fellowship at the Center for Family Intervention Science at Children's Hospital of Philadelphia.

18 Mirisse Foroughe, Prakash Thambipillai, Adapting Emotion Focused Therapies for Online Delivery

Mirisse Foroughe, Ph.D., is a Clinical Psychologist and Director of Clinical Training and Research at the Family Psychology Centre. She has over 20 years of experience providing assessment and treatment to children, adolescents, and families and has expertise in Emotion Focused Therapy (EFT), Cognitive Behavioural Therapy (CBT), Dialectical Behaviour Therapy (DBT), Emotion Focused Family Therapy (EFFT), Family-Based Treatment (Maudsley FBT), and Motivational Interviewing (MI). Dr. Foroughe currently oversees clinical services at the Family Psychology Centre, providing training and supervision to the clinical team, as well as directs the Emotion Transformation Institute, a clinical research lab.

Prakash Thambipillai is a M.Sc candidate in Clinical Psychology at Queen's University. He worked closely with Dr. Mirisse Foroughe studying the effectiveness of Emotion-Focused Family Therapy interventions at the Family Psychology Centre. His research interests are related to the physiological basis of emotion regulation, and the role of trauma and the family system in the emotion socialization process.

19 Shoshana Hellman, Don Cole, Arnon Rolnick, Gottman Method: Assessment and Treatment in the Age of Online Therapy

Shoshana Hellman, Ed.D. is a psychologist, licensed couple and family therapist and the first Certified Gottmn couple therapist,consultant and trainer in Israel. She works in private practice both in Israel and US, after many years of experience in the Psychological services of the Ministry of Education in Israel and being a faculty at the University of Wisconsin Madison.

Don Cole, D. Min., is the Clinical Director for The Gottman Institute and a licensed mental health counselor in the state of Washington. As a Certified Gottman Method Couples' Therapist and a member of the Gottman Relationship Institute and a master trainer in Gottman Method Therapy, he teaches all levels of the Gottman Method Certification Program. Dr. Cole has written numerous workshops and articles based on the Gottman Method of couples therapy.

20 Kalanit Ben Ari, Healing Through the Screen: Using Imago Relationship Therapy Online.

Kalanit Ben-Ari, Ph.D., is a psychologist, psychotherapist and author. She has worked as a senior family and couples therapist for over 20 years and has a private clinic in London. Kalanit is also the Chair of Imago Relationship Therapy UK since 2013, trainer, an international speaker, supervisor, and she is an Associate member of the Imago International Training Institute.

21 Bob and Rita Resnick, Online Contemporary Couples Gestalt Therapy "Two Become One" - and Then There are None!

Rita F. Resnick, Ph.D. Gestalt Therapist since 1974 and Gestalt Trainer since 1986. Faculty Chair since 1997 of the premier annual European Summer Residential Gestalt Therapy Training program with over 125 participants from 30 different countries with an amazing return rate of 80%. In addition to her private practice, Rita is actively training psychotherapists in the United States, Australia, Europe, and Central Asia in both Gestalt and Couples Therapy.

Robert W. Resnick, Ph.D. Trained, (Passed away as this book went to press) mentored and certified by Fritz Perls the co-developer of Gestalt Therapy. Chosen by Perls in 1969 to introduce Gestalt Therapy to Europe where he spent several months each year for almost fifty-five years where there are now tens of thousands of Gestalt Therapists. Awarded the APA Division 29 (Psychotherapy) 2019 Distinguished Award For the International Advancement Of Psychotherapy.

Section IV Specific Populations

22 Mary V. Tipton, Josh Brenner, Jennifer Crumlish, Melinda Moore & David A. Jobes, Online Suicide-Focused Treatment: The Telehealth Use of CAMS.

Mary Tipton is a clinical psychology doctoral student at The Catholic University of America (CUA). She is a graduate research assistant in the Suicide Prevention Lab run by Dr. David A. Jobes at CUA. Mary has clinical and research interests in the prevention of suicide death in young children, adolescents, and youth adults.

Josh Brenner is a clinical psychology doctoral student at The Catholic University of America (CUA), and he is a research assistant in the Suicide Prevention Lab ran by Dr. Dave Jobes at CUA. Josh has both clinical and research interests in suicide and trauma within active-duty military and veteran populations.

Jennifer Crumlish, Ph.D., in clinical psychology at The Catholic University of America and is Board Certified in Clinical Psychology by the American Board of Professional Psychology. Dr. Crumlish is the Assistant Director of the Suicide Prevention Lab at the Catholic University of America. Dr. Crumlish is a Senior Consultant for CAMS-care, where she has conducted training for clinicians employed in several state correctional facilities, military behavioral health centers and community mental health centers. Dr. Crumlish also maintains a private practice as a partner at the Washington Psychological Center (WPC) where she works with adolescents, adults and couples.

Melinda Moore, Ph.D., is an Associate Professor in the Department of Psychology at Eastern Kentucky University in Richmond, Kentucky, and part of the core faculty for the Clinical Psychology doctoral program. She routinely trains clinicians in the suicide focused treatment framework, Collaborative Assessment and Management of Suicidality, and is in private practice in Lexington, Kentucky.

David Jobes, Ph.D., is a Professor of Psychology, Associate Director of Clinical Training, and Director of the Suicide Prevention Laboratory at The Catholic University of America. He is the creator of the Collaborative Assessment and Management of Suicidality (CAMS), which is an evidence-based, suicide-focused, clinical intervention supported by extensive clinical trial research. He has published six books on clinical suicidology and numerous peer-reviewed articles in suicide prevention and mental health ethics and risk management

23 Mooli Lahad, Miki Doron, Dori Rubinstein, Reactivating playfulness online for PTSD treatment

Mooli Lahad, Ph.D., full professor of Psychology Tel Hai College, has two PhDs. Founder and president of the Community Stress Prevention Center (CSPC). One of the world leading experts on the integration of the artsform therapies and psychotrauma /coping with disasters Author and co-author of 35 books, recipient of six national and international awards.

Miki Doron, senior psychologist. Formerly Chief Mental Health Officer at the IDF. Head of Israeli association of focused psychotherapy. Coordinator of the program for resilience in Israel's ministry of justice. Co-founder of SEE FAR CBT clinical protocol (with Prof. Mooli Lahad). Author of the book Trauma and its Treatment.

Dori Rubinstein Ph.D. Faculty of Health Sciences, Ben-Gurion University of the Negev. Research in the field of Imagination and PTSD. Clinical Psychologist, lecturer at Tel-Hai Academic College. Head of research department and clinical development - Community Stress Prevention Center (CSPC), Kiryat Shmona, Israel. Clinical adviser and teacher of clinical oriented topics (including SEE FAR CBT, trauma and resilience programs).

24 Kristen Holderle, Jeffrey Iler, Online ACT: Adapting Focused Acceptance and Commitment Therapy for Individuals with Childhood-Onset Medical and Developmental Disabilities.

Kristen Holderle, Ph.D., is a licensed psychologist and Assistant Professor of Psychiatry and Pediatrics at the University of Rochester Medical Center in Rochester, NY. She specializes in the use of ACT-based interventions for individuals with co-occurring medical and psychiatric concerns.

Jeffrey Iler, M.D. is an assistant professor of clinical psychiatry at the University of Rochester in Rochester, NY. He completed medical school at the University of Toledo College of Medicine and Life Sciences, residency at Dartmouth-Hitchcock Medical Center, and fellowship at Yale-New Haven Medical Center. Dr. Iler works embedded in the primary care network at the University of Rochester, assisting primary care providers to meet the needs of their patients outside of traditional mental health settings.

25 Brian Keating, Diving into the World of Online Play Therapy

Brian Keating, M.A. LPC is a licensed professional counselor providing telehealth services to Colorado residents through his private practice Deep Listening Psychotherapy, LLC. As a Certified Synergetic Play Therapist and Certified Group Psychotherapist, Brian enjoys working with patients of all ages. Previously working as a professional musician for 12 years, he is grateful that his skill and appreciation for deep listening has been an asset in both fields.

Introduction

Haim Weinberg, Arnon Rolnick, and Adam Leighton

Why Another Book on Online Therapy?

In the midst of 2019, a few months before the outbreak of the COVID-19 pandemic, two of the editors of this book (Weinberg & Rolnick) published their needed and well-received book "Theory and Practice of Online Therapy", which since has been translated into multiple languages. What's happened since then that necessitates a new book?

The quick answer is the COVID-19 pandemic. During the pandemic there was a mass transition of therapists to online therapy, according to one survey an estimate of 98% of therapists used online therapy during the pandemic (Sampaio et al., 2021). This vast amount of health care professionals working online have created a huge body of experience, knowledge, research, and academic articles. The number of research studies about online therapy jumped exponentially in the past two years. This book attempts to share a carefully chosen part of this accumulated knowledge.

The massive transition to online therapy and online work in general has indirectly influenced other aspects. Online therapy is rapidly becoming more available due to improvements in technology, user experience, and slowly reduced internal barriers (such as our fears and ambivalent approach). Although there are still barriers, as you will read in Lou Agosta's chapter (Chapter 3), they are rapidly diminishing, therefore the scope and boundaries of what is perceived as possible in online therapy are changing. Our "online comfort zone" may still be presently limited by client characteristics, such as age or suicidality (Chapters 25 by Keating & 22 by Tipton, Brenner, Crumlish, Moore & Jobes), and possibly by therapeutic modality (can you really perform online hypnosis? Biofeedback? EMDR? Read Chapters 15 by Meyerson, 14 by Ehrenreich, Rolnick & Leighton, and 13 by Oren and Meignant).

Our previous book, mentioned above, was divided into four parts, relating to working online with individuals, couples, groups, and even organizations. In this book we go even further: we tried to address most of the main approaches and schools of psychotherapy that are prevalent in the therapeutic field nowadays, and to explore how each of them adjust to online therapy.

DOI: 10.4324/9781003205029-1

What are the main challenges and obstacles unique for each approach and how do leading experts of those approaches overcome these challenges? Without a deliberate intent, we also created a collection of the most practiced therapeutic approaches in this book. It was not easy to choose the methods to be represented in the book. There are hundreds of methods of different psychological modalities (Wikipedia for example counts approximately 200 different approaches. Other sources present even higher numbers). We received dozens of suggestions and abstracts, from which we selected those who were able to describe the modality and its adaptation to remote work.

At first glance, one might think that dynamic psychotherapy and especially the intersubjective approach – is only partially represented. However, at closer look, the question of the therapeutic relationship appears in almost every chapter, again some chapters dealing with more general issues come from a dynamic orientation.

Describing their proposed framework, Process Based Therapy, Hayes and Hoffman (2021) wrote: "While useful knowledge has emerged from each of these eras, it is time to focus on a set of organizing principles that will allow what is most important in our knowledge base to be used by all researchers and practitioners interested in evidence-based care. For that to happen, we need to reconsider what evidence-based care even is." (p. 368)

We believe that the transition to online therapy offers another opportunity to reexamine psychotherapy in general and our own practice specifically and we believe that this book will facilitate this process. We hope that this book will furthermore help mental health professionals responsibly explore and expand their own "online comfort zone."

How do We Define Online Therapy and What is Included in this Book?

Online therapy is a broad term and can be interpreted in many ways. We have chosen to focus on video-based human-facilitated psychotherapy, that is to say psychotherapy sessions online, similar to those carried out in face-to-face sessions in a clinic.

This is not to say that other forms of online are less valid. There are various hybrid platforms offering text-based sessions combined with computer-assisted interventions, which provide considerable value to their users. We have examined AI-based text bots providing for example CBT-based sessions. In our epilog, we briefly describe additional technologies which may support remote therapy. However, our key interest is how the transition to online therapy may and can impact therapeutic elements of "traditional" psychotherapy sessions.

For those seeking to learn about the "mechanics" of online therapy, specifics regarding legal issues, ethical dilemmas, or detailed descriptions of setting or software platform, we suggest either reading through "Theory and Practice of Online Therapy" or additional books available on the topic.

Flexibility and Creativity as the Main Factors:

Keywords: Flexibility and Creativity

"The secret of change is to focus all of your energy not on fighting the old, but on building the new" – Socrates.

We asked the authors of the chapters for this book, each of them representing a different approach to therapy, to clarify the main challenges for shifting their frame of reference to online therapy. Reviewing the many different approaches to therapy throughout the book, we found out that many of them related to factors pointed out in our first book (in Weinberg & Rolnick 2020: introduction to the book): mainly the questions of presence, the disembodied environment, and the loss of the ability to construct the setting and to create the holding environment. Some of the authors expand and elaborate on these factors beyond what we have written in the first book, and we join them, adding some more thoughts about these factors in this introduction.

However, we also noticed that some of the writers emphasized, directly or indirectly, another factor: the question of flexibility, which is probably one of the main factors that impacts the outcome of online therapy. Once we stop being obsessed with the question how similar online therapy is to in-person therapy (still a common error which we warned against in our previous book) and acknowledge that it is NOT the same as in-person therapy, that the setting is not controlled and structured by the therapist, that failures of communication are inevitable, that it's difficult to establish conditions of safety and a holding environment – we have to flex the usual rigid boundaries and rules of conservative psychotherapy. Perhaps this is the main threat for more traditional therapists, since immediately the question that might pop up is: "how flexible should we become?"

Here is an example: A client in online meetings seemed quite constrained and quiet for a long time in the sessions. When the therapist inquired what is happening to him and why he is so quiet and passive, he revealed that he is having serious problems in his marriage, but since he is connecting from home and the walls in his house are thin, he does not feel that it's safe to talk about his intimate issues and difficulties in his relationship with his wife when she is behind the wall. The therapist suggested that the patient will go to his parked car and connect from there.

This simple example shows that if we want to adjust ourselves to the new conditions of online therapy, we must be flexible, especially regarding the setting and boundaries of the sessions. This flexibility negates the long tradition of psychodynamic psychotherapy, which assumes that the therapist should establish rigid boundaries in order to guarantee a better holding environment. Since we should be aware that online, at least half of the setting is determined by the clients (they choose a quiet room with privacy), we cannot strictly attach to the old notion that the therapist is the only one controlling the setting. It means that we share responsibility with the clients for creating a safe environment, recruiting their ego functions and strength, and preventing some deeper regression.

Together with the need to become flexible when working online, comes the need to be more creative in finding solutions to the inherent obstacles. If you are an art therapist, how do you encourage your client to create their art piece, and how do you participate in the process of this creation? If you work with children, how do you set the boundaries from afar to keep them safe, and how do you join their spontaneous playing at home? If you are a psychodynamic oriented therapist, how do you use the personal information revealed through your natural home background (assuming that you decided not to use the virtual background or the blurred one), to advance the therapy and explore transference issues? All these examples and questions require creative answers. You can find some examples and creative ways for these questions in Galit Mor's (chapter 10), showing how to create a shared experience online, or in Brian Keating's chapter (Chapter 25) manifesting how he used his own countertransference in therapy. Using creativity, we can also overcome the challenge that is inherent in remote therapy: How to create a mutual shared experience when the therapist and the client are in different locations (see Mor, no. 10 and Ehrenreich, no. 14)

More About the Therapeutic Setting

Setting is an important concept in psychotherapy and is related to the "technical laws" according to Freud. Triest (2011) writes about the changes this concept went through along the history of psychoanalysis, creating different types of setting. He defines the setting as the characteristics of the framework and system of laws that are set a priori to ensure the environmental conditions necessary for the existence and effective conduct of the treatment. The therapist creates and maintains the setting in order to advance the work of treatment, ensure and secure it as much as possible from disturbances, "noises," and bruises, whether conscious or unconscious.

Trieste refers to two principal conceptions of the setting: The formal aspects ("the law of the father"): Meeting time, duration, frequency, payment, and method of payment. The basic rules included neutrality, anonymity, and abstinence of the therapist. They were emphasized by Freud's successors, and heightened the rigid aspect of the therapeutic setting, dictated by a rigid and forbidding father figure. In fact, most of those rigid elements of the setting do not change in online therapy (or can easily be obtained) and sometimes they are even strengthened by the new paradigm (e.g., abstinence).

With the formulation of object relations theory through the writings of Melanie Klein and later Winnicott, the concept of the treatment framework became more affected by the mother figure: The holding environment was conceived as a womb, warm, safe, containing, and protected from the outside world. This aspect is usually the one that psychoanalytic-oriented therapists are concerned about while moving online. When we take care of this holding environment, instead of the patient being required to adapt to reality, reality (at least the interpersonal one) is required to adapt to the patient.

This interesting idea, of changing the reality to meet the patient's needs, is very relevant to the changes of the setting following the shift to online therapy. Clearly, the online setting is different from the traditional one in our office. In our previous book (Weinberg and Rolnick, 2020) we related to the fact that the therapist cannot control the conditions on the patients' side of the screen and should educate them how to create a safe environment. This is an important issue that should be emphasized again and again: prepare your patient for the online meeting, and instruct them how to keep privacy, stay focused, etc. Many of the chapters in this book teach us how to do that from different theoretical schools' perspectives. However, this is not the only aspect of setting that changes online: The entire physical framework is different, including the fact that therapists and patients sit in two different rooms. The question is how much we should try to replicate the situation occurring in our office, and to what degree we should accept that this is a different modality with different settings and different rules. Instead of trying to adapt ourselves and the setting to "reality" perhaps we accept virtual reality as a given and learn how to benefit from it. Various chapters in this book struggle with this dilemma as some of its answers are based on the theoretical frame of reference.

Harris and Tylim (2018) note that the concept of the framework has undergone far-reaching changes as social, cultural, and **technological** forces had a decisive influence on the concept of setting. In the case of online therapy, technology affects the setting tremendously. For example, the place of the camera affects our ability to appear looking directly at the patient.

Belcher (1967/2018) describes how the frame sometimes carries denied aspects of the patient as well as of the analyst. Changes in the framework, under certain conditions, can be catastrophic in their results. However, paying attention and discussing the materialistic aspects, the quality of light and sound, the location of the armchairs or the decoration, all of these can contribute to the positive effects of the frame. It is often the work of re-stabilizing the framework that enables the occurrence of a powerful change. Although he related to in-person therapy, taking this idea to our online setting, the main conclusion is that discussing the technical changes, obstacles, difficulties, and challenges can be the right thing to do in order to re-create a safe and holding environment. Belcher argues that the normal, quiet, ongoing presence of the setting offers the patient an opportunity for a body-level relationship that restores early symbiosis of the baby with its mother. As long as the setting is not disturbed, it remains imperceptible. The implications for the psychotherapeutic technique are that the setting itself must undergo analysis. These implications are especially true in on Cyberspace.

Online Therapeutic Alliance: Is Online Therapy Effective?

Therapeutic approaches can be classified as emphasizing one of the two axes: Those who emphasize the therapeutic techniques (CBT therapies) vs. those who emphasize the therapeutic relationship (psychodynamic-oriented therapies). The chapters in this book represent both of those approaches. When reading the chapters dealing with techniques (e.g., no.14 and 15), and the tips that the writers add at the end of their articles, it became clear that those approaches have little difficulty in moving the techniques to the online environment. For example, Lahad and Doron (Chapter 23) present the SEE FAR CBT model, using imagination as their main tool of intervention. There is no problem in instructing clients to use their imagination online, since it doesn't necessitate the therapist's presence in the same room, and the online setting poses no challenge to the therapeutic process since it's a protocol-based therapeutic method. The only problem is how to use the therapeutic cards online, and this is an easy to solve problem.

However, approaches emphasizing the relationship between the therapist and the client are concerned whether we can create the same kind of relationship online. It is well established through research that the therapeutic or working alliance is the best predictor for positive outcomes in all psychotherapies (Horvath & Symonds, 1991; Martin et al., 2000). If this is the case, it is imperative that we explore whether this alliance can be transferred to online relationships. In order to do so, we should check the ingredients of the therapeutic alliance to find out whether all these ingredients can be established online. Bordin (1979) analyzed three components composing the therapeutic alliance: 1. The therapist and client agree about the goals of therapy. 2. They also agree about the tasks (how to achieve these goals). 3. The quality of the relationship that develops in therapy. This analysis was confirmed later by Norcross and Lambert (2018) and Flückiger et al. (2018). The first two factors (agreeing on the goals and tasks) can easily be achieved online by discussing the goals and tasks before beginning the group (usually, in the online first meeting or the intake). As for the question whether the same kind of relationships can be developed online as in-person, reviewing studies that measured therapeutic alliance in video conference meetings, Simpson and Reid (2014), found that "studies overwhelmingly supported the notion that therapeutic alliance can be developed in psychotherapy over video conference." Cook and Doyle (2002) compared the working alliance between in-person and online therapy and found no significant difference. Following the massive use of videoconferencing in COVID-19 time by therapists, Simpson et al. (2021) summarized (p. 409): "Historically, the uptake of videotherapy has been hindered by psychotherapist expectations of inferior therapeutic alliance and outcomes, in spite of considerable research evidence to the contrary. Research suggests that videotherapy provides a powerful pathway for clients to experience enhanced opportunities for self-expression, connection and intimacy." This conclusion is echoed by Frye et al. (2021) finding that pediatric patients rated a high level of therapeutic alliance following psychological services provided through either telehealth via video-conferencing or in-person modality. Kaiser et al. (2021) in their meta analysis concluded that therapeutic alliance and outcome are significantly correlated in internet-based therapy.

So, is online therapy using videoconferencing effective? In a meta analysis examining pre-post changes within Video Delivered Psychotherapy (VDP) and comparing the outcomes with In-Person Psychotherapy (IPP), Fernandez et al. (2021) concluded (p. 1535): "Substantial and significant improvement occurs from pre- to post-phases of VDP, this in turn differing negligibly from IPP treatment outcome. The VDP improvement is most pronounced when CBT is used, and when anxiety, depression, or PTSD are targeted, and it remains strong though attenuated by publication bias. Clinically, therapy is no less efficacious when delivered via videoconferencing than in-person, with efficacy being most pronounced in CBT for affective disorders."

Beyond therapeutic alliance, there is enough research using randomized control trials showing that VDP is equally effective as face-to-face psychotherapy in many dimensions, such as overall treatment outcome (Kingsley & Henning, 2015; Sucala et al., 2012) and client satisfaction (King et al., 2014; Simpson & Reid, 2014). These results have been found positive for a variety of disorders such as anxiety (Backhaus et al., 2012; Chavooshi et al., 2016), depression (Berryhill et al., 2019; Giovanetti et al., 2022), and addictions (Backhaus et al., 2012; King et al., 2014), but also for personality disorders, such as Borderline type (Zimmerman et al., 2021).

However, we should also pay attention to a critical commentary by Smith et al. (2021) reminding us that research results on online therapy depends on how video therapy is defined. They conclude that while the current evidence whether video therapy is effective, and whether the working alliance and therapeutic relationship functions in video counseling is promising, it is limited in quantity and applicability and hence generalisability.

This book examines the important factors that construct the therapeutic relationship and how they are manifested online: Intimacy (Magaldi & Trub, Chapter 2; Chatjoulis & Ntali, Chapter 4, Eherenreich et al., Chapter 4), presence (Geller, Chapter 1), trust (Mor-Ofek, Chapter 6), empathy (Agosta, Chapter 3), holding and containing (Ben Ari, Chapter 20; Meyerson, Chapter 15, Mor, Chapter 10), etc.

Rupture and Repair: The Online Challenge

Lately, there has been an increase in the number of articles relating to the topic of rupture and repair in therapy (Larsson et al., 2018; Miller-Bottome et al., 2019; Humer et al., 2021; Dolev-Amit et al., 2022). Some of the articles connect this topic to the therapeutic alliance claiming that a rupture is "a deterioration in the therapeutic alliance, manifested by a disagreement between the patient and therapist on treatment goals, a lack of collaboration on therapeutic tasks, or a strain in their emotional bond" (Eubanks et al., 2018, p. 508). In our opinion, since human beings are prone to make mistakes, there will always be some ruptures in our therapeutic alliance, and the important issue is not to be perfect, trying to prevent them, but to focus on repairing them when they happen. Focusing on repairing empathic failures and mistakes in therapy can become more powerful in the therapeutic process than intellectual interpretations, since they touch a deep unconscious wish that our care-givers acknowledge and apologize for their mistakes and unattuned responses from our childhood. Incidentally, frequently, apology is not enough to repair a deep rupture since it can be expressed or perceived as lip service or social norm with no deep meaning.

Moving to online therapy, the therapist immediately faces an abundance of challenges, many of them seem technical. Interrupted Internet connections, freezing video, time gap between lips movement and the voice, and difficulties to focus and be present, are some of the obstacles that affect online therapy. The failing technology is tiring, distracting, disappointing, and frustrating. However, if we look at it as another kind of psychological rupture, we can change our view about these failings and see them as opportunities for repair. In fact, the online modality may allow for more opportunities to work on repairing ruptures than face-to-face meetings.

The question to follow is when is repair impossible? Beyond a possible psychological answer to this question (e.g., when the patient is too hurt by the therapist's comments and is only seeking revenge), from a technical aspect, there is of course a moment when the internet connection cannot be resumed as it breaks down. However, the therapist can still bring the topic of failure to discussion in the next session, exploring the impact of this rupture and finding a way to make amends. We recommend that the therapist will use this technique every time that a technological rupture occurs online, thus enriching the opportunities to work on repairs.

Dolev-Amit, Leibovich and Zilcha-Mano (2021) provide detailed guidelines for therapists on how supportive techniques developed in traditional face-to-face treatment can be effectively used in telepsychotherapy to resolve alliance ruptures. They point out that confrontation ruptures (characterized by overt expression of anger and dissatisfaction) are easier to detect both online and offline, but withdrawal ruptures (moving away from the therapist through avoidance or detached behavior) that can go unnoticed by therapists in face-to-face treatment, are even more challenging in telepsychotherapy. This is due to both the disembodied environment and the technical failures. In the transition to telepsychotherapy, identifying ruptures, especially withdrawal ruptures, may be challenging. They suggest that therapists create an appropriate setting and basic technical conditions and pay greater attention to the nuances of the patients' in-session behavior. With online therapy, we need to work even harder to make sure our clients see us as completely engaged.

Is Online Therapy Suitable for All?

It is a common myth that certain disorders and situations are not suitable for online therapy; however, there is sparse solid research that supports this belief. Many therapists believe that online therapy is suitable only for less severe cases (Richards & Viganó, 2013), and that severe depression (especially with suicidal threats), borderline personality disorders, and PTSD cases, should not be treated online. This belief stems mainly from the assumption that such cases need the physical presence of the therapist, and an ability to reach out in person in case of emergency. However, as in some of our book chapters (Chapters 22 and Chapter 23, Tipton et al; Lahad, Doron and Rubinstein, respectively) you will read that online therapy is particularly relevant for working with suicidal patients or those dealing with PTSD. As mentioned before, Fernandez et al. (2021) found in their meta-analysis of research studies that Videoconference therapy outcomes are positive when anxiety, depression, or PTSD are targeted. In fact, the high availability of online therapy in many ways makes it particularly suited for such extreme and urgent situations. While editing this book we were surprised to find out that these assumptions of ours were faulty. Client age is also frequently mentioned as an important criterion. This book covers online therapy for all age groups including younger children (25, Keating).

Barker and Barker (2021) found that "The effectiveness of online therapy was more strongly associated with client characteristics and treatment approaches than with diagnoses and treatment goals" (p. 66). Although their study examined effectiveness rather than suitability, we believe that client characteristics possibly offer more criteria for online therapy suitability. Clients who are "physical-oriented," who are very sensitive to bodily cues (theirs or of others), who use all their senses (including smell) in their communication – might find the online connection too difficult. Clients who are easily distracted by intrusive stimuli, might also feel that the online meeting is not for them, since they cannot stay present. Fisher et al. (2021) add: "Transition to VCP [Video Conference Psychotherapy] requires a stance of willingness to change flexibly to adapt to a changed external reality, and a sense that such a transition is, or will be, of personal benefit, even if this is not entirely clear at first." (p. 513).

Another question the reader may ask is whether online therapy is suitable for all therapists. Although we do not cover this question directly in the book, a consistent understanding of many of the authors in this book (examples can be found in the chapters of Athena Chatjoulis & Evdokia Ntali, Lou Agosta, Vered Bar, Galit Mor) is that therapists' attitude towards technology in treatment can have considerable effect on the treatment itself. Furthermore, this attitude can also predict the likelihood of the therapist to adopt technology in their treatment plans (Bagarić & Jokić-Begić, 2020). Bekes et al. (2021) similarly found that therapists' *perceived* obstacle regarding connectedness during online therapy predicted their negative view of online therapy and its effectiveness. As discussed below, inclusion of training for online therapy psychotherapy training programs is crucial in order to reduce therapists' objections and difficulties. We will outline what is needed in such training in the next section.

Since we question the myth of who cannot benefit from online therapy, we dare say that some patients benefit MORE from remote treatment. One of the advantages of the COVID-19 pandemic is that it enabled a comparison of pre (doing only in person therapy) and post (moving online), almost the classical conditions of a scientific study. Comparing pre and post sessions, therapists discovered, to their surprise, that some of their clients do BETTER in the virtual environment. Possibly, for those patients, who felt more overwhelmed when meeting the therapist in the same room, the computer screen provided a barrier that reduced their anxiety and allowed them to make better use of therapy. In general, it seems that those patients were using an avoidant-dismissive attachment style, which helped them withdraw from being too emotionally invested in the therapeutic relationship. Our experience shows that patients with social anxiety disorders, some with borderline personality disorders, and some who suffered from PTSD, felt more protected when we shifted to online meetings at the outbreak of the pandemic (Weinberg, 2021). They became more self-disclosing, more communicative, and less defensive online.

Are We Psycho-Technologically Proficient?

Imagine visiting a dentist who is renowned for his professionalism, the best dentist in the region. As he is about to use his drill, a jet of water shoots out soaking your shirt. The dentist apologetically explains that it is the latest motor drive system, and he has just received it. He approaches you and as he is about to apply the pressure, the dental light switches off. How would you feel at this stage? Do you believe the hypothetical dentist is in a position to deliver the best care at the given moment? His lack of technical skills in this case impedes his ability to deliver his core skills. It would be reasonable to say that in this case – his ability to operate his equipment is in fact a core skill.

All schools of psychotherapy require that the therapist has certain basic skills. The minimally required skill set may include empathy, rapport, communication skills, or flexibility.

We suggest that a basic requirement for online therapists is "psycho-technological proficiency."

Merriam Webster Dictionary – Psychotechnology (Merriam-Webster, n.d.): 1. the practical application of psychological principles, as in economics, sociology, and business. 2. the application of psychological principles to alter or control the behavior of an individual.

We choose this term to emphasize that this is not a purely technical aspect. This skill requires understanding how to use the technology and its relevant application and implications in the clinical setting.

The therapist who is not comfortable with the video conferencing software may find his attention partly focused on the software, possibly at the expense of the attention towards his client. If we do not arrange the setting properly (e.g., camera location, lighting), the session will be directly affected (see Weinberg & Rolnick, 2020). If we do not feel comfortable sharing a video on the screen, we probably will not do it – even if it offers a great opportunity for the therapeutic process. If I sit too close to the camera, how can I lean forwards compassionately? If my internal laptop microphone is not sensitive – how can I sit at the suitable distance? As we shall discuss, if we can't use the latest immersive features of Zoom, we are certainly missing out on opportunities to improve the therapy itself.

We should remember that being somehow techno-knowledgable and advising/directing the patient how to overcome technological difficulties, is interpreted as taking care of the client and providing the holding environment. Many of us did not become therapists expecting to be required to develop technological abilities, however, we believe that psycho-technological proficiency is now a basic required skill. Just as we attempt to stay updated with the latest reading on the modalities we work with, we now need to accept that staying up to date with psycho-technological development is also necessary. We have passed the point where being a "technophobe" is an acceptable reason for not developing these crucial skills. Or to paraphrase Lou Agousta (Chapter 3) "you are definitely the help desk!".

The Pandemic and Its Consequences

The Covid pandemic, already with us for more than two years when writing this introduction, created havoc globally, affecting the world of psychotherapy as well. Therapists had to shift to "virtual" meetings without any preparation or training within days. The danger of physical proximity because of the virus, and the lockdown that followed the epidemic in many countries, forced therapists to shift to "screen relations" (Russell, 2015). Therapists who in their worst nightmare never imagined they would even attempt to treat patients online found themselves doing it daily. Many of our colleagues vehemently objected to online therapy, claiming that it is impossible to create the same connections, presence, transference, and dynamics online as it occurs offline. The only caveat was that they never experienced it. Their resistance was based purely on their fantasy.

When the pandemic erupted, therapists were pushed to meet their clients over the Internet. Indeed, in some countries authorities and health insurance companies doubted whether this modality is secure or effective enough. However, in most countries, therapists who shifted to therapy on the screen were surprised to find out that it is no less powerful than in-person meetings.

In our opinion, even when (or if) the vaccine for COVID-19 eliminates the pandemic and life returns to what is considered normal – online therapy is here to stay. Its legitimacy increased dramatically following the world crisis, and although it has some limitations, some of the advantages (e.g., the comfort of connecting from home, no traffic jams, the fact that the therapist does not have to be local and can have clients from other places) are very tempting. In the coming future more therapy sessions would be conducted online, and more specific research would be carried out about them. The pandemic clearly legitimized online therapy and it's probably going to stay as another equal modality for providing therapy, and not a less valued one.

Dynamic Aspects of Remote Therapy

While we structured this book around different therapeutic approaches and schools of thoughts, asking each writer to explain what challenges their approach faces online, we do not want to lose the broader psychodynamic view of online therapy and the challenges that working online pose to this approach. Psychoanalytic psychodynamic approaches include many schools nowadays, such as object relations, ego psychology, self psychology, and relational approaches. One way to define and understand what unifies all psychodynamic approaches is to point out that they all focus on transference and resistance. However, Shedler (2010) suggested seven factors that include these dimensions and go beyond them. We will explore how these factors can be applied online:

1   Focus on affect and expression of emotion: Psychodynamic therapy fosters inquiry and discussion of the patient's emotions. The therapist assists the patient to articulate emotions in words, including recognizing feelings that the patient initially may struggle to identify.

   In order to help patients to express their emotions online, the therapist should help them overcome the screen barrier, and their tendency to use it to distance themselves. Asking questions that focus on feelings, noticing facial expressions and bodily gestures that might hide emotions and being curious about those expressions can help overcome this barrier.

2   Exploration of attempts to avoid distressing thoughts and feelings: In order to avoid stress and pain, people use (consciously and unconsciously) defense mechanisms and resistance. These may appear in more obvious behavioral manners, such as canceling sessions, patients using mobile phones during sessions, or lashing out at the therapist. They may take more subtle forms such as changing the topic when certain issues are discussed, focusing on others' behaviors, or shifting to intellect to avoid talking about emotions.

   In addition to the usual forms of avoidance and defense, online, it can be challenging to distinguish between real technical difficulties and those that point to a deeper resistance. When the patient is late for a Zoom meeting it can be a result of an Internet failure and not a sign of avoidance. When the communication is terminated abruptly, it can mean that the computer crashed and not that the patient ended the session in order to avoid the topic and the pain involved. A more careful examination and exploration of each situation is needed online in order to be sure that resistance is involved.

3   Identification of recurring themes and patterns: People frequently repeat their maladaptive behaviors or respond to certain triggers in the same problematic way. Psychodynamic therapists work to identify and explore recurring motifs and patterns in patients' internal experiences and external behaviors. This factor can easily be explored in online treatment since the repeating patterns are either reported verbally by the patient or are easily noticed in the behavior during the meetings. There are some recurring behaviors, containing some emotional meaning, that are specific to the online interactions (e.g., pushing the chair away from the screen) and the therapist should pay attention to them as well. The fact that the session is often carried out in the patient's own home may even increase the likelihood that certain patterns may present themselves in the session.

4   Discussion of past experiences (developmental focus): Our past experiences influence our current interpretation of the situation and behavior. Early experiences of attachment figures impact how we relate and experience the present. Psychodynamic therapy helps the patient examine early experiences in order to develop the understanding of how they affect the patient's present. The purpose of this examination is to allow the patient to live more fully in the present.

Since this factor is explored through discussion, the transition to online is straightforward. The therapist should be aware that it is easier to discuss past experience online in a distant/non-involved manner, and take measures to avoid this intellectualization.

5   Focus on interpersonal relations: Object relations and attachment are central in psychodynamic therapy. When interpersonal patterns prevent a patient from fulfilling his/her emotional needs, psychological suffering is frequently the outcome.

We can certainly help our patients to explore interpersonal patterns when carrying out therapy online. Relational oriented therapy is particularly powerful in a virtual context because it allows us to be subjective and use our subjectivity in ways that have the potential to bridge the technological separation.

6   Focus on the therapy relationship: A special position is given to the relationship between the patient and the therapist – the transference. The repetitive themes in a person's relationships and manner of interacting, mentioned above, tend to emerge in some form in the therapy relationship. These themes appearing in the therapy relationship (transference and countertransference) allow the therapist to help the patient examine and develop new ways of interacting during the here and now of the therapy session.

Perhaps this is the main question that psychodynamic therapists ask themselves: Is the transference online "the same" as the transference when we meet in-person? In our previous book (Weinberg and Rolnick, 2020), Gily Agar discussed in length transference phenomena online, and distinguished between modalities that can be attributed to "one person psychology" (e.g., transferential modalities that stem from the technical characteristics of the medium) and "two person psychology." She concludes that: "The transference that occurs in video therapy is therefore characterized by duality. On the one hand, projective and phantasmatic transference qualities of 'one-person psychology' occur, and on the other hand, there are qualities of mutuality and a rich encounter with the therapist's subjectivity in 'two-person psychology' terms. These two poles do not cancel each other out, but coexist, providing a unique dualism from an early stage of the relationship." (p. 76).

Hickey et al. (2022) focused on Davanloo's intensive short-term dynamic psychotherapy asking how technology impacts psychodynamic psychotherapy in general and transference in particular. They note that this approach makes use of a close, emotionally intimate relationship with the therapist. They concluded that "Even without the face-to-face sessions, mobilization can be achieved with the proper application of Davanloo's techniques by applying the maximum pressure within the patient's capacity to tolerate anxiety and painful affects and thereby removing resistance …" (p. 129).

7   Exploration of fantasy life: Psychodynamic therapy by definition is unstructured, the patient is urged to freely share his/her thoughts. As patients learn to do this, the emergence of desires, emotions, memories, fantasies, and dreams may occur. The content shared by the patient can provide important insight and understanding about the patient's unconscious world ultimately facilitating his or her attempt to reduce emotional suffering and live a more satisfying and meaningful life. Fantasy life is an inner phenomenon and occurs whether we are in the office or behind the screen. Creating a safe space for the patient to speak about their dreams, fantasies, inner thoughts, and images, can be achieved in online therapy, albeit the difficulties. It might take more time. Since one of our recommendations for the online therapist is to use his/her imagination, and to encourage the patients to use theirs, it can help us open the road to use this factor.

How to Read this Book

After the reader may likely start his journey through the book by reading the chapter describing the modality he or she usually works with, we would like to suggest a journey through the "scenic route." As with any other journey, reading about the background always makes the journey more interesting and richer. The first part of the book describes underlying theoretical aspects of therapy and specifically online therapy. Reading this part first will certainly add to the rest of the route. Follow the scenic route through the variety of different modalities. Each will offer a different angle, another view. Examine how this scenic route with its fascinating views can contribute to how you, our reader, experience your home modality of which we all know the perfect place to finish any journey is where you started – at home.

We have worked hard planning the route, covering a diversity we believe is relatively unique, offering not just practical information on enhancing on-line therapy but also an opportunity to visit modalities outside the comfort of our own neighborhood.

References

Agar, G. (2020). The clinic offers no advantage over the screen, for relationship is everything. In H. Weinberg, & A. Rolnick (Eds.), *Theory and Practice of Online Therapy: Internet-delivered Interventions for Individuals, Families, Groups, and Organizations* (pp. 66–78). New York: Routledge.

Backhaus, A., Agha, Z., Maglione, M. L., Repp, A., Ross, B., Zuest, D., & Thorp, S. R. (2012). Videoconferencing psychotherapy: A systematic review. *Psychological Services*, *9*(2), 111–131.

Bagarić, B., & Jokić-Begić, N. (2020). Measuring therapists' attitudes toward in-tegration of technology in psychotherapy and predicting their use of technology. *Journal of Clinical Psychology*, *76*(6), 1151–1172.

Barker, G. G., & Barker, E. E. (2021). Online therapy: Lessons learned from the COVID-19 health crisis. *British Journal of Guidance & Counselling*, *1–16*, 66.

Békés, V., Aafjes-van Doorn, K., Luo, X., Prout, T. A., & Hoffman, M. D. (2021). Psychotherapists' challenges with online therapy during COVID-19: Concerns about connectedness predict therapists' negative view of online therapy and its perceived efficacy over time. *Frontiers in Psychology*, *12*, 3036.

Berryhill, M. B., Culmer, N., Williams, N., Halli-Tierney, A., Betancourt, A., Roberts, H., & King, M. (2019). Videoconferencing psychotherapy and depression: A sys-tematic review. *Telemedicine and e-Health*, *25*(6), 435–446.

Bickman, L. (2020). Improving mental health services: A 50-year journey from ran-domized experiments to artificial intelligence and precision mental health. *Administration and Policy in Mental Health and Mental Health Services Research*, *47*(5), 795–843.

Bleger, J. (1967/2018). Psychoanalysis of the psychoanalytic setting. In A. Harris, & I. Tylim (Eds.), *Reconsidering the Moveable Frame in Psychoanalysis. Its Function and Structure in Contemporary Psychoanalytic Theory* (p. 22). New York: Routledge.

Bordin, E. (1979). The generalizability of the psychoanalytic concept of the working alliance. *Psychotherapy*, *16*, 252–260.

Chavooshi, B., Mohammadkhani, P., & Dolatshahi, B. (2016). A randomized double-blind controlled trial comparing Davanloo intensive short-term dynamic psy-chotherapy as internet-delivered vs treatment as usual for medically unexplained pain: A 6-month pilot study. *Psychosomatics*, *57*(3), 292–300.

Cook, J. E., & Doyle, C. (2002). Working alliance in online therapy as compared to face-to-face therapy: preliminary results. *Cyberpsychology Behavior*, *5*, 95–105

Dolev-Amit, T., Leibovich, L., & Zilcha-Mano, S. (2021). Repairing alliance ruptures using supportive techniques in telepsychotherapy during the COVID-19 pandemic. *Counselling Psychology Quarterly*, *34*(3–4), 485–498. 10.1080/09515070.2020.1777089

Eubanks, C. F., Muran, J. C., & Safran, J. D. (2018). Alliance rupture repair: A meta-analysis. *Psychotherapy, 55*(4), 508–519. 10.1037/pst0000185

Fernandez, E., Woldgabreal, Y., Day, A., Pham, T., Gleich, B., & Aboujaoude, E. (2021). Live psychotherapy by video versus in-person: A meta-analysis of efficacy and its relationship to types and targets of treatment. *Clinical Psychology & Psychotherapy, 28*(6), 1535– 1549. 10.1002/cpp.2594

Fisher, S., Guralnik, T., Fonagy, P., & Zilcha-Mano, S. (2021). Let's face it: Video conferencing psychotherapy requires the extensive use of ostensive cues. *Counselling Psychology Quarterly, 34*(3–4), 508–524. 10.1080/09515070.2020.1777535

Flückiger, C., Del Re, A. C., Wampold, B. E., & Horvath, A. O. (2018). The alliance in adult psychotherapy: A meta-analytic synthesis. *Psychotherapy, 55*(4), 316–340.

Frye, W. S., Gardner, L., & Mateus, J. S. (2021). Utilising telemental health in a pediatric outpatient psychology clinic: Therapeutic alliance and outcomes. *Counselling and Psychotherapy Research*, 1–9. 10.1002/capr.12450

Giovanetti, A. K., Punt, S. E., Nelson, E. L., & Ilardi, S. S. (2022). Teletherapy versus in-person psychotherapy for depression: A meta-analysis of randomized controlled trials. *Telemedicine and e-Health, 28*(8). 10.1089/tmj.2021.0294

Harris, A. & Tylim, I. (2018). Introduction: The frame. In A. Harris, & I. Tylim (Eds.), *Reconsidering the Moveable Frame in Psychoanalysis. Its Function and Structure in Contemporary Psychoanalytic Theory* (pp. 1). New York: Routledge.

Hayes, S. C., & Hofmann, S. G. (2021). "Third-wave" cognitive and behavioral therapies and the emergence of a process-based approach to intervention in psychiatry. *World Psychiatry, 20*(3), 368.

Hickey, C., Schubmehl, J. Q. & Beeber, A. (2022), Technology, transference, and COVID-19 — With reference to Davanloo's intensive short-term dynamic psychotherapy. *British Journal of Psychotherapy, 38*, 116–135. 10.1111/bjp.12693

Horvath, A. O., & Symonds, B. D. (1991). Relation between working alliance and outcome in psychotherapy: A meta-analysis. *Journal of Counselling Psychology, 38*, 138–149.

Humer, E., Schramm, E., Klein, J. P., Härter, M., Hautzinger, M., Pieh, C., & Probst, T. (2021). Effects of alliance ruptures and repairs on outcomes. *Psychotherapy Research, 31*(8), 977–987.

Kaiser, J., Hanschmidt, F., & Kersting, A. (2021). The association between therapeutic alliance and outcome in internet-based psychological interventions: A meta-analysis. *Computers in Human Behavior, 114*, 106512.

King, V. L., Brooner, R. K., Peirce, J. M., Kolodner, K., & Kidorf, M. S. (2014). A randomized trial of web-based videoconferencing for substance abuse counseling. *Journal of Substance Abuse Treatment, 46*(1), 36–42.

Kingsley, A., & Henning, J. A. (2015). Online and phone therapy: Challenges and opportunities. *The Journal of Individual Psychology, 71*(2), 185–194.

Larsson, M. H., Falkenström, F., Andersson, G., & Holmqvist, R. (2018). Alliance ruptures and repairs in psychotherapy in primary care. *Psychotherapy Research, 28*(1), 123–136. 10.1080/10503307.2016.1174345

Martin, D. J., Garske, J. P., & Davis, M. K. (2000). Relation of the therapeutic alliance with outcome and other variables: a meta-analytic review. *Journal of Consult Clinical Psychology, 68*, 438–450.

Merriam-Webster. (n.d.). Psychotechnology. In Merriam-Webster.com medical dictionary. Retrieved March 21, 2022, from https://www.merriam-webster.com/medical/psychotechnology

Miller-Bottome, M., Talia, A., Eubanks, C. F., Safran, J. D., & Muran, J. C. (2019). Secure in-session attachment predicts rupture resolution: Negotiating a secure base. *Psychoanalytic Psychology*, *36*(2), 132–138. 10.1037/pap0000232

Norcross, J. C., & Lambert, M. J. (2018). Psychotherapy relationships that work III. *Psychotherapy*, *55*(4), 303–315. 10.1037/pst0000193

Richards, D., & Viganó, N. (2013). Online counseling: A narrative and critical review of the literature. *Journal of Clinical Psychology*, *69*(9), 994–1011.

Russell, G.I. (2015). *Screen Relations: The Limits of Computer-Mediated Psychoanalysis and Psychotherapy* (1st ed.) Routledge.

Shedler, J. (2010). The efficacy of psychodynamic psychotherapy. *American Psychologist*, *65*(2), 98–109.

Simpson, S. G., & Reid, C. L. (2014). Therapeutic alliance in videoconferencing psychotherapy: A review. *Australian Journal of Rural Health*, *22*(6), 280–299.

Simpson, S., Richardson, L., Pietrabissa, G., Castelnuovo, G., & Reid, C. (2021). Videotherapy and therapeutic alliance in the age of COVID-19. *Clinical Psychology & Psychotherapy*, *28*(2), 409–421. 10.1002/cpp.2521

Smith, K., Moller, N., Cooper, M., Gabriel, L., Roddy, J., & Sheehy, R. (2021). Video counselling and psychotherapy: A critical commentary on the evidence base. *Counselling and Psychotherapy Research*, *22*, 1–6. 10.1002/capr.12436

Sucala, M., Schnur, J. B., Constantino, M. J., Miller, S. J., Brackman, E. H., & Montgomery, G. H. (2012). The therapeutic relationship in e-therapy for mental health: A systematic review. *Journal of Medical Internet Research*, *14*(4), 175–187. 10.21 96/jmir.2084

Triest, Y. (July 2, 2011). *Between "law" and "lap" - reflections on border patrol and issues of containment*. Hebrew Psychology. Retrieved February 27, 2022, from https://www.hebpsy.net/articles.asp?id=2622

Weinberg, H. (2021). Obstacles, challenges, and benefits of online group psychotherapy. *American Journal of Psychotherapy*, *74*(2), 83–88. 10.1176/appi.psychotherapy.20200034

Weinberg, H., & Rolnick, A. (Eds.). (2020). *Theory and Practice of Online Therapy: Internet-delivered Interventions for Individuals, Groups, Families, and Organizations* (1st ed.). Routledge. 10.4324/9781315545530

Zimmerman, M., Ward, M., D'Avanzato, C., & Tirpak, J. W. (2021). Telehealth treatment of patients with borderline personality disorder in a partial hospital setting during the COVID-19 pandemic: Comparative safety, patient satisfaction, and effectiveness of in-person treatment. *Journal of Personality Disorders*, *36*(3), 1–19.

Section I

Theoretical Aspects of Online Therapy

1 Being Present and Together While Apart: Therapeutic Presence in Telepsychotherapy

Shari Geller

In the face of drastic and unprecedented change caused by the COVID-19 pandemic, psychotherapists across the globe showed a great deal of resilience and creativity in adapting their psychotherapy practice to telepsychotherapy. Public health recommendations, including physical distancing and working from home, required a quick shift to developing therapeutic relationships in an online setting, with many therapists having minimal prior experience or training. Physical health and safety superseded the psychological and emotional safety, as well as the privacy and security, characteristic of traditional in-person sessions. Psychotherapy increasingly transformed into being together, yet apart, with therapists and clients separated by two screens. Creating strong and enduring therapeutic relationships online was the new challenge.

Substantial research demonstrates that the therapeutic relationship and alliance are the most consistent predictors of therapeutic change (Norcross & Lambert, 2011, 2019). Yet, much less is known about the relational factors contributing to the cultivation of strong therapeutic relationships and a positive alliance. Therapeutic presence is one quality, or common factor, that is foundational to creating safety for clients, strengthening the therapeutic alliance, and improving therapy effectiveness (Geller, 2017; Geller & Greenberg, 2012; Geller et al., 2010; Geller & Porges, 2014; Hayes & Vinca, 2011, 2017; Pos et al., 2011). Presence generates psychological and emotional safety, which in turn strengthens the working alliance between therapists and clients (Geller & Porges, 2014). It naturally follows that cultivating and communicating therapeutic presence in teletherapy is a necessary step to creating effective therapeutic relationships.

Psychotherapy training programs have only recently begun developing training in therapeutic presence, despite the knowledge that therapists' inner work is integral to relating with presence (Geller, 2017; Geller & Greenberg, 2012). This training emphasizes how to be present with clients as a foundation to effective use of therapeutic interventions and a strong therapeutic alliance. It encourages a sense of groundedness and attunement within therapists, which is key to attuning with clients (Siegel, 2007). This commitment to

DOI: 10.4324/9781003205029-3

self-growth and relational skill building has a myriad of benefits; however, online therapy is different from sitting in the room with a client and involves more than simply conveying the same live therapeutic approach and relationship through the screen. The potential for online therapy to continue successfully even past the pandemic calls for service enhancement rooted in therapeutic presence (Rathenau et al., in press).

This chapter expands on therapeutic presence as a precondition to strong therapeutic relationships, with a focus on presence in online therapy. Research on the efficacy of therapeutic presence and the therapeutic relationship in online therapy are explored and a discussion is followed on specific challenges involved in cultivating online therapeutic presence. Finally, suggestions will be offered to help support both therapists and clients to remain present during telepsychotherapy sessions.

What is Therapeutic Presence?

Therapeutic presence is a way of *being* with clients that enriches the *doing* or therapeutic approach and techniques that therapists offer in therapy. In this context, therapists bring their whole self to session and become deeply rooted in the moment on a physical, emotional, cognitive, relational, and spiritual level (Geller, 2017; Geller & Greenberg, 2002, 2012; Geller et al., 2010). Therapeutic presence can be viewed as a common factor, or trans-theoretical approach across various psychotherapeutic approaches (Geller, 2017, 2020; Geller et al., 2012).

Embodying and conveying presence in encounters with clients helps therapists stay grounded and centered when dealing with difficult emotions. Therapists become attuned within themselves, while also remaining open, attuned, and responsive to their clients' moment-to-moment verbal and nonverbal experiences (Geller, 2017, 2019). Clients can perceive this presence in a way that evokes safety, "feeling felt" (Siegel, 2010), met, and understood. Ultimately opening a portal for optimal engagement in therapeutic work (Geller, 2017; Ogden, 2018).

Therapists' self-care is also an integral part of the model of therapeutic presence (Geller, 2017; Geller & Greenberg, 2002, 2012). The ongoing practice of presence in therapy demands much of a therapist's personal resources and active engagement. Practicing presence outside of session, in one's life and personal relationships, helps build the neural pathways for presence to be able to be experienced in the session with clients. As well, the intentional aspect of self-care is a necessary part of lowering the risk of burnout and increasing the ability to sustain presence in session with clients. (Geller, 2020)

Therapeutic Presence as a Foundation for Creating Safety

How therapeutic presence evokes change is rooted in safety. According to polyvagal theory, our nervous systems are constantly communicating bidirectionally with the nervous systems of others (Geller, 2017, 2018; Geller & Porges, 2014; Porges, 1998, 2011, 2018; Thompson, 2018). When therapists approach clients from a present-centered state of receptiveness and attunement, clients receive a neurophysiological message that they are being heard, met, felt, and understood (Geller & Porges, 2014; Geller, 2017, 2018). This exchange establishes "a neuroception" of safety for both therapist and client, and strengthens the therapeutic alliance (Badenach, 2018; Dana & Grant, 2018; Geller, 2017, 2018; Geller & Porges, 2014; Ogden, 2018; Porges, 1998, 2011). A mutual sense of safety in the therapeutic environment can support clients in developing new neural pathways, repairing attachment injuries, and engaging in positive social interactions that promote health and neural growth (Allison & Rossouw, 2013; Rossouw, 2013). It also allows clients to engage in the necessary therapeutic work, while bringing awareness to the limits of their window of tolerance (Geller, 2017, 2018; Siegel, 1999).

Therapists' presence is known to have a co-regulating effect on clients' emotions (Geller, 2019). This regulation is facilitated by attuned right brain to right brain communication to nonverbal communication through body posture, vocal expressions, facial expressions, and gestures (Quillman, 2012; Schore, 2009, 2012; Siegel, 2010). When working with clients who have experienced trauma, it is important to recognize that safe situations may not be perceived as such (Geller & Porges, 2014; Gray, 2018). Their heightened state of fear and self-protection, coupled with arousal of the sympathetic nervous system (SNS) or over-arousal of the dorsal vagal wing of the parasympathetic nervous system (PNS), can evoke a shut-down or freeze response (Dana & Grant, 2018). In these moments, a therapists' soothing presence can help activate the clients' social engagement system and ventral vagal wing of their parasympathetic nervous system.

Over time, repeatedly journeying back to this state of safety through co-regulation, with a present centered therapist, creates an optimal environment for clients to express their emotional vulnerabilities, pain, traumas, and fears, and eventually feel safe in other relationships (Geller, 2018; Geller & Porges, 2014; Ogden, 2018). This requires skill to embody presence, stay attuned to clients and their own moment to moment experience, and authentically convey presence to the client in a way that is well received. The question of interest for this chapter is whether therapeutic presence can be experienced and received in an online setting.

What Does the Research Say? Therapeutic Presence and Relationships in Telepsychotherapy

Although some researchers contend that clients have a preference for in-person rather than online therapy (i.e., Berle et al., 2014), a literature review indicated that clients are open to both modalities, and it does not hinder the development of an alliance (Simpson & Reid, 2014). In fact, online therapy calls for creativity in forming strong therapeutic relationships founded on deeper therapeutic intimacy, all while overcoming access barriers and serving a diverse range of clients (Chen et al., 2020; Varker et al., 2019; Weinberg & Rolnick, 2019). For example, seeing the face so closely and meeting in this engaged way online, can allow therapists to read and attune to clients' emotional expression in a more fine-tuned way than live therapy.

There is growing research suggesting that teletherapy is effective for clients with various disorders (Varker et al., 2019). However, the negative perceptions held by therapists can get in the way. Whether it stems from inexperience, limited resources (e.g, training, literature), or fear of challenges to attunement (Hafermalz & Riemer, 2016; Sjöström & Alfonsson, 2012), therapists' negative bias can impact their ratings of alliance and inhibit the potential to strengthen therapeutic relationships online (Rees & Stone, 2005). Despite therapists' negative perceptions toward online therapy (Jerome & Zaylor, 2000; Rees & Stone, 2005; Wray & Rees, 2003), this modality can be beneficial to clients and the development of a positive working alliance (Cook & Doyle, 2002; Reynolds et al., 2006).

Research suggests that therapists who feel less competent providing online therapy and those who experience more perceived difficulties, tend to experience decreased presence (Rathenau et al., in press). Considering the significant role of presence in the therapeutic alliance, these effects require further attention to help improve online therapy and therapeutic presence in this context.

Oshni Alvandi (2019) outlined three modules of counselling presence to enhance cybertherapeutic engagement – cognitive, counselling, and emotional. Cognitive presence refers to empathizing with clients, counselling presence reflects listening, building trust, and expressing compassion to help clients feel heard and understood, and finally emotional presence involves feeling emotions with the client and supporting them in their ability to express and manage emotions. Although the author mentions that missing nonverbal cues online can negatively affect therapists' expressed presence, it is still possible to convey facial cues, gestures, and prosodic vocal tone online. In online therapy, this supports ventral vagal activation and clients' feeling safe and calm.

Nursing literature offers some examples where presence can be expressed and received online (Hafermalz & Riemer, 2016; Tuxbury, 2013). Following semi-structured interviews with six telehealth nurses, Tuxbury (2013) found that nurses are able to provide care as well as attain personal and relational presence through non-video calls. Presence can be generated in online therapy if nurses are trained and accustomed to the equipment and the technology (Hafermalz & Riemer, 2016). They can then focus on the relationship and engage aspects of presence by expressing care, being present, and experimenting with visualization of patients' experiences and mirroring of gestures. In this context, they experience being in the same room, even when at a distance, a term known as co-presence or telepresence.

It is helpful to distinguish telepresence from therapeutic presence, as they have similar qualities yet are qualitatively different. Telepresence is broad in scope of its applications (e.g., customer service, education), and often viewed as a key component of online therapy as it involves feeling the presence of someone in a different physical space as if they are together (Fink, 1999). Telepresence is experienced as therapists' absorption in the moment and feeling in the same room with their client, forgetting about the physical distance. It is deemed an important factor for establishing a therapeutic bond online (Bouchard et al., 2000, 2007) and is made possible based on the quality of therapist-client exchanges and client sharing (Haddouk, 2015b). Although both forms of presence are complementary and may reciprocally influence one another, therapeutic presence specifically originated within the context of therapy and goes beyond just the feeling of being together. It is an active process of attuning to self, client, and the relationship and responding to the clients' moment-to-moment experience, while building safety in the therapeutic encounter.

Therapists offering different therapeutic modalities can access a sense of presence that transcends the distance and helps them forget they are not actually physically together (Bouchard et al., 2007; Prenn & Halliday, 2020). Psychotherapy research with CBT for the treatment of panic disorder with agoraphobia, suggests therapist and client can feel they are together when online, reflecting the concept of telepresence (Bouchard et al., 2007). Fishkin et al. (2011) recognize that online psychodynamic therapy maintains the standard principles of face-to-face therapy. These authors share that there is a level of intimacy, comfort, vulnerable sharing, and deeper therapeutic work that is possible in online settings. Therapists' reflections during the pandemic also illuminated that Accelerated Experiential Dynamic Psychotherapy (AEDP), grounded in psychodynamic therapy, is highly suitable for online delivery (Prenn & Halliday, 2020). AEDP therapists' fundamental approach is flexible, adaptive, willing, attentive, kind, present, and self-aware for the benefit of their clients; techniques include making the implicit explicit, cultivating therapeutic presence before and during session, as well as using imagination as a tool to envision being together (Prenn & Halliday, 2020). While therapeutic presence is an important transtheoretical approach to strengthening effective therapeutic relationships, there are specific challenges to being present in virtual therapy.

Challenges of Therapeutic Presence in Telepsychotherapy

Therapists will inevitably encounter technological difficulties in an online setting, yet they must also navigate the challenges of cultivating presence and safety to establish effective relationships with clients. Below are some common challenges described in research conducted prior and largely in response to the coronavirus pandemic.

A lack of physical contact can provide a challenge to expressing therapeutic presence online. A major component of therapeutic presence involves using full body to body non-verbal cues such as prosodic vocal tone, leaning forward, gesturing, an open posture, and soft facial expressions (Geller, 2017, 2018; Geller & Porges, 2014; Ogden & Goldstein, 2019). Similarly, building trust is heavily influenced by the synchronization of bodily movements and physiological rhythms such as entrained breathing, mutual eye gaze, and mirroring of gestures and expressions (Geller, 2017; Marci et al., 2007; Marci & Orr, 2006; Ramseyer & Tschacher, 2011, 2014). The bidirectional communication of nervous systems and co-regulation that occurs when therapists offer a calm and grounded presence can facilitate safety, emotional stability, and connection in the therapeutic relationship (Butler & Randall, 2013; Geller, 2017). However, the physical distance and limited nonverbal cues in telepsychotherapy can complicate the way therapists communicate presence or attune to clients' emotions and experiences (Oshni Alvandi, 2019; Sjöström & Alfonsson, 2012). Combined with more pronounced delays and fragility of trust in video and telephone conferencing (Bos et al., 2002), working toward a positive therapeutic alliance online requires more intentional effort from the therapist.

Another challenge is the possible increased likelihood of therapists' countertransference and vicarious traumatization. Therapists in the pandemic reported moderate levels of vicarious traumatization activated by clients' simultaneous exposure to trauma, with higher levels accounted in therapists who were younger and had less clinical experience (Aafjes-van Doorn et al., 2020).

Increased fatigue also occurs for therapists working online (Aafjes-van Doorn et al., 2020). Excessive screen time can lead to disconnection and exhaustion if not balanced with breaks, outdoor activities, and face-to-face connections for the restoration of well-being (Dodgen-Magee, 2018).

Clients may struggle to feel safe in expressing their emotional vulnerabilities when the therapist is not physically present with them (Geller, 2020). It is important to recognize that their home environment may exacerbate this inhibition due to the close physical proximity of others with whom they experience conflict or complex relationships. Therapists must explore creative ways to express their presence, ensuring clients can sense and feel it.

Technological challenges, glitches, and a lack of training can also impact therapeutic presence and the alliance in online therapy (Brahnam, 2014; Geller, 2020; Markowitz et al., 2020; Oshni Alvandi, 2019). Clients may mistake delays or glitches in the technology for a therapist's characteristics or lack of presence (Schoenenberg et al., 2014). The inevitable technological challenges are then amplified for therapists who are less familiar with technology and lacking sufficient training to conduct online therapy (Hafermalz & Riemer, 2016; Schoenenberg et al., 2014). The attention provided to technological aspects when therapists are not comfortable with this medium, may also compromise their ability to be fully present.

Suggestions for Cultivating Therapeutic Presence Online

Despite the challenges and missing aspects of embodied interaction online (i.e., body to body communication) it is possible to cultivate presence online (Geller, 2020). Weinberg and Rolnick (2019) emphasize becoming present and attuned to clients online simply demands more time, investment, energy, and effort to stay focused and unmoved by distraction. An extensive list of tips and suggestions for cultivating online presence can be found in Geller (2020). Below are some highlights from that article.

Prior to Session

Great care is required by therapists to create online spaces which reflect the sensory, affective, and embodied experiences characteristic of in-person settings. This can include preparing your virtual space to resemble your in-session space so it feels warm, comfortable, and private to ensure confidentiality (Geller, 2020). Taking time before your therapy day and prior to each session is helpful to optimize your presence. Suggestions include walking around the block (to arrive at your "virtual office"), stretching, practicing mindful breathing, or inviting gentle movement with a grounding yoga posture. Simpson and Reid (2014) discuss a potential association between improved clinical outcomes and therapists' tendencies to settle into themselves before entering their "virtual therapy office."

Supporting clients in finding safe places within the home is critical to their engagement in therapeutic work. Prepare a tip sheet for clients to support them in creating a safe, supportive, and non-disruptive space to engage in online therapy. This includes having a tissue box nearby and any other emotion regulation tools (e.g., weighted blanket, ice, sensory balls) and therapeutic props (e.g., chairs for EFT, thought records for CBT, diary cards for DBT). Empower clients to voice their privacy needs with members of their household, and encourage them to reduce distractions (e.g., notifications).

In-Session

Find an optimal distance between yourself and the screen for clients to feel connected with you. Collaborate with clients by experimenting with different distances to find what feels safe and comfortable for them. Maintain mutual eye gaze to enhance a state of synchrony and connection (Geller, 2020; Marci et al., 2007). This does not require you staring at the camera – if you have the camera at eye level yet look directly at your client, it will correct for this.

Expressing your presence online requires the same in person communication, such as prosody of voice, soft facial expression, nonverbal cues of presence and gestures, with more emphasis given the virtual setting (Geller, 2017, 2020). For example, placing a hand on your heart to reflect your feeling with clients in their pain can be helpful. Verbal comments can help express presence such as "uh huh," "I am here with you," "feel me with you," "I am breathing with you," "I feel moved by what you are saying." Utilizing more overt and purposeful verbal responses as well as asking questions to clarify clients' nonverbal gestures and cues is important given the physical distance in online therapy (Prenn & Halliday, 2020; Simpson & Reid, 2014). Enhance clients' experience of your presence by being explicit in your communication. Ask clients if they feel your presence, how the distance is, what they are experiencing.

Attune to clients through attending to micro-expressions of emotions in facial expressions (Ekman, 2004). Given the direct face-to-face contact in online therapy, reading emotions through the eyes, mouth, and voice can be more available to therapists.

Attune to yourself by staying connected to your own emotional experience, resonance with clients' experience, and verbal/nonverbal cues of presence or absence (Geller, 2017; Ogden & Goldstein, 2019). Enhance co-regulation by mirroring clients' expressions, gaze, vocal tone, and breath to invite co-regulation, enhance interpersonal synchrony, and evoke a felt sense of safety and connection (Geller, 2017, 2020; Imel et al., 2014; Marci & Orr, 2006; Ramseyer & Tschacher, 2014).

When you notice challenges in being present, such as anxiety-inducing resonance with clients' experience, or technical difficulties and self-doubt causing distress, name your experience within yourself (and to the client if this is helpful). Engage a self-compassion or emotion regulation practice to return to the moment, such as long exhalations, grounding, and PNR (pause, notice, return) practices (see Geller, 2017 for more). Frank (2020) recommends therapists soothe their own anxiety over what the distanced client may be feeling "over there," by repeatedly attuning to what is occurring "here" in their own bodies.

Therapeutic presence can serve as a supportive approach for therapists to navigate inevitable ruptures, repair alliances, and contribute to greater growth and connection in the therapeutic process all while compensating for the lack of physical presence (Dolev-Amit et al., 2020). If instances of countertransference arise, intentionally put them aside in session and take care of yourself and return to the issues out of session (in supervision, therapy, etc.). If your internet is dropping, transition to a feasible backup plan such as the phone for clear audio, while maintaining the video (if possible) online. Most importantly, be compassionate with yourself when confronting challenges in the online therapy environment as they are bound to occur.

Hold space for a dialogue with clients around any concerns for online therapy. Discuss with clients what they need to help transition out of sessions and back into their home, work, or social life.

Post-Session

Caring for yourself post-session and outside of your therapy day is especially important in the context of online therapy where increased screen time can feel more draining than in-person interactions. Set aside time to transition between sessions and end your online therapy day, through intentionally completing notes, closing your computer, taking a walk, or whatever self-care supports you to decompress, including affirming your own work/life boundaries.

Conclusion and Implications for Training

Online therapy has been used for decades by psychotherapists. Yet its usage expanded dramatically because of the coronavirus pandemic when therapists had to quickly adapt to this modality (Geller, 2020; Weinberg, 2020). Despite the devastating impact of the pandemic, we learned a great deal about online therapy – particularly its effectiveness and value for both therapists and clients globally. Whether offering teletherapy ongoing or engaging in a hybrid therapy practice with face-to-face and online counselling, many therapists and clients have recognized the benefits of accessibility, ease, and connection. Telepsychotherapy is here to stay, so it would be beneficial to develop user-friendly technology and expand training in cultivating therapeutic presence and effective therapeutic relationships online.

Research shows that training and support increase the likelihood for therapists to move their practice online, and it can help develop skills to strengthen therapeutic relationships (Geller, 2020; Pierce et al., 2020). Research and training in presence is important then to further investigate ways to build cohesion, cultivate therapeutic presence online, and express it effectively through a screen (Geller, 2020; Weinberg, 2020). Training in online therapy generally can increase the potential for therapists to use tele-health, allowing access to therapy to a much broader community (i.e., clients who live in rural communities, have physical, cognitive, or emotional limitations hindering in person visits, or those who would like to see a geographically distant therapist). Training in the logistics, equipment, and expression of therapeutic presence, would further increase this likelihood. The foundational suggestions offered in this chapter and in Geller (2020) can be used as part of the development of this envisioned training program.

Therapeutic presence training includes preparing for presence – through intention before and during session as well as self-care post-session to offer balance in online work. Embodying presence is also trained through grounding, centering, and tapping into sense of calm with exercises that activate the ventral vagal nervous system. Enhancing the process of presence and relational engagement through attuning to clients and therapists' own experience can serve to understand clients' experience through the virtual setting and to strengthen the therapeutic alliance. Given the challenges in online therapy, there is greater possibility for therapeutic ruptures. Training can help therapists to recognize countertransference, therapeutic ruptures, or interpersonal responses, and to attend to them by softening their expression with presence and communicating directly with clients about challenges that arise. Recognizing therapeutic ruptures also allows therapists to focus on repairing these ruptures, thus strengthening the therapeutic alliance. Also, training should include becoming aware of the impact of technology-related issues (glitches, screen freezing, or pixelating) on expressed presence (therapists' facial expression displaying frustration) and perceived presence (clients believing the therapist is upset with them).

Training therapists to communicate their presence online is essential. In fact, the most important aspect of presence and emotional expression (i.e., facial cues, prododic voice, and upper body) is accessible and can be used to create safety (Geller, 2020; Oshni Alvandi, 2019; Weinberg & Rolnick, 2019). Gesturing and verbal expressions of presence need to be more heightened in online therapy to allow clients to feel and receive the presence of their therapist (Prenn & Halliday, 2020; Simpson & Reid, 2014). Cultivating and training therapeutic presence in telepsychotherapy can support therapists in learning how to explicitly express presence, helping clients to experience emotional and psychological safety, and allowing both to feel together, even from a physical distance.

References

Aafjes-van Doorn, K., Békés, V., & Prout, T. A. (2020). Grappling with our therapeutic relationship and professional self-doubt during COVID-19: Will we use video therapy again? *Counselling Psychology Quarterly*, *34*(3-4), 1–12. 10.1080/09515 070.2020.1773404

Aafjes-van Doorn, K., Békés, V., Prout, T. A., & Hoffman, L. (2020). Psychotherapists' vicarious traumatization during the COVID-19 pandemic. *Psychological Trauma: Theory, Research, Practice, and Policy*, *12*, S148–S150. 10.1037/tra0000868

Allison, K. L., & Rossouw, P. J. (2013). The therapeutic alliance: Exploring the concept of "safety" from a neuropsychotherapeutic perspective. *International Journal of Neuropsychotherapy*, *1*(1), 21–29.

Badenach, B. (2018). Safety is the treatment. In S. Porges, & D. Dana (Eds.), *Clinical applications of the polyvagal theory: The emergence of polyvagal-informed therapies* (pp. 73–88). W.W. Norton & Company.

Berle, D., Starcevic, V., Milicevic, D., Hannan, A., Dale, E., Brakoulias, V., & Viswasam, K. (2014). Do patients prefer face-to-face or internet-based therapy? *Psychotherapy and Psychosomatics*, *84*(1), 61–62.

Bos, N., Olson, J., Gergle, D., Olson, G., & Wright, Z. (2002). Effects of four computer-mediated communications channels on trust development. Proceedings from SIGCHI '02: *Conference on Human Factors in Computing Systems*. New York, NY: ACM Digital Library. 10.1145/503376.503401

Bouchard, S., Payeur, R., Rivard, V., Allard, M., Paquin, B., Renaud, P., & Goyer, L. (2000). Cognitive behavior therapy for panic disorder with agoraphobia in video-conference: Preliminary results. *Cyber Psychology & Behavior*, *3*(6), 999–1007.

Bouchard, S., Robillard, G., Marchand, A., & Riva, P. R. (2007). Presence and the bond between patients and their psychotherapists in the cognitive-behavior therapy of panic disorder with agoraphobia delivered in videoconference. https:// astro.temple.edu/~lombard/ISPR/Proceedings/2007/Bouchard,%20Robillard, %20Marchand,%20and%20Riva.pdf

Brahnam, S. (2014). Therapeutic presence in mediated psychotherapy: The uncanny stranger in the room. In G. Riva, J. Waterworth, & D. M. De Gruyter (Eds.), *Interacting with presence: HCI and the sense of presence in computer-mediated environments* (pp. 123–138). De Gruyter.

Butler, E. A., & Randall, A. K. (2013). Emotional coregulation in close relationships. *Emotion Review, 5*(2), 202–210.

Chen, C. K., Nehrig, N., Wash, L., Schneider, J. A., Ashkenazi, S., Cairo, E., Guyton, A. F., & Palfrey, A. (2020). When distance brings us closer: Leveraging tele-psychotherapy to build deeper connection. *Counselling Psychology Quarterly. 34*(3-4). 554–567. 10.1080/09515070.2020.1779031

Cook, J. E., & Doyle, C. (2002). Working alliance in online therapy as compared to face-to-face therapy: Preliminary results. *CyberPsychology & Behavior, 5*(2), 95–105.

Dana, D., & Grant, D. (2018). The polyvagal playlab: Helping therapists bring polyvagal to their clients. In S. Porges, & D. Dana (Eds.), *Clinical applications of the polyvagal theory: The emergence of polyvagal-informed therapies* (pp. 185–206). W.W. Norton & Company.

Dodgen-Magee, D. (2018). *Deviced!: Balancing life and technology in a digital world.* Rowman & Littlefield Publishers.

Dolev-Amit, T., Leibovich, L., & Zilcha-Mano, S. (2020). Repairing alliance ruptures using supportive techniques in telepsychotherapy during the covid-19 pandemic. *Counselling Psychology Quarterly.* 10.1080/09515070.2020.1777089

Ekman, P. (2004). *Emotions revealed: Recognizing faces and feelings to improve communication and emotional life.* Henry Holt and Company.

Fink, J. (1999). *How to use computers and cyberspace in the clinical practice of psychotherapy.* Aronson.

Fishkin, R., Fishkin, L., Leli, U., Katz, B., & Snyder, E. (2011). Psychodynamic treatment, training, and supervision using internet-based technologies. *Journal of the American Academy of Psychoanalysis and Dynamic Psychiatry, 39*(1), 155–168.

Frank, R. (2020). Developing presence online. *The Humanistic Psychologist, 48*(4), 369–372. 10.1037/hum0000208

Geller, S. (2020). Cultivating online therapeutic presence: strengthening therapeutic relationships in teletherapy sessions. *Counselling Psychology Quarterly, 34*(3-4), 1–17.

Geller, S. M. (2017). *A practical guide to cultivating therapeutic presence.* American Psychological Association.

Geller, S. M. (2018). Therapeutic presence and polyvagal theory: Principles and practices for cultivating effective therapeutic relationships. In S. Porges, & D. Dana (Eds.), *Clinical applications of the polyvagal theory: The emergence of polyvagal-informed therapies* (pp. 106–126). W.W. Norton & Company.

Geller, S. M. (2019). Therapeutic presence: The foundation for effective emotion-focused therapy. In L. S. Greenberg, & R. N. Goldman (Eds.), *Clinical handbook of emotion-focused therapy* (pp. 129–145). American Psychological Association.

Geller, S. M., & Greenberg, L. S. (2002). Therapeutic presence: Therapists' experience of presence in the psychotherapy encounter. *Person-Centered & Experiential Psychotherapies, 1*(1–2), 71–86.

Geller, S. M., & Greenberg, L. S. (2012). *Therapeutic presence: A mindful approach to effective therapy.* American Psychological Association.

Geller, S. M., & Porges, S. W. (2014). Therapeutic presence: Neurophysiological mechanisms mediating feeling safe in therapeutic relationships. *Journal of Psychotherapy Integration, 24*(3), 178.

Geller, S. M., Greenberg, L. S., & Watson, J. C. (2010). Therapist and client perceptions of therapeutic presence: The development of a measure. *Psychotherapy Research, 20*(5), 599–610.

Geller, S. M., Pos, A. W., & Colosimo, K. (2012). Therapeutic presence: A common factor in the provision of effective psychotherapy. *Society for Psychotherapy Integration, 47*, 6–13. Psychotherapy Bulletin.

Gray, A. (2018). Roots, rhythm, reciprocity: Polyvagal-informed dance movement therapy for survivors of trauma. In S. Porges, & D. Dana (Eds.), *Clinical applications of the polyvagal theory: The emergence of polyvagal-informed therapies* (pp. 207–226). W.W. Norton & Company.

Haddouk, L. (2015a). Presence at a distance. *Annual Review of Cybertherapy and Telemedicine, 13*, 208–212.

Haddouk, L. (2015b). Presence in telepsychotherapy: towards a video-interview framework. International *Journal of Emergency Mental Health and Human Resilience, 17*(4), 712–713.

Hafermalz, E., & Riemer, K. (2016). Negotiating distance: "presencing work" in a case of remote telenursing. Proceedings from ICIS '16: *The International Conference on Information Systems*. Dublin, Ireland: AIS Electronic Library. https://www.researchgate.net/publication/313794397_Negotiating_Distance_Presencing_Work_in_a_Case_of_Remote_Telenursing

Hayes, J. A., & Vinca, M. (2017). Therapist presence, absence, and extraordinary presence. In L. G. Castonguay, & C. E. Hill (Eds.), *How and why are some therapists better than others?: Understanding therapist effects* (pp. 85–99). American Psychological Association.

Hayes, J., & Vinca, J. (2011). Therapist presence and its relationship to empathy, session, depth, and symptom reduction. Proceedings from SPR '11: *The 42nd Annual Meeting for Society for Psychotherapy Research*. Bern, Switzerland.

Imel, Z. E., Barco, J. S., Brown, H. J., Baucom, B. R., Baer, J. S., Kircher, J. C., & Atkins, D. C. (2014). The association of therapist empathy and synchrony in vocally encoded arousal. *Journal of Counseling Psychology, 61*(1), 146.

Jerome, L. W., & Zaylor, C. (2000). Cyberspace: Creating a therapeutic environment for telehealth applications. *Professional Psychology, Research and Practice, 31*(5), 478.

Marci, C. D., & Orr, S. P. (2006). The effect of emotional distance on psychophysiologic concordance and perceived empathy between patient and interviewer. *Applied Psychophysiology and Biofeedback, 31*(2), 115–128.

Marci, C. D., Ham, J., Moran, E., & Orr, S. P. (2007). Physiologic correlates of perceived therapist empathy and social-emotional process during psychotherapy. *The Journal of Nervous and Mental Disease, 195*(2), 103–111.

Markowitz, J. C., Milrod, B., Heckman, T. G., Bergman, M., Amsalem, D., Zalman, H., Ballas, T., & Neria, Y. (2020). Psychotherapy at a Distance. *The American Journal of Psychiatry*. 10.1176/appi.ajp.2020.20050557

Norcross, J. C., & Lambert, M. J. (2011). *Psychotherapy relationships that work II* (Vol. 48, pp. 4). Educational Publishing Foundation.

Norcross, J. C., & Lambert, M. J. (Eds.). (2019). *Psychotherapy relationships that work: Volume 1: Evidence-based therapist contributions*. Oxford University Press.

Ogden, P. (2018). Polyvagal theory and sensorimotor psychotherapy. In S. Porges, & D. Dana (Eds.), *Clinical applications of the polyvagal theory: The emergence of polyvagal-informed therapies* (pp. 34–49). W.W. Norton & Company.

Ogden, P., & Goldstein, B. (2019). Sensorimotor psychotherapy from a distance: Engaging the body, creating presence, and building relationship in videoconferencing. In H. Weinberg, & A. Rolnick (Eds.), *Theory and practice of online therapy* (pp. 47–65). Routledge.

Oshni Alvandi, A. (2019). Cybertherapogy: A conceptual architecting of presence for counselling via technology. *International Journal of Psychology and Educational Studies*, *6*(1), 30–45.

Pierce, B. S., Perrin, P. B., & McDonald, S. D. (2020). Demographic, organizational, and clinical practice predictors of U.S. psychologists' use of telepsychology. *Professional Psychology, Research and Practice*, *51*(2), 184–193.

Porges, S. W. (1998). Love: An emergent property of the mammalian autonomic nervous system. *Psychoneuroendocrinology*, *23*(8), 837–861.

Porges, S. W. (2011). *The polyvagal theory: Neurophysiological foundations of emotions, attachment, communication, and self-regulation (Norton Series on Interpersonal Neurobiology)*. W.W. Norton & Company.

Porges, S. W. (2018). Polyvagal Theory: A primer. In S. Porges, & D. Dana (Eds.), *Clinical applications of the polyvagal theory: The emergence of polyvagal-informed therapies* (pp. 50–69). W. W. Norton & Company.

Pos, A., Geller, S., & Oghene, J. (2011). Therapist presence, empathy, and the working alliance in experiential treatment for depression. Proceedings from SPR '11: *The 42nd Annual Meeting for Society for Psychotherapy Research*. Bern, Switzerland.

Prenn, N., & Halliday, K. (2020). See Me, Feel Me: An AEDP Toolbox for Creating Therapeutic Presence Online. *Transformance: The AEDP Journal*, *20*(1). https://aedpinstitute.org/transformance-volume-10-therapeutic-presence-halliday-prenn/

Quillman, T. (2012). Neuroscience and therapist self-disclosure: Deepening right brain to right brain communication between therapist and patient. *Clinical Social Work Journal*, *40*(1), 1–9.

Ramseyer, F., & Tschacher, W. (2011). Nonverbal synchrony in psychotherapy: Coordinated body movement reflects relationship quality and outcome. *Journal of Consulting and Clinical Psychology*, *79*(3), 284.

Ramseyer, F., & Tschacher, W. (2014). Nonverbal synchrony of head-and-body-movement in psychotherapy: Different signals have different associations with outcome. *Frontiers in Psychology*, *5*, 979.

Rathenau, S., Sousa, D., Vaz, A., & Geller, S. (in press). The effect of attitudes towards online therapy and difficulties perceived in the online therapeutic presence. *Journal of Psychotherapy Integration*.

Rees, C. S., & Stone, S. (2005). Therapeutic alliance in face-to-face versus video-conferenced psychotherapy. *Professional Psychology, Research and Practice*, *36*(6), 649–653.

Reynolds, D. A. J., Stiles, W. B., & Grohol, J. M. (2006). An investigation of session impact and alliance in internet-based psychotherapy: Preliminary results. *Counselling and Psychotherapy Research*, *6*(3), 164–168.

Rossouw, P. J. (2013). The end of the medical model: Recent findings in neuroscience regarding antidepressant medication and the implications for neuropsychotherapy. *Applied Neuropsychotherapy*. http://www.neuropsychotherapist.com/the-end-ofthe-medical-model/

Schoenenberg, K., Raake, A., & Koeppe, J. (2014). Why are you so slow? — Misattribution of transmission delay to attributes of the conversation partner at the far-end. *International Journal of Human-computer Studies*, *72*(5), 477–487.

Schore, A. N. (2009). Right-brain affect regulation: An essential mechanism of development, trauma, dissociation, and psychotherapy. In D. Fosha, D. J. Siegal, & M. F. Solomon (Eds.), *The healing power of emotion: Affective neuroscience, development & clinical practice* (pp. 112–144). W. W. Norton & Company.

Schore, A. N. (2012). *The science of the art of psychotherapy (Norton series on interpersonal neurobiol ogy)*. W.W. Norton & Company.

Siegel, D. J. (1999). *The developing mind*. Guilford Press.

Siegel, D. J. (2007). *The mindful brain: Reflection and attunement in the cultivation of well-being*. W. W. Norton & Company, Inc.

Siegel, D. J. (2010). *The mindful therapist: A clinician's guide to mindsight and neural integration (Norton Series on Interpersonal Neurobiology)*. W.W. Norton & Company.

Simpson, S. G., & Reid, C. L. (2014). Therapeutic alliance in videoconferencing psychotherapy: A review. *The Australian Journal of Rural Health, 22*(6), 280–299.

Sjöström, J., & Alfonsson, S. (2012). Supporting the therapist in online therapy. Proceedings from ECIS '12: *The 20th European Conference on Information Systems*. Barcelona, Spain: AIS Electronic Library. https://www.researchgate.net/ publication/289165884_Supporting_the_therapist_n_online_therapy?enrichId= rgreq-71f42d9094fd1dd4ca7034c64b671e45-XXX&enrichSource=Y292ZXJQY WdlOzI4OTE2NTg4NDtBUzo0NDA3NTg5MTUzNDIzMzdAMTQ4MjA5Nj- UyMjkzNw%3D%3D&el=1_x_2&_esc=publicationCoverPdf

Thompson, G. (2018). Brain-empowered collaborators: Polyvagal perspectives on the doctor-patient relationships. In S. Porges, & D. Dana (Eds.), *Clinical applications of the polyvagal theory: The emergence of polyvagal-informed therapies* (pp. 127–148). W.W. Norton & Company.

Tuxbury, J. S. (2013). The experience of presence among telehealth nurses. *Journal of Nursing Research, 21*(3), 155–161.

Varker, T., Brand, R., Ward, J., Terhaag, S., & Phelps, A. (2019). Efficacy of Synchronous telepsychology interventions for people with anxiety, depression, posttraumatic stress disorder, and adjustment disorder: A rapid evidence assessment. *Psychological Services, 16*(4), 621–635.

Weinberg, H. (2020). Online group psychotherapy: Challenges and possibilities during COVID-19—A practice review. *Group Dynamics: Theory, Research, and Practice, 24*(3), 201–211. 10.1037/gdn0000140

Weinberg, H., & Rolnick, A. (2019). Introduction. In H. Weinberg, & A. Rolnick (Eds.), *Theory and practice of online therapy* (pp. 1–10). Routledge.

Wray, B. T., & Rees, C. S. (2003). Is there a role for videoconferencing in cognitive–behavioural therapy. Proceedings from AACBT '03: *The 11th National Conference on Australian Association for Cognitive and Behaviour Therapy*. Perth, Australia.

2 Finding Closeness while Socially Distant: Clinical Considerations for the Therapeutic Frame and Process in Teletherapy

Danielle Magaldi and Leora Trub

Clinical Considerations for the Therapeutic Frame and Process in Teletherapy

Prompted by the COVID-19 outbreak, for the first time in psychotherapy's history, therapy was almost universally conducted outside of the consulting room as patients and therapists met over screens and phones from their own homes. Pets, partners, children, or roommates might be right outside the door (and sometimes even inside the room). Initially and as a fairly new phenomenon, teletherapy was slowly finding its place in our field with therapists engaged in teletherapy based on their own comfort and at their own pace (Perle et al., 2011), until teletherapy became the sole means of outpatient and private practice treatment during the COVID-19 pandemic. Now, the practice of psychotherapy has changed and the clinical implications of this abound.

Over the past 15 years, social media and smartphones have fundamentally altered the way we relate. With those changes, therapists had to consider competing realities – that communication technologies could offer progress and opportunities for emotional wellbeing, while also threatening to reduce complex emotional expressions to limited characters and emojis on a screen. With the advent of teletherapy, the debate continued, with therapists considering whether to stress the importance of in-person encounters or to adopt new communication technologies for therapeutic use. One measure of the field's confusion regarding how to negotiate this new modality can be detected in the bevy of terms used to describe teletherapy: E-mental health, internet therapy, e-therapy, online counseling, cyber counseling, remote treatment, distance therapy, virtual therapy, all as practices under the umbrella of online therapy or telehealth (Barak et al., 2009). While some therapists may have felt hesitant to embrace therapy over a screen and lose the rich clinical information derived from feeling one's body in the consulting room, the necessity of conducting therapy over a screen in a time of social distancing protocols quickly made obvious the benefits and affordances of teletherapy.

DOI: 10.4324/9781003205029-4

Regardless of previous experience with this modality, understanding and effectively practicing teletherapy is now an ethical imperative for all psychotherapists. An empirically supported discussion of the practice of teletherapy is essential. We understand that communication enacted online is different from face-to-face meetings (Finkel et al., 2012). While there are good reasons for both in-person and teletherapy models, the field until the present time, had focused much of its energy on in-person encounters. Psychotherapy had long privileged face-to-face, in-person sessions. But we now recognize that screens offer connection. Teletherapy brings patients into treatment who would otherwise be excluded. It is convenient, increasing access for patients who live in rural areas or who have decreased mobility because of physical limitations or mental health conditions that limit traveling, like agoraphobia. It allows for flexibility, and keeps patient and therapist connected when breaks in continuity might be counterproductive for treatment. Some patients experience lowered inhibitions, allowing them to say things to their screen therapist that they would have difficulty saying in person (Reynolds et al., 2013).

The current outbreak is an extreme version of the very dynamic which has most commonly motivated therapists to engage in remote treatment – necessity and circumstance (Trub & Magaldi, 2017). But experiencing teletherapy as something that is unavoidable or even compulsory may create the conditions where therapists avoid thinking deeply about the meanings behind its use for a given treatment. Even before COVID-19 forced us all into remote treatment, the reasons for engaging in teletherapy were already expanding – many therapists were offering remote sessions when they themselves (rather than their patients) were on a vacation. The sudden onset of remote treatment prompted by COVID-19 now has lasting effects. The following chapter offers practical clinical considerations for teletherapy based on data generated from a Grounded Theory study that engaged 28 therapists in their impressions of teletherapy and what changes in the clinical encounter over a screen (Magaldi & Trub, 2020; Trub & Magaldi, 2021; Trub, Berler, & Magaldi, 2022). Based on those findings and clinical cases of the authors, practical considerations in two categories – modification to the therapeutic frame and therapeutic processes are suggested. The present moment in psychotherapy requires immediate consideration of best practices. Importantly, these considerations are aligned with and support previous clinical writing and research on the differences that both therapists and patients experience when moving treatment online (see Bayles, 2012; Isaacs Russell, 2015; Sabbadini, 2014; Tao, 2015).

Clinical Considerations

Phone Versus Screen

There are two basic options when conducting remote sessions – phone or screen. Both patients and therapists may have a clear preference. In our interviews, some therapists preferred the screen for the added visual domain, and for its ability to simulate greater closeness and intimacy. They valued seeing the patient's face, and the option to be invited into the patient's surroundings. Others, however, described feeling distracted and overstimulated and disliked being unable to modulate the distance between themselves and their patients. One therapist described the visual set-up of screen sessions as "intrusive," and found working over a screen made her feel "not human." Another therapist described feeling "jarred" by the image of himself on screen, and wished to turn the video off so he could focus better on the patient's voice. Some therapists felt more able to focus on what the patient said and on their own thoughts, reactions, intuitions, and states of reverie via the phone.

Such negative responses are an outgrowth of doing therapy in a modality for which almost nobody has been trained. Therapists' feelings of incompetence, inexperience, or resentment can interfere with the ability to be fully present. When therapist and patient preferences clash, therapists must decide how to proceed – to defer to a patient's wishes or suggest their own. Therapists should weigh the wish to be flexible and accommodating against their own capacity to operate in a certain domain. Oftentimes, therapists may not know what modality is best until they have used it. As treatment progresses, therapists can invite discussion of progress, with the knowledge there is always the option to move to a different domain.

The following considerations are relevant to practice of teletherapy, and provide an opportunity for therapists to consider the clinical differences when practicing over this modality.

Modifications to the Frame

In teletherapy, we lose our ability to cultivate the shared experience of sessions. We cannot keep the tissues stocked. Nor can we strategically situate ourselves at the right distance from the patient – to be present but not invasive. We do not choose the wall hangings and ornaments of the patients' environment. This loss of control marks a significant shift in our work. Our tendency is to deal with this by ignoring it or compensating, which shortchanges the clinical process (Essig, 2015b). Instead, we can attempt to neither deny, nor try too hard to correct for, the differences in experience between remote and in-person treatment. To assert that they are not the same is not a matter of judgment, it is a statement of fact. We might instead tune into the differences, explore them, and allow them to hold meaning (Weinberg & Rolnick, 2020).

Creating a New Frame

Screens are used for countless tasks and encounters, making it easy for patients to unwittingly transmute and confuse the rules of engagement for social networking and other online communication to teletherapy. This can be true for many patients, while even more so for adolescents and young adults, who are digital natives (Magaldi et al., 2019). Therapists must seriously take on changes to the therapeutic frame when therapy moves from the office to the screen so that patients still feel the encounter is curated with thoughtfulness and clinical intention (Trub, 2021).

The commute to the therapy office for both the patient and the therapist provides an essential transition from one space to the next. Now, patient or therapist might be responding to email, FaceTiming a family member, scrolling through a dating app, online shopping for groceries, even watching pornography, moments before they click over to their therapy session. Teletherapy requires we now discuss with our patients about how best to set up the encounter from their end. Patients have long relied on therapists to be in charge of creating the ideal conditions for sessions. We can help patients discuss the physical and emotional space needed for teletherapy: finding privacy, locking the door, turning off notifications, playing music or running a fan for sound insulation, and setting up time before and after session for transitions. In our study, it was not uncommon for therapists to describe patients sitting in a parked car doing remote treatment. While some may not have a choice about this, others have chosen it simply because they have not seriously considered their needs or options. Therapists can help facilitate such conversations, and must help a patient consider their needs in creating the therapeutic frame for themselves.

Time and Space

Time and space are foundational parts of the therapeutic frame. Patients and therapists might be seeing each other in different time zones and times of day, morning for one and evening for the other, raining for the therapist, and sunny for the patient. The clashing of realities has the potential for new levels of disorientation. In a teletherapy session, a therapist described a session in which she found her very depressed adolescent patient fast asleep. Since the beginning of treatment a couple of months earlier, the therapist had struggled to connect with the girl, who presented with a flat, depressed affect and had little to say. The therapist tried to wake the patient up by speaking to her, but to no avail. She considered her options – contacting the mother would risk allowing an intrusion into the session, but not contacting her might result in the patient missing the entire session despite being there. At first somewhat disoriented and paralyzed on how to proceed, she then decided to spend the time observing the patient and considering the clinical meanings of this moment, including her own difficulty staying on this task and "with" the patient as she slept. Eventually she entered into a sort of reverie state where she felt a deep warmth towards the sleeping girl for the first time. When the patient woke up 15 minutes later, the session took a different course from previous sessions. For the first time, the patient was able to put words to a deep emptiness that plagued her, and from which she often used to sleep to escape. In this moment, the screen transformed from something that kept patient and therapist distant and separated to allow for a connection that led to the deepening of therapy.

Teletherapy also splits therapeutic space into two – one room for the therapist and another for the patient. We find ourselves in our patients' spaces, in their bedrooms and kitchens, partners or children or parents within a short distance (hopefully not within earshot). Some patients may want to give us a tour of their home, or retrieve an art project that before they could only have described. These shifts in the time and space and session present some challenges that are somewhat unprecedented when it comes to the frame and therapeutic boundaries. Where do we draw the line? Do we conduct sessions with patients while they are lying in bed? The benefits of allowing a patient to give us a tour of their house and their favorite things, even other family members, might outweigh the risks of rejecting such a request. But this calculus changes when a patient casually mentions that their partner or friend is actually in the room, listening to the session. Or when a patient decides to conduct a session while driving a car. These changes to the frame can take the therapist by surprise, as our training has never addressed these possibilities. But now that teletherapy is a therapeutic norm, we can be prepared to speak with our patients about the frame of remote therapy, and to process the increased flexibility and convenience – both its benefits and its consequences.

The same considerations exist in regard to our own spaces. While we may have an expanded view of the patient's space, their view of our space shrinks. If we are working in an office where we have had co-present sessions, there may be no mystery. Otherwise, our patients are left in the dark about what surrounds us. Teletherapy creates intrigue, as our patients know we too have retreated into our private spaces, which may not always be our offices. As we invite our patients into our homes, there will be questions – both those they ask and those that remain unspoken. Our patients may be used to knowing where we are; are we prepared to share that information when using teletherapy? How important is it to maintain consistency in our background from one session to the next? How does our actual space impact our ability to convey to patients we are still right there with them? While these changes in the frame may feel acceptable, recognizing their importance and impact for each treatment will be necessary for preserving the safety and relational benefits of maintaining a consistent frame. Going further, would we consider a new, common virtual space that is co-created through technology tools like Zoom Immersive Mode or Teams Together Mode? This would allow the therapist and patient to include shared elements in their physical background.

Privacy

Teletherapy now must consider how privacy changes for therapist and patient alike when therapy is conducted outside the confines of the closed doors of the consulting room. If therapists choose not to work from an office, they lose a degree of anonymity working from home or other remote locations. They may be unable to shield patients entirely from the sounds of a baby crying in the next room or the dog barking to go out. External cues may offer clues of our surroundings. Theoretical orientation influences decisions around how to respond. A classical approach suggests remaining silent and waiting for the patient to ask questions, absolving the therapist of directly addressing a patient's possible desire to know more of a therapist's whereabouts (Lane & Hull, 1990). A relational model suggests the therapist might self disclose more openly about their new venue. Cognitive behavioral therapists may openly disclose as a means of modeling and reinforcement (Goldfried et al., 2003). For patients, privacy is a serious concern as well. Patients may unconsciously restrict topics or emotional expression if their own privacy is not ensured or conversely, may be triggered to engage topics because of proximity to people and situations experienced in the moment. A therapist's attunement to this will help in noticing whether a patient has the privacy needed to freely engage the work, and how the work may be impacted by factors in a patient's home environment.

A psychologist from the research study reported on a woman in her 20s who started a relationship just before the COVID-19 pandemic. The new romantic partner was immediately let go from his job and had to move out of his home, which prompted her to invite him to stay with her for a while, giving them the opportunity to feel out their relationship. The patient lived in a one-bedroom apartment and conducted sessions in the bedroom while he was in the living space. The therapist quickly noticed that the patient had become somewhat more hesitant and guarded when talking about the partner, and wondered about the authenticity of the patient's portrayal of how great things were going. It became clear that the patient was somewhat afraid of her new partner, who seemed rather controlling despite a charismatic and convincing presentation of himself as gentle and flexible. However, attempts to engage her in discussion were undermined by the patient's fear of being heard, even when she had taken several steps to ensure that he could not hear her, and she would not ask him to leave for fear of giving the impression that anything was wrong in the relationship. The therapist felt much more stymied in her ability to facilitate a conversation with the patient than she would have if they were together in person, separate from the boyfriend. Ultimately, the therapist took an assertive stance in insisting that the patient leave her own home to conduct sessions outside, and only then were they able to start having more honest conversations about the state of affairs in this new partnership.

Until COVID, the patient's living situation had helped her establish boundaries with her romantic partners, and she used therapy effectively to work through dysfunctional dynamics. But the situational and psychological realities of COVID led her to open her home to a partner, which cost her a safe space where she was free to consider her own needs. Similar to her home life as a child, she found herself unable to find respite from a controlling, intrusive but also caregiving individual. This situation undermined the therapist's effectiveness in helping her explore the dynamics of her relationship and consider what she wanted. But as the screen was the only portal through which the therapist could offer any assistance, the therapist felt compelled to be quite directive in setting up the sessions to best ensure a sense of safety for the patient. This was a departure from the more collaborative way they had worked previously, which the therapist understood to be a representation of how working remotely created unique vulnerabilities for this patient, which had to be managed in a unique way.

Maintaining Professionalism

Finally, our patients have the right to the same professionalism online as they experience in our consulting rooms. Therapists do find themselves cheating in a variety of ways, and with varying degrees of intentionality: Forgetting to turn off sounds from other programs, reading notifications that pop up on the screen, responding to texts outside of a patient's view. Multitasking may be an enigma to the therapy environment, but it is part and parcel of technology use; as such, the temptations may be powerful (Carr, 2010). The perception of oneself as a luddite does not absolve a therapist of her responsibility to prepare for this encounter, just as she would prepare the consulting room by straightening the office, making sure the white noise machine was working, and removing unnecessary distractions. Configuring the computer to minimize distraction, choosing to use the full-screen mode, being dressed for our professional interaction, and deciding how to deal with one's own image on screen are essential to the process.

Therapeutic Processes

Silence and Affect

Therapists and patients alike have noted that silences are shorter and less frequent in remote sessions, with longer silences leading to anxiety about having lost the internet connection – hardly an ideal way to follow up the emergence of meaningful material or deep affect. To avoid this, we fill spaces with words that before we had trusted to silence (Isaacs Russell, 2015). Now, we can take close notice of changes in the pace and frequency of words as well as silences. Notice shifts in affect – is it easier for the patient to cry? Harder? One therapist noticed that it was hard for her to convey safety over a screen. The gentle, subvocal sounds she might make to signal she was listening felt distracting over the screen. Without our bodies to lean forward or our three-dimensional facial expressions, communicating empathy can feel strained. We might make adjustments over a screen by purposely sitting further from the camera so that we can lean in at times. But, when we lose the live presence and emotional resonance of in-person treatment, we find ourselves operating without our usual toolbox. One therapist described "sitting at my desk with my laptop there and I could see her and she could see me but it just felt like we were missing a lot."

Intersubjectivity

The intersubjective dimension refers to the meeting or overlap between the subjectivities of two people (Benjamin, 1995; Stolorow et al., 1987). While the concept is most commonly linked to relational psychoanalysis, the ideas behind it are relevant to any psychotherapy which privileges the interpersonal context and considers this dimension essential to good therapeutic outcomes (e.g., IPT; see Lipsitz & Markowitz, 2013). Working over a screen can make it harder to attend to subtleties of body language and other implicit forms of communication which are core to identifying attachment dynamics and the emergence of maladaptive relational patterns (Bruschweiler-Stern et al., 2002).

This echoes IsaacsRussell's (2015) assertion that in teletherapy the analyst's main tools are compromised as a function of having to attend more intensely to the patient, while losing the ability to pay attention to the self. In that process, as one therapist in our study noted, it can be particularly challenging to "hold on to the intersubjective space … which I really find uncomfortable."

The screen can also exacerbate certain relational dynamics. One therapist described a feeling of being taken advantage of when the patient situated the therapy time into their personal schedule in precisely the way they wanted, while she was walking around her home drinking some tea: "there's something about the quality of switching on and off - she's sipping her tea and talking to me and she's not always in the same room. I'm always in the same room … she values Skype because even if she's in the middle of what she calls a crisis, she can talk to me … so it's enabled her to bring that really broken down self to a therapist … [but] I have to muck around my therapy times to talk to her – I have to accommodate to her more than I usually would."

When we have the opportunity to see a patient both on screen and in person, we have the benefit of being able to compare the experiences. How does resistance manifest itself differently in each context? We might also notice differences in the quality of our attention. Are we attending more to make up for some loss? Are we experiencing less reverie, which can offer insight into enactments or other subtle aspects of the treatment? When treatment is entirely remote we can consider these dynamics nonetheless, and allow ourselves space to notice

Eye Contact

Eye contact is but one component of remote treatment that impacts intersubjectivity. When we are meeting by screen, where do we look? Whether we look at the camera or the screen, there is no way to truly hold eye contact with our patients. How might we find ourselves compensating for this? We understand from early childhood development how the reciprocal gaze is one of our earliest forms of communication, creating a sense of safety (Beebe, 2005). The therapeutic encounter similarly uses eye contact to communicate between patient and therapist, helping a patient feel emotionally seen and held. But teletherapy changes that and requires an adjustment, as noted by one therapist, "When you're using Skype the distance between the camera and where the person's face is, means that if I'm looking at their face, then they're not getting my eyes." Teletherapy must contend with discovering new ways to hold patients over a screen.

Content of the Session

The disembodied experience of meeting over a screen, with a two-dimensional image of our heads or bodies from the waist up, can have some patients feeling disconnected to the therapist while others feeling more freedom to connect. It may be helpful to consider the content of the session and what may have changed as treatment moves over a screen. Some patients will keep the content lighter and more superficial, as they feel unmoored by the loss of physical and emotional containment over a screen (Isaacs Russell, 2015). Others may go deeper or discuss topics they didn't broach before, as they feel less inhibited without the physical presence of the therapist in the room. In one treatment that moved over a screen, the patient felt free to share her anxiety and shame surrounding her confession that she had never masturbated. Together she and the therapist took up the meaning underneath this, but also engaged how she was feeling too self conscious to engage with her therapist in-person on feelings around her body and sex.

Conclusion

In an increasingly globalized world, digital technology allows people to stay connected to one another even while people are more mobile than ever for both work and leisure. Therapists and their patients are no exception to this. Deep therapeutic work can and does take place over a screen. Ideally, at least according to some (see Essig; Isaacs Russell), this work happens best when we are aware of the limitations of the screen, when we hold in mind the inherent contradiction of transitioning the subtle and intimate nature of our work to a distant and unreliable medium.

The conflicts and challenges presented by remote treatment prior to March 2020 was flipped on its head when a global pandemic made it unsafe to see our patients in person, which took the choice of whether or not to engage in remote sessions away from individual therapeutic dyads. No longer having to hold these conflicts internally, many therapists took the news of this fate with some mixture of displeasure and anxiety. There was little time to prepare, and no training on how to move entire clinical practices to the computer and the phone.

Two years later, perceptions of teletherapy have largely transformed from a tolerated necessity to a fully viable form of treatment. But the way we use technology to facilitate psychotherapy requires deep consideration so that we can engage it in the most authentic and meaningful way while maintaining a commitment to the therapeutic process and frame. Technology use outside of the consulting room is paradoxical in nature, often simultaneously engendering feelings of connection and disconnection, empowerment and enslavement, and independence and dependence (Jarvenpaa & Lang, 2005; Trub & Barbot, 2016; Trub & Magaldi, 2019; Turkle, 2011). Similarly, there are paradoxes inherent in teletherapy. Patients may feel untethered over a screen, producing feelings of freedom on the one hand and loss and anxiety on the other. Therapists may be grateful for the adaptability screens offer to our livelihood, even while feeling resentful for always being within reach of our patients. Patients and therapists may appreciate maintaining connection but might also experience this connection as an invasion of privacy. Teletherapy requires we actively and intentionally consider these paradoxes while evaluating how changes in the frame, eye contact, silence, privacy, and intersubjectivity will impact treatment.

References

Aguilera, A., & Muñoz, R. F. (2011). Text messaging as an adjunct to CBT in low-income populations: A usability and feasibility pilot study. *Professional Psychology: Research and Practice, 42*(6), 472–478.

Aron, L. (1996). *A meeting of minds — mutuality in psychoanalysis.* London: The Analytic Press.

Barak, A., Klein, B., & Proudfoot, J. G. (2009). Defining internet-supported therapeutic interventions. *Annals of Behavioral Medicine, 38*(1), 4–17.

Bayles, M. (2012). Is physical proximity essential to the psychoanalytic process? An exploration through the lens of Skype? *Psychoanalytic Dialogues, 22*(5), 569–585.

Beebe, B. (2005). Mother-infant research informs mother-infant treatment. *The Psychoanalytic Study of the Child, 60*(1), 7–46. 10.1007/s10615-009-0256-7

Berler, M., Trub, L. , & Magaldi, D.(in press). Evolving Public Self in a Digitally Disrupted Marketplace. *Journal of Psychotherapy Integration.*

Benjamin, J. (1995). *Like subjects, love objects: Essays on recognition and sexual difference.* New Haven, CT: Yale University Press.

Bruschweiler-Stern, N., Harrison, A. M., Lyons-Ruth, K., Morgan, A. C., Nahum, J. P., & Tronick, E. Z. (2002). Explicating the implicit: The local level and the microprocess of change in the analytic situation. *International Journal of Psychoanalysis, 83*(5), 1051–1062.

Carr, N. (2010). *The shallows: What the internet is doing to our brains.* WW Norton & Company.

Clough, B. A., & Casey, L. M. (2015). The smart therapist: A look to the future of smartphones and health technologies in psychotherapy. *Professional Psychology: Research and Practice, 46*(3), 147–153. 10.1037/pro0000011.

Essig, T. (2015a). The "full training illusion" and the myth of functional equivalence. *Round Robin Newsletter, 30*(2). Retrieved July 16, 2017 http://internationalpsy choanalysis.net/wp-content/uploads/2015/05/RoundRobin2Essig2015FINAL

Essig, T. (2015b). The "full training forms" mother-infant treatment. *Psychoanalytic Study of the Child, 60,* 7–46.

Finkel, E. J., Eastwick, P. W., Karney, B. R., Reis, H. T., & Sprecher, S. (2012). Online dating: A critical analysis from the perspective of psychological science. *Psychological Science in the Public Interest, 13*(1), 3–66. 10.1177/1529100612436522.

Goldfried, M. R., Burckell, L. A., & Eubanks-Carter, C. (2003). Therapist self-disclosure in cognitive-behavior therapy. *Journal of Clinical Psychology, 59*(5), 555–568.

Isaacs Russell, G. (2015). *Screen relations: The limits of computer-mediated psychoanalysis and psychotherapy.* London: Karnac Books Ltd.

Jarvenpaa, S. L., & Lang, K. R. (2005). Managing the paradoxes of mobile technology. *Information Systems Management, 22*(4), 7–23.

Lane, R. C., & Hull, J. W. (1990). *Self-Disclosure and classical psychoanalysis.* In G. Stricker, & M. Fisher (Eds.), *Self-Disclosure in the Therapeutic Relationship.* Boston, MA: Springer.

Lemma, A., & Caparrotta, L. (2014). *Psychoanalysis in the technoculture era.* New York, NY: Routledge.

Lipsitz, J. D., & Markowitz, J. C. (2013). Mechanisms of change in interpersonal therapy (IPT). *Clinical Psychology Review, 33*(8), 1134–1147. doi: 10.1016/j.cpr.2013.09.002.

Magaldi, D., & Trub, L. (2020). Staying Close while Social Distancing: Lessons for Teletherapy from a Grounded Theory Study. *The Integrative Therapist, 3*(6), 19–20.

Magaldi, D., Appel, R., & Berler, M. (2019). Adolescence and Social Media Use. In S. Hupp, & J. Jewell (Eds.), *The Encyclopedia of Child and Adolescent Development.* Hoboken, NJ: Wiley-Blackwell.

Markowitz, J. C., Lipsitz, J., & Milrod, B. L. (2014). Critical review of outcome research on interpersonal psychotherapy for anxiety disorders. *Depression and Anxiety, 31,* 316–325.

Perle, J. G., Langsam, L. C., & Nierenberg, B. (2011). Controversy clarified: An updated review of clinical psychology and telehealth. *Clinical Psychology Review, 31*(8), 1247–1258.

Reynolds, D. J., Jr., Stiles, W. B., Bailer, A. J., & Hughes, M. R. (2013). Impact of exchanges and client-therapist alliance in online-text psychotherapy. *Cyberpsychology, Behavior and Social Networking, 16*(5), 370–377. 10.1089/cyber.2012.0195. Epub 2013 Mar 26.

Rizvi, S. L., Hughes, C. D., & Thomas, M. C. (2016). The DBT coach mobile application as an adjunct to treatment for suicidal and self-injuring individuals with borderline personality disorder. *Psychological Services, 13*(4), 380–388. 10.1037/ser0000100.

Sabbadini, A. (2014). New technologies and the psychoanalytic setting. In A. Lemma, & L. Caparrotta (Eds.), *Psychoanalysis in the technoculture era* (pp. 23–32). New York, NY: Routledge.

Stolorow, R. D., Brandchaft, B., & Atwood, G. E. (1987). *Psychoanalytic treatment: An intersubjective approach.* Hillsdale, NJ: Analytic Press.

Tao, L. (2015). Teleanalysis: problems, limitations, and opportunities. In J. S. Scharff (Ed.), *Psychoanalysis online 2: Impact of technology on development, training, and therapy* (pp. 105–120). London: Karnac Books Ltd.

Trub, L. (2021). Playing and digital reality: Treating kids and adolescents in a pandemic. *Psychoanalytic Perspectives: An international Journal of Integration and Innovation, 18*(2), 208–225. 10.1080/1551806X.2021.1896308

Trub, L., & Barbot, B. (2016). The paradox of phone attachment: Development and psychometric properties of the attachment to phone scale. *Computers in Human Behavior, 64*, 663–672.

Trub, L., & Magaldi, D. (2017). Left to our own devices. *Psychoanalytic Perspectives, 14*(2), 219–236. 10.1080/1551806X.2017.1304118

Trub, L., & Magaldi, D. (2019). Digital dialectics: navigating technology's paradoxes in online treatment. In H. Weinberg, & A. Rolnick (Eds.), (2020) *Theory and practice of online therapy: Internet-delivered interventions for individuals, families, groups, and organizations.* New York: Routledge.

Trub, L., & Magaldi, D. (2021). Secret powers: Acts of googling in the therapeutic relationship. *Journal of Clinical Psychology, 202*, 1–18. 10.1002/jclp.23107.

Trub, L., Berler, M., & Magaldi, D. (2022). Collisions and collusions with new norms: Renegotiating therapeutic boundaries in the digital age. *Journal of Psychotherapy Integration, 32*(1), 64–82. 10.1037/int0000272.

Turkle, S. (2011). *Alone together: Why we expect more from technology and less from ourselves.* New York, NY: Basic Books.

Van der Kolk, B. A. (2015). *The body keeps the score.* New York, NY: Penguin Books.

Weinberg, H., & Rolnick, A. (Eds.) (2020). *Theory and practice of online therapy: Internet-delivered interventions for individuals, families, groups, and organizations.* New York: Routledge.

3 Reflections on Empathic Presence in Online Therapeutic Relations

Lou Agosta

Definitions and Context: Empathy and the Digital Divide

A rigorous definition allows that empathy exists across the screen-mediated conversation in online relations. Empathy is rigorously defined in this essay as the four-fold process of receptivity to the other person's emotions ("bottom up," *affective* empathy), understanding of the other person as a possibility, seeing matters from the other individual's perspective, i.e., taking a walk in the other's shoes (with the other's shoe size, not yours ("top down," cognitive empathy)), and empathic responsiveness in an articulate, expressive communication, providing recognition and acknowledgment of the other's struggle and humanity (see Agosta, 2010, 2015, 2020). Empathy is not a mere psychological mechanism; empathy is a practice, a way of relating, communicating, and being with the other person. Nothing in this definition limits the context to shared physical space provided one includes communication technology as part of the presence and relatedness (transference).

An expanded definition of empathy, consistent with the above, allows that empathy is understood as being fully present with another person without judgment, evaluation, or anything else added. Being present with another person in the same physical space (such as a therapist's office) is the traditional approach (e.g., see Russell (2015), discussed below). However, if we apply a non-traditional approach, we can say that the genie is out of the bottle. The genie is online therapy.

In my own work on empathy, published the same year as Gillian Isaacs Russell's book on *Screen Relations* (2015), my preface concludes with the ontological definition of empathy as "being in the presence of another human being without anything else added" – anything else such as judgment, evaluation, memory, desire, hostility, and the many factors that make us unavailable to *be* in a relationship (Agosta, 2015; see also 2010). Gillian Isaacs Russell is a noted psychoanalyst who has engaged in a penetrating and incisive discussion of doing online therapy (2015). Though Russell uses the word "empathy" in a specific psychological sense, I would argue that her work on "presence" is consistent with and contributes to an enlarged sense of empathic presence that builds relatedness.

DOI: 10.4324/9781003205029-5

It means: The digital divide creates discontent for everybody. No exceptions. Indeed the digital divide creates magical thinking, new kinds of parapraxes, and motivated coincidences regardless of one's level of technological sophistication. New technologies call forth new challenges. To err is human; really to stumble requires the Internet!

Empathy Both Divides and Connects as Does Screen Relations

Amid a storm of uncertainties, one thing is for sure. Empathy is one of the things in the world that a person cannot do all alone. People have to relate to each other to bring forth empathy. Even though a person has empathy for her/himself, such relatedness is derivative on the individual in question having received empathy from empathic others, such as parents and caretakers. Empathy is the foundation of community as people work, play, and relate in families and society.

Transference has always and without exception included the safe and private setting, context, and frame. Transference needs a safe space. The frame for therapy is largely invisible as long as it functions as designed. The frame becomes visible when there is a breakdown. The outer door to the consulting room is locked or the schedule gets mixed up or the client loses his/her job and can no longer afford the service as agreed. The frame does not hold and the therapy breaks down. What is new, disruptive, disturbing, and even possibly inspiring about online therapy is that the frame now includes communication software and client friendly interfaces.

Online therapy reduces the list of breakdowns in some ways and expands the list of breakdowns in other ways. One does not get stuck in traffic on the way to one's session; but computer breakdowns are abundant. The communication network is invisible unless the network "goes down." A whole new world of breakdowns and ruptures emerge, as the client and/or therapist are "old school" or lack basic computer literacy. Getting therapy previously did not require computer literacy. How do you feel about the fact that therapy now requires computer literacy? Very ambivalent! Many empathic therapists I know are going to be discontented by computer anxiety, which, arguably, may be added to the list of treatable disorders.

Whether empathy – spontaneous relatedness – is a subset of transference or vice versa has never been adequately addressed as an issue. Empathy is also closely related to projective identification; but the point is that empathy is not a mere psychological mechanism but an authentic form of human interrelations (for a detailed discussion, see Agosta, 2014). At the current state of the debate, the value lies in the very idea of authentic interrelatedness, not the circular dance of the many psychological distinctions.

Freud encountered *Einfühlung* (the word "empathy" in German) in the works of Theodor Lipps (Freud, 1905), for whom empathy was a form of aesthetic projection of the animate life of the one person's psyche onto nature and other persons. Freud expanded the use of this psychological mechanism without fully appreciating its potential, and, even today, empathy's possibilities are still expanding in transforming human stuckness and suffering. Nevertheless, whenever two human beings encounter one another, whether online or in-person or via the written word in a novel, empathy is the foundation of relatedness. A case can be made (Russell, 2015) that empathy is privileged in the person-to-person encounter in shared physical space, but I note without contradicting her, empathy is possibly present when and wherever people try to relate to one another.

Empathy Confronts Screen Relations

When the pandemic hit in Chicago, USA, in March 2020, I had three clients who were severely challenged by the transition from in office to online therapy.

For example, Mr Joe (imaginary name), a 20-something worker in logistics, did indeed have a family computer at home, but he was living at home in genteel poverty, sharing a room with his younger brother. That was not a problem at first, since he was able to visit me in-person in the office for a confidential conversation. But with the pandemic, we were unable to do that – and he had no privacy at home. He tried taking the video session call at the job in what he hoped would be a private space. It was not as private as hoped. He tried walking around the block using Facetime video on his smart phone. The March wind is blowing, the client is walking, and the image is bouncing up and down.

I am thinking to myself: "Do I ask him to stand still, please, as I am getting motion sickness?" My empathy is disrupted. Do not confuse cause and effect. Lack of empathy is a consequence here – of lack of financial and computer resources. I am not saying a person cannot get into a state of reverie while walking. Indeed Aristotelian philosophers were famous for being peripatetic – doing philosophy while walking. Yet, with this individual, it was not working.

With a second individual, she asserts that she does not have privacy at home or at work and she sets up her video smart phone in the car and there is the image, her behind the steering wheel. I am thinking: "Okay—if the client is in enough stress to meet this way—from her auto—I am not going to stop listening or present a logistical obstacle." Yet I wonder how deep we can go? Once again, my empathy is disrupted. Some CBT perhaps, but the milieu does not seem conducive to a psychodynamic reverie.

Another therapist may object: "I did not have any problem having many sessions with a client who was in a parked car." It happens. We meet the client where she or he is at. With this client, with this car, with my skills, this did not work for me as well as I might have hoped. Maybe there are über-therapists (a super-therapist, not someone who is also driving an Uber because of skimpy insurance reimbursements) out there for whom this would not be an issue. They jump seamlessly between online and physical environments. I study at their knee. But for myself, a merely above-average therapist, I struggled. I acknowledge your experience – and your mileage – may differ.

With the third client, the family had a computer but, technically speaking, it was a "clunker" – not able to sustain an online conversation for fifty minutes. We fall back to having a conversation on the phone. It is not bad – it is workable in the short-term, but is it sustainable over the long term?

My training is in-person. Still, I work reasonably well on the phone. Yet I am persistently troubled by losing touch with this engaging though dis-embodied voice. The empathy is leaking away, becoming thinner and atte-nuated. I wonder if the other person is feeling the same way. I feel like I am giving – or want to give – a Ted Talk – a lecture – to fill in the empty space. It is too much like a radio play – the "dead air" once again ends up resem-bling the unresponsive emotionally dead mother – the empathy is significantly disrupted.

One may object: "Why empathy? Isn't it focus and presence that leak away? The answer is direct: Why does one think it is either/or? Both focus and empathic presence are at risk. Lack of focus "takes down" empathy and vice versa. I hasten to add this was my experience. Perhaps there are über-therapists for whom this would not be an issue. Once again, for myself, a merely above-average therapist, I struggled.

Therapists are already dealing with what Marsha Linehan calls "therapy interfering behaviors" (Linehan, 1993: 138–141). Especially with the see-mingly ever-growing segment of my practice living in genteel poverty, fi-nances and scheduling are perennial issues. Now add the requirement that the person needs an upgrade to his/her computer. Now add the challenging requirement that the person needs a home office or an uncompromising private space.

We can go as far as our empathy allows us to go. If we cannot build rapport online with a deeply regressed patient who is struggling to find words, then it is necessary to meet in person, though that is no guarantee as to the outcome. It is necessary for the therapist to learn to dance in the chaos or at least the rapidly shifting dynamics. In the face of breakdowns in the technology enabling screen relations, our empathy is willing to go farther than the technology glitches allow us to go.

Against the expectation that the therapist can provide a gracious and generous listening, if the screen-mediated relationship is faulty, the con-versation is in breakdown. So is the empathy.

I informed a client I was not operating the Computer Help Desk; but then I immediately had the thought, "Maybe I am!" If I have to explain the joke, it is not funny. The humorous edge to this otherwise uncomfortable truth: Where else would the client turn with a technical problem if not to the person, in this case, the therapist, with whom s/he is working?

The practical technical help creates a holding environment. Even if you are working in an institution that has a formal computer help desk function, it is unlikely that it will be responsive in a timely way. This is a breakdown in holding and, thereby, another breakdown in empathy. Is this yet another encounter with the unresponsive "dead" mother of André Green fame? If you are a sole practitioner, working alone, then you are definitely the help desk. This is significantly different than giving a new client geographic directions to the office. Most people have learned how to navigate by car or public transit and are good at it. Most people are *not* good at debugging computers and networks. This impacts therapists who may not realize the future of online therapy is now, and, in so far as we are online, we are on television, and need to take our screen relations game up a level to fulfill our commitment to empathy and vice versa.

Answering the Devil's Advocate Before Canonizing Online Therapy

The debate is joined. Online therapy is better than nothing. And yet is it better than anything else? There are trade-offs in abundance.

One of the most articulate voices expanding the practice of empathy and denouncing the unthinking use of online practices is Sherry Turkle. Professor Turkle has written widely on technology and psychoanalysis (see 1976, 2017; see also Agosta 2022).

Turkle pushes back on endorsing online therapy for the reason that it is "better than nothing" (Turkle et al., 2017). The slippery slope here is that "better than nothing" becomes "better than anything." Online therapy starts as good enough and allegedly becomes better than anything.

According to Turkle, the smart phone and text messaging are significant disruptors to one's ability to be present with oneself and with others. One of the main effects of the digital revolution in everything is that, as noted, we as a community have an "acquired attention deficit" due to device interruptions. Surely we can agree with that – but neither psychoanalysis nor online therapy caused that – nor will they readily fix it. The fix? Hit the off button. Easier said than done.

We have ample evidence that babies and children of tender age require "hands on" involvement from their parents, teachers, and caretakers. They require people who babies are able to breathe on and who can breathe on them in the same contiguous space of possibility in order to activate key aspects of their humanity – cognitive, affective, and practical.

Adult clients who are struggling with social awkwardness, introversion, inhibitions that put them on the isolating schizoid spectrum require a "hands on" approach in shared physical space. Such clients are already "remote." They may benefit most from the empathic presence in an office.

The screen can provide a barrier and a defense. The screen can also create the classic issue of a secondary gain, enabling the patient to avoid the issues that bring him to therapy. If you feel your head is spinning or this is a roller-coaster ride, then try to enjoy it.

Empathy Online: A Phenomenology of Online Presence

Turkle scores a point: One cannot have eye contact over Zoom/Skype, because one is looking at the "green dot" (camera) to simulate eye contact. This is controversial, but the point cannot be dismissed.

Part of one's training as a therapist includes the distinction the client's "eye contact is furtive." Key term: Furtive. It is diagnostically relevant regarding the client's mental status and ability to *be* present that s/he looks around anxiously.

Meanwhile, as we are debating how online therapy affects eye contact, we have the compelling assertion that Freud started using The Couch so that he would *not* have to be looked at all day long (Freud 1913: 134). Then Freud discovered the couch had other advantages, inducing a mild state of reverie and free association, useful in working through emotional complexes. I am a strong advocate of using the couch, because I have seen people lie down for the first time and have a breakthrough in the work that needed doing. They get in touch with their feelings and thoughts at a deeper level.

One thing is for sure – there is no eye contact between the person on the couch and the person sitting behind the person lying down. Instead, there is a rich physical presence, listening to the other person breathe or listening to their stomach gurgle.

The point is the rich physical presence of the other person. From an empathic point of view, such techniques may dial down the client's empathic interpretation and cognitive empathy – so called "top down" empathy – while expanding the empathic receptivity and responsiveness – "bottom up," affective empathy – of the therapeutic pair.

A lot of distance exists on the spectrum between "better than nothing" and "better than everything else." If this is Turkle's position (2017), then it is logically and rhetorically flawed – perhaps to make her point about the loss of our ability to be present with one another – since most of the work we aim to do in addressing human suffering is to reduce suffering across all available media. The vast majority of good therapy gets done in the area of "let not perfection be the enemy of the good." We now turn to the intermediate, "between" area.

Transference is Transference: The Irreality is Coming from the Therapy

The genie – online therapy – has escaped from the lamp. Indeed a live, real-time video call is an "in-person" meeting, albeit one that is mediated by a screen and network connection. When the in-person encounter is mediated in this way, what are the effects on free association and the ability to engage in the kind of imaginative reverie – key term: Reverie – that many consider to be the most powerful and transformative aspect of the therapeutic encounter?

This struggle is especially acute with clients described as being not self-expressed, communicating non-verbally in body language, and struggling with words, lacking words, to get in touch with their feelings and themselves (and others).

I hasten to add that such a difficult individual client presents challenges even for standard psychoanalysis or self analysis, which take place within shared space as a talking cure. There is no substitute for being in physical proximity to such a person to get in touch with what they are feeling. A bold statement of the obvious: A person whose mental status is remote in a shared physical space does not overcome emotional distance by inviting another level of remoteness in going online.

I am firm in my conviction and commitment that such individuals whose trauma is preverbal can and do benefit from psychoanalysis. Psychoanalysis can do things that no other intervention can accomplish; and yet and yet … If one becomes preverbal enough, then sometimes something else is required – art therapy, play therapy, music therapy, Dialectical Behavior Therapy. See the reflections by Marion Milner below, which, not for the faint of heart, accounts an authentically heroic psychoanalysis of a significantly disordered client – a person remote even when one is in the same shared space – struggling with lack of verbal self-expressive capabilities.

The criticism (that the online approach is insufficiently real) fails not because the online media is "unreal" or, strictly speaking, real in a different way than in shared physical space. Rather the criticism fails because the physical, in-person psychotherapy encounter is shot through-and-through with the imaginary, with symbolism, fantasy and irreality. The "irreal" includes the symbolic, the imagined, the fictional, the part of reality which is distinct from the real but includes the past and the future and the imaginary, which are not really present yet influence reality.

In psychotherapy in all contexts, the encounter is precisely about the symbolic and the imagined – the transference. The irreality is coming from the therapy.

Many therapists were sitting there in physically shared space being "the voice of reality," reasoning with their clients, problem solving, worrying about "the facts," while overlooking the imaginary nature of the entire enterprise. I hasten to add that I am not suggesting, "be irrational," but this particular therapeutic conversation is not a rational process the way one has an ordinary talk. All other things being equal, talking online works almost as well as talking in-person. Many readers will have studied Winnicott's "good enough" mother (Winnicott, 1965). Talking online is often a "good enough" solution.

In psychotherapy, the encounter is precisely about the symbolic and the imagined – the transference. The irreality is coming from the transference not from the online therapeutic frame as such.

Let us grant for the moment that going online is sufficiently real. But is it sufficiently safe, secure – able to engage with and demonstrate "survivability"? Here we call as a witness and devil's advocate Gillian Isaacs Russell (2015).

Demonstrating Survival and Safety Online

Isaacs Russell and others are adamant that the ability of the therapist to survive, in Winnicott's sense (1965), cannot be properly tested in the online context (see Isaacs Russell, 2015; Sayers, 2021). If this ability to demonstrate survivability could be significantly tested, then much written about inadequate, unworkable online presence would be invalidated or significantly reduced.

For example, Isaacs Russell, quoting a client (2015: 181), makes much of the potential to "kiss or kick" the other person in shared physical space (acting out seduction or aggression); and while it is true that such acting out rarely occurs, what is needed is the *potential* for its occurring.

Still, what has been overlooked is that such acting out bodily is not the only way of testing the separation and survival of the therapist. Many examples exist in which the client tests the limits speech act (Austin 1955/1962) - including seductive or aggressive language. Speech is physical and would not occur without sound waves impacting the biology of the ear. This is not a mere technicality. The distinction online versus physical is not exclusive. Tone of voice, rhythm, and timing are *present* online.

Recall that Winnicott's point is that when the client acts out – in this case verbally – the therapist demonstrates his/her survival skill by not retaliating. Thus, s/he remains in integrity as a "good enough" partner in empathic relatedness and the client's independence grows. The client's integrity and power expands.

If the therapist retaliates – say, by moralizing or withdrawing or blaming or becoming aggressive or seductive – then the treatment is at risk of derailment. Absent significant repair, the relationship ends, even if the conversation continues in an impasse.

Deleting confidential details, for example, I recall an instance where, being with a new online client, who was vulnerable in a way that I did not appreciate, I clumsily triggered a challenge to survival. It was a toxic combination of panic, retraumatizing flashback, and upset, that resulted in an extended and seemingly automatic combination of verbal abuse. It threatened me professionally and the safety of the client such that I seriously thought of sending emergency services to the client's address. The screen was no protection against the impact of the hate.

So while the client might not have been able to throw a pencil at me (to use Isaacs Russell's example), the individual would have been able to inflict self-harm in a way that would do more damage to me than a kick in the shins (another Isaacs Russell example (2015: 181)). Never underestimate the ability of clients to innovate in acting out around the constraints of an apparently solid therapeutic framework.

The client survived. Without making any commitments I couldn't keep, by a combination of soothing statements, self-depreciating humor, apologetic words, and de-escalating suggestions, I kept my wits about me, and was able to restore the integrity of the therapeutic process. S/he agreed to continue the conversation. I survived and so did the relationship. It actually was a break-through, and, without everything being wonderful, the client demonstrated capabilities not previously expressed.

Thus, my counter-example: Survival was tested online, not by physically throwing a pencil, but in reciprocal speech and the enactment of presence in speech acts, a physical media not to be underestimated. One learns that the environment is safe when safety breaks down. The potential for non-survival was engaged and transformed, survival and safety engaged and expanded.

The conclusion? The client can – can indeed – test the capacity to survive and do so online. "Kissing or kicking" is a special case of acting out. Such behaviors occur in abundance both online and off.

Positively expressed, evidence is available that the analyst's survival can indeed be tested in an online session and s/he may survive or not. Ultimately even "kiss and kick" can be enacted as verbal abuse online, perpetrating boundary violations with hostility or seduction that can be grave and survival threatening, either in imagination or reality, including the survival of the therapist as a professional and the therapy itself.

Physical In-Person Therapy Remains Indispensable in Selected Cases

The connection to empathy is direct: If one understands an empathic holding environment as the context for therapy, then the advantage in selected (to be detailed) cases to physical presence for empathic relatedness is direct. Consider the following cases.

Some cases are indeed unsuited for online engagement. Marion Milner engaged in a long and famous analysis of a deeply disturbed and regressed client, in which the client was silent for long periods of time (Milner, 1969). The client finally was able to recover significant aspects of her humanity in producing hundreds of drawings and sketches that expressed a therapeutic process of pre-verbal recovery. Though these were visual artifacts, and pre-sumably might have been communicated remotely, the client herself was al-ready so "remote" from reality that another layer of virtuality was not going to work (nor was it possible mid-20th century).

Heinz Kohut has provided a celebrated example that Kohut presented in a lecture a few days before his death (Strozier, 2001: 367–377). Kohut was working with a deeply regressed and suicidal client. The client comes in, lies down, and says she feels like the coffin lid has closed shut over her. In a desperate moment, Kohut offered to let the client, lying on the couch, behind which he was sitting in his customary straight-backed wooden chair, hold two of the fingers of his hand. The point of this potentially life saving (and boundary testing) gesture was Kohut's association to the client's desperate grasp with her hand being like that of a toothless infant sucking on a nipple. An empty nipple or a life giving one? Powerful stuff, which would be impossible online. Far be it for me to be the voice of reality, nevertheless, these two cases of Milner and Kohut are two from a hundred cases, outliers, albeit deeply moving ones, that are completely consistent with the sensitive and dynamically informed application of online remote analysis.

Though the uses of extended moments of online silence should not be underestimated or dismissed, Milner's and Kohut's cases were ones that privileged physical presence. One thing is for sure: Whether it was the couch or mere physical presence, the patient could not have held Kohut's two fingers (like the "empty nipple") if they had not been in the same physical space. This in no way refutes the power or potential of online engagement. What we are missing are criteria for telling the difference. No easy answers here, but the rule of thumb is: Do what furthers the treatment in the proper professional sense of the words. What is going to sustain and advance the conversation for possibility in the face of the client's stuckness? Do that. Winnicott has been mentioned, and rightly. He spoke of the "good enough" mother. Here we have the "good enough" therapeutic framework including the online one.

Comparing Online and Physical Transcripts

Isaacs Russell reports (2015) on online psychoanalytic training with colleagues in China. There are few psychoanalysts in China, so in addition to and despite significant culture and language challenges, such remote work would not be possible without online analytic sessions and supervision. The unanimous consensus is that this work is "functionally equivalent" or in other ways "just the same as" work done physically in-person. The evidence?

Neutral observers are asked to evaluate transcripts of sessions where the online versus physical feature and descriptive details have been masked. The result? They can't tell them apart. What more do we need to say?

Quite a bit. With dynamic psychotherapy and related forms of talk therapy, if you can tell the difference between an online and an in-person meeting (other than comments about traffic or Internet misconnections), then you are doing it wrong. Abstinence is easier online – no hugs. But if we are talking boundary violations, some people – exhibitionists – may be tempted to take off their clothes on camera. This has not happened to me – yet. Anonymity – just as one's office has clues as to one's personal life, so too does the background on camera. Neutrality – being on camera suddenly causes one to adopt an exhibitionistic point of view on social media or politics or nutrition or economics or education? Interpretations and conversations are useful in all these instances.

However, what Isaacs Russell does not discuss is the "other" transcript – the unwritten one, which is only available as a thought-experiment. There is another transcript different than the verbatim account of what was said or even what a webcam could record. It is a transcript that is just as important as the recording of the conversation, and why verbatim recordings are less useful than one might wish. Both participants may consciously "forget" that the session is being recorded, but the unconscious does not.

The unexpressed or indirectly expressed transcript of what the participants are thinking and experiencing *lives* as the subtext. Such an aspect of the countertransference – a thought transcript – is harder to access and includes the therapist's countertransference. That is why this remains a "thought experiment": The delta between the online and physical therapies contains thoughts and feelings that escape from the recording transcript(s).

Though technically impossible, add to the unexpressed transcript, the subtext of the therapist's countertransference. Add the reaction to the patient and the framework. Then the differences between online and physical presence would stand out boldly. This is an important aspect of the empathic relatedness that is present in both the physical and online therapies, though in different ways. How so?

When empathy provides the context, then both a physical encounter and an online encounter via a video session are ways of implementing, applying, and bringing forth relatedness. As a general rule of thumb, the online context provides less resistance to cognitive, "top down" empathy; whereas the physical context provides less resistance to affective, "bottom up" empathy. However, for the experienced practitioner, this rule has many exceptions. For example, I have a high functioning online client for whom long silences and reverie are relatively easy. I check in with her periodically in the online moment, "Checking in—what are you present to?" Works quite well.

A New World of Parapraxes, "Freudian" Slips and Acting Out

The online environment and the imaginary thought transcript present new forms of client resistance and therapist countertransference.

Moving therapy to online opens up a new world of symptomatic acts, parapraxes, "Freudian" slips, and acting out. A single example must suffice.

I had one online client who stood up in the middle of a session to check on what she had cooking in the oven, carrying the camera-enabled device along. Was I amazed? Indeed.

I acknowledged to the client that clients sometimes have mixed feelings about their therapists, and nothing wrong about that as such. Yet I was wondering did she believe I was perhaps half-baked? Key term: Half-baked. Further discussion occurred of whether this client was expressing her unconscious hostility towards me – while, of course, also preparing a baked dish for dinner.

The breakdown in empathy may be a thoughtless remark by the therapist, a mix up in the schedule, or a failure of the computer network. The empathy – and transmuting internalization working through it – *LIVEs* in restoring the wholeness and integrity of the relatedness. Empathy lives as spontaneous relatedness, a form of transference and vice versa. This is not limited to psychoanalysis versus psychodynamically informed psychotherapy. This is not limited to online versus in-person therapy in a shared space. We call out the many shortcomings of online remote therapy and go off to our online sessions.

The pandemic has taught us: we humans are a species that likes to breathe on one another. This should be heard literally, though it is also a metaphor. That is what has been so hard about a disease that is communicated through the air – we cannot get physically close to one another and breathe the same air. We humans seem to want to do that – indeed need to do that – and here we are with all these necessary rules about social distancing.

The point is: It is as misguided to require therapists exclusively to perform in-person therapy, as it would be for everyone exclusively to perform online therapy. Turning back the clock is not possible. The shift is from sounds of stomach gurgling, smells of body odor or cologne, literally bodily warmth in the in-person physical encounter to high definition close ups of the imperfections of people's facial complexion. The shift is from empathic receptivity to empathic understanding, from "bottom up" affective empathy to "top down" cognitive empathy. To be sure, both are needed and in both environments.

The genie is out of the bottle and online therapy will continue to grow and contribute to clients' recoveries. Abundant space exists between "better than nothing" and "better than anything" for both online and in-person office-based therapies to coexist as "good enough" therapies, helping clients get unstuck using empathy both in unmediated physical relations and online.[1]

Practical Considerations and Tips

Online therapy tends to dial up empathic interpretation and cognitive, "top down" empathy; whereas physical shared space therapy tends to dial up empathic receptivity (affective, "bottom up" empathy). For experienced practitioners, this rule of thumb has many exceptions.

The therapist claims s/he is not the Computer Help Desk, then it turns out s/he really is.

Online therapy presents new forms of "Freudian" slips, parapraxes, and acting out. Our empathy guides us in addressing them.

It is as misguided to require therapists exclusively to perform in-person physical therapy, as it would be exclusively to perform online therapy.

Clients whose mental status is "remote" even in-person in a physical, shared space are not initially a good choice to work with remotely online.

"Better than nothing" versus "better than anything" is a choice that needs to be declined: Both online and in-person physical therapy coexist and help clients flourish using empathy to bridge the gap between physical presence and screen-mediated relatedness.

Note

1 **An earlier version of this work with significant differences of emphasis was published as** Empathy: A bridge across the digital divide," *Psychoanalytic Review*, 109(4), December 2022. The author gratefully acknowledges the editors of *Psychoanalytic Review* for their support and permission.

References

Agosta, L. (2010). *Empathy in the Context of Philosophy*. London: Palgrave Macmillan.

Agosta, L. (2013). A rumor of empathy: Reconstructing Heidegger's contribution to empathy and empathic clinical practice. *Medicine, Health Care and Philosophy: A European Journal.* DOI: 10.1007/s11019-13-9506-0

Agosta, L. (2014). *A Rumor of Empathy: Rewriting Empathy in the Context of Philosophy.* Springer. pp. 4–8.

Agosta, L. (2015). *Reclaiming Conversation*. New York: Penguin.

Agosta, L. (2015).*A Rumor of Empathy: Resistance, Narrative, and Recovery*. London: Routledge.

Agosta, L. (2018). *Empathy Lessons*. Chicago: Two Pears Press.

Agosta, L. (2020). Empathy in cyberspace: The genie is out of the bottle. In H. Weinberg, & A. Rolnick (Eds.), *Theory and Practice of Online Therapy: Internet-delivered Interventions for Individuals, Groups, Families, and Organizations* (pp. 34–46). London: Routledge.

Agosta, L. (2022). Review: The Empathy Diaries by Sherry Turkle, Psychoanalysis, Self and Context, 17:2, 237-241, Feb 11, 2022 (online) and April 2022 (hardcopy). 10.1080/24720038.2021.1990297.

Austin, J. (1955/1962). *How To Do Things With Words*. Oxford, UK: Oxford University Press.

Freud, S. (1905).Jokes and Their Relation to the Unconscious.*The Standard Edition of the Complete Psychological Works of Sigmund Freud [hereafter SE]. James Strachey (ed.). Volume VIII: 1–247*

Freud, S. (1913).On Beginning the Treatment (Further Recommendations on the Technique of Psycho-Analysis I). SE XII: 121–144.

Linehan, M. (1993). *Cognitive-Behavioral Treatment of Borderline Personality Disorder.* New York: Guilford Press.

Milner, M. (1969). *The Hands of the Living God: An Account of a Psycho-analysis* (2010). London: Routledge.

Russell, G. I. (2015). *Screen Relations*. London: Karnac Books.

Sayers, J. (2021). Online psychotherapy: Transference and countertransference issues. *British Journal of Psychotherapy*, *37*(2), 223–233. DOI: 10.1111/bjp.12624.

Strozier, C. (2001). *Heinz Kohut: The Making of a Psychoanalyst*. New York: Farrar, Straus, and Giroux.

Turkle, S. (1976). *Psychoanalytic Politics: Freud's French Revolution* (1981). Cambridge, MA: MIT Press.

Turkle, S., Essig, T., & Russell, G. I. (2017). Afterword: Reclaiming psychoanalysis: Sherry Turkle in conversation with the Editors. *Psychoanalytic Perspectives*, *14*(2), P241.

Winnicott, D. W. (1965). *The Maturational Processes and the Facilitating Environment.* London: Hogarth Press.

4 "The Untouched – Touched": Intimacy and Intersubjectivity Online

Athena Marouda - Chatjoulis and Evdokia Ntali

Introduction

This chapter aims to give an overview of the impact that new technologies and online communication have on how people relate and on the concepts of intimacy and intersubjectivity created and their effect on psychoanalytic psychotherapeutic interactions.

Online communication along with the features of online interactions, such as immediacy, issues of privacy, and personal data security, contribute to the transformation of relationships (Attwood et al., 2017; Baym, 2010; Miguel, 2018). Relationships formed online are no longer limited by physical presence. Instead, the use of the Internet promotes the buildup of close relationships even between strangers, mainly on the basis of sharing common needs and mutual feelings (Attwood et al., 2017; Castells, 2001; Koch & Miles, 2020; Nebeling Petersen et al., 2018). In this new social paradigm, current social relationships as well as the interactions that take place, involve the exchange of images and are highly visualized. As a result, this visualization changes several aspects of communicating and interacting and especially the way intimacy is experienced (Lobinger et al., 2021).

The ubiquitous presence of online environments has also affected psychological interventions, leading to a growing trend to use Internet-based communication in psychotherapy. Especially in the era of COVID-19, the psychotherapeutic settings are characterized by the use of online video platforms. As a result, a wealth of online therapeutic methods, defined as "any type of professional therapeutic interaction that makes use of the Internet to connect qualified mental health professionals and their clients," have been developed and are used worldwide (Dowling & Rickwood, 2013, p.3).

Significant research has been carried out examining online psychotherapy, however, there are still differing opinions regarding the matter. Some believe that online sessions can be psychologically equivalent to face-to-face encounters (Agar, 2019), and are considered preferable for clients who have difficulties seeing the psychotherapist in a face-to-face setting (Kocsis & Yellowlees, 2018). Others disagree and point out that online psychotherapy lacks the quality, richness, and intimacy of human contact generated during

DOI: 10.4324/9781003205029-6

the in-person sessions and creates instead a gap in the therapeutic relationship (Isaacs Russell, 2015). More recently, the issues of transference and countertransference within the psychodynamic setting and the context of the new online psychotherapeutic environment have been considered. Particular emphasis has been placed on the concepts of containment and the need for empathetic mirroring (Sayers, 2021), the psychoanalytic setting (Lemma, 2020), and the disembodied environment as well as on the question of presence (Weinberg, 2020).

Taking the above into consideration, the possible ways that the transformation of relationships affect intimacy and intersubjectivity in psychotherapeutic online interactions, are discussed throughout this chapter by exploring the manners in which online interactions facilitate the process of self-disclosure. In addition, the question whether the "new intimacy media encounter" creates a new transitional space or not for online psychotherapy is explored.

The Transformation of Relatedness and Intimacy in the Realm of Online Interactions

Modern times have been characterized by a shift in the nature of relationships, which have become more "intimate" than social (Jamieson, 1998), with greater focus on kinship and friendship. Intimacy has been associated with privacy, individualism, and the home realm as opposed to being associated with civil society, community, and the public (Heath, 2004). Intimacy, according to Zelizer (2009), is three-dimensional composed of physical, informational, and emotional elements that are interconnected and defined by the act of privately sharing one's inner thoughts and feelings with another (Giddens, 1992; Marar, 2012). However, the emergence of the Internet and the use of e-mail and online apps have changed the rituals of communication since they have removed the element of "physical presence" required for building up intimacy, and thus they have blurred the dichotomy between private and public. As a result, new privacy concerns have arisen regarding online interactions in social networking sites. On the one hand, users feel more willing to disclose personal information and relinquish their personal privacy although information sharing in online social networks can lead to privacy and security violations (Benson et al., 2015).

Intimate online interactions are perceived in real time without physical co-presence. Intimacy, therefore, is constructed and experienced subjectively. Furthermore, even if the various aspects of mobile lives such as networks, new digital technologies, and consumerism are used (Elliott & Urry, 2010), the development of intimate connections continue to require certain basic components, such as sharing attention, mutual attention, emotion, and behavior (Battich & Geurts, 2021; Campos-Castillo & Hitlin, 2013). Sharing attention enables the integration of the knowledge, beliefs, and experiences of each participant in joint attention to an object/event (Battich & Geurts, 2021). Mutual attention (Roth, 2014) promotes the emergence of a mutual emotion (arising through empathy), which results in automatic and intentional behavior referred to as "the Chameleon Effect" that makes possible the establishment of a subjective closeness (Campos-Castillo & Hitlin, 2013). There can be cases, however, when the individual, although in contact with many other people, at the same time may feel alienated – "being alone together" (Turkle, 2011, p.14).

Psychoanalysts, particularly, need to be intersubjective and relational, and so they must be able to harness these intimate online connections to bring change through the establishment of a therapeutic relationship. However, recent research shows that the online psychoanalysis has difficulties with transference, countertransference, and other aspects of therapy (Sayers, 2021), even when the experienced "joint virtual presence" promotes the development of a feeling of "togetherness" in sharing and mutual attention (Agar, 2019; p.67). It is important, therefore, to understand whether online sessions affect the therapeutic aspect of psychotherapy and transform fundamentally the analytic frame and work. Online psychotherapy cannot be considered simply a new technological platform where the psychotherapeutic processes take place through a different medium. To understand the implications, we must look at how changes in communication brought about by the online technologies, affect intimacy in the psychotherapeutic context.

Facilitating Self-Disclosure

In online textual communication, users are substantially less inhibited in displaying behaviors and/or feelings, and in using verbal expressions that are not socially acceptable (Casale et al., 2015; Cheung et al., 2020). This is due to the characteristics of cyberspace use, including anonymity, lack of visibility and visual contact, neutralization of the individual's status, and the asynchronous and written nature of communication. Because individuals are more relaxed when communicating online, they feel less restrained in expressing themselves openly, a behavior that has been described as "the disinhibition effect" (Suler, 2004). The sense of control of the duration and type of online contact functions as a "release filter" of thoughts, behavior, and description of events that are difficult to share or display in offline environments with such intensity or frequency (Singleton et al., 2016).

According to Suler's (2004) due to the "online disinhibition effect," textual communication expands to all modalities of online interactions. As reiterated by Scharff (2020), the online session gives patients "freedom to access negative transference that they had not been able to express in the analyst's office" (p. 586). Clients no longer need to use their social "masks" that inhibit the establishment of close therapeutic relationships, especially at the start of therapy. Instead, they are more willing to reveal deeper dilemmas, conflicts, and difficulties with which they are trying to cope. The therapist's simultaneous absence (physical body) and presence (image on screen) as a significant other, appears to create a safe place for the client, lessening his/her resistance.

The effectiveness of the "online disinhibition effect" – known also as the "distance medium" in media psychology (see Roesler, 2017) – is supported by clinical evidence, which has demonstrated that it enables both positive and negative material to arise and be processed. In psychotherapy, this disinhibition effect promotes the client's therapeutic expression and self-reflection much earlier than in face-to-face therapy. Indeed, Simpson et al. (2020) highlight how online sessions may "lead to greater disinhibition and openness as a result of a heightened sense of safety" and "more neutral power balance" (p.412). In addition, Svenson (2020) concludes that the "medium magnifies the dynamics" (p. 448) of psychotherapy, allowing painful experiences to be confronted. This calls into question claims such as that of White (2020) that online work can have a "distancing" effect enabling some patients to hide their needs. Even Gutierrez (2017), who is very critical of online psychotherapy, acknowledges that videoconferencing might allow unpleasant topics such as issues of love or hate to be addressed in the transference.

Patients with a high level of shame or an increased need to control things or with avoidant coping styles may find that online sessions provide the environment they need to develop and maintain a more positive therapeutic alliance (Martin et al., 2020). Scharff (2013, p.71), in her paper on teleanalysis, stresses that voice-based therapy may be beneficial for patients with trauma-related dissociation. According to media psychology research, the "distance medium" lessens inhibitions and lowers the threshold for discussing potentially shameful content, thus allowing clients with problems like trauma and sexual disorders to begin treatment. Such examples demonstrate that "disinhibition" can be clinically useful in enabling suppressed material to arise and thus it is not a negative phenomenon in and of itself.

This tendency toward "disinhibition" in an online psychotherapeutic framework, may scare therapists. They may be concerned about losing control in front of the screen because of personal transferences to technology as a separate object or because of feelings confined by the need to remain in view (Svenson, 2020; p. 448). Hence, some therapists may react defensively to online therapy and reject it as less valuable and more susceptible to analytical error than in-person analysis. In this case, they may need instead to investigate the relevance of their own responses to the online medium, in addition to that of the patient's. Analysts, therefore, may be able to facilitate more positive outcomes if they are to take into consideration the potential, limitations, and boundaries associated with online communication in their work.

The Effects of Disembodiment: The Untouched-Touched

Reading facial expressions for identifying emotional indicators or paying attention to gestures and posture to comprehend clients' emotional states are all part of the accepted need for the presence of the therapist in psychotherapy

(Geller, 2018; Ogden & Goldstein, 2019). In addition, the therapists' ability to express their presence using their whole body (prosody, open body posture, gestures, and mirroring clients' movement in real time), are considered important for emotional attunement, the conveyance of trust, and for a sense of safety (Geller, 2020).

However, in online psychotherapy, some of these means of communication may be absent. Depending on the online method used, communication cues may be lost due to the absence of kinesthetics (posture and gestures), visualization of the lower part of the body, and clear facial features (Sfoggia et al., 2014; Oshni Alvandi, 2019). In this case, clients may not feel nearly as comfortable sharing personal information and, as a result, free associations may be limited. Furthermore, this may result in the transformation of the interaction between the therapist and the client, and as a result clients may find themselves in an "untouched-touched" position. Aspects of the therapeutic-mediated relationship may need to be reinforced, facilitating the process of transference. In addition, other aspects of the therapeutic relationship may be hindered due to the modified body images of both therapist and patient. For example, the presence of a magnified head – representing intellectual processes – and a well-hidden lower body – may leave impulsive forces related to the latter in the realm of imagery.

In particular, those who are critical about the effectiveness of online therapy emphasize that a "real" therapeutic relationship needs to contain both verbal and non-verbal elements. If there is only verbal communication, therapeutic relationships may become highly intellectualized. For example, in traditional "discourse linguistic" methods used to examine micro-processes in analytical (and other) psychotherapies, one needs the nonverbal aspects of the transference-countertransference connection that define the features of the therapeutic relationship. These features may be lost or distorted in technologically mediated interactions, thus undermining the quality of the relationship with the client (Roesler, 2017). Under such circumstances, the intersubjective encounter is perceived as more intellectual than emotional. Winnicott's (1960) calls this "intellectual defense"; that is the mind concentrates on "the False Self," thus dissociating intellectual activity (the mind) from the rest of the body (p. 144). Furthermore, the impoverished quality of the analytic material due to a "tendency to literalism and disaffection typical of banalization" (Gutierrez, 2017; p. 1109), may result in a kind of concretization that inhibits regression. On the other hand, this limited presence of non-verbal cues is not very different from the traditional psychoanalytic therapeutic context. According to Freud's technique of putting the patient on the couch, the absence of eye contact between therapist and client, and a limited intimacy were required to facilitate the free association process. Today, online psychotherapy seems to incorporate these elements by minimizing the impact of bodily presence during the session (Aryan, 2013).

This new kind of bodily presence online also affects the clinicians, who seem to be more susceptible to exhaustion (Isaacs Russel, 2020). The loss of subtle non-verbal cues while trying to concentrate and focus while on line, may increase anxiety and result in hypervigilance (Isaacs Russell, 2020; p.368). After conducting interviews with analysts working online, Trub and Magaldi (2017) concluded that when analysts see themselves on screen during a session, they become self-conscious and may feel less at ease with their bodies. This may result in self-monitoring, loss of spontaneity in interventions, and the need to display an "ideal" behavior, which can contribute to "de-naturalization" of the therapists' behavior (Gutierrez, 2017; p. 1108).

The novel bodily presence in online sessions, also requires the need to avoid transferring face-to-face techniques directly to online work (Isaacs Russell, 2020). Since technology-related issues can affect one's expressed and perceived presence in online therapy (Geller, 2020), therapists need to be trained on how to communicate in the context of their Internet presence. Modification of approaches to be followed when on screen, should be explored and adopted to improve therapeutic alliances. Such approaches could include: The provision of more intentional and apparent nonverbal responses; exaggeration of the tone of voice, gestures, and mannerisms as well as the use of more questions to prevent misunderstandings (Martin et al., 2020). Therefore, online analysis needs to combine aspects of physical and virtual settings. These two settings should not replace one another. Instead, they should complement each other, and either be used simultaneously or alternatively (Corbella, 2020) with the analyst making the necessary adjustments.

Between Presence and Absence: The Transitional Space

When individuals seek psychological support, they are searching for a relationship with another, who can respond directly to their needs but, at the same time, for the freedom to distance themselves without much psychological cost. Within the online psychotherapeutic context, the paradoxical coexistence of proximity and distance forms a unique online transitional space. This space creates a sense of alienation and of closeness, a sense of dependence, and of independence simultaneously (Turkle, 2011; Weinberg, 2014). It promotes a constant dialogue between self and other, between omnipotence and limitations set by the reality principle and between similarities and differences. Within the context of online psychotherapy, the "intimacy media encounter" can then be described as an experience in an intermediate "private" space of the screen, which is at a distance ("away from me"), but at the same time uniquely personal ("in me").

According to Neumann (2013), by extending traditional notions of what constitutes time and space to the realm of psychic reality, we can say that patients and their analysts interact in a setting that transcends physical space and linear time, regardless of time zone or place of residence. That is, during the analytic hour online, the patient and analyst are sharing the same time and space, which may or may not coincide with either party's physical location.

Under such conditions, unconscious dynamics may still arise and, therefore, cyberspace can be regarded to have the properties that are akin to the potential space of the therapeutic interactions and thus provide the transitional space appropriate for identity exploration and growth. (Fischbein, 2010; Lingiardi, 2008). As Gabbard (2001) has pointed out: "Virtual space has a lot in common with transitional space, in the sense that it is not truly an internal realm but lies somewhere between external reality and our internal world" (p. 734). Turkle (2011) suggests that this transitional area that arises in the virtual environment allows the individual in front of the screen to feel safe and unburdened by expectations. At the same time, the individual has the impression that he/she is not alone because of the possibility of instantaneous interaction. Even experienced users who are aware that electronic conversations can be saved, give in to the illusion of privacy in this strange social realm. Turkle (2011) best describes this as being "Alone with your thoughts, yet in contact with an almost tangible fantasy of the other, you feel free to play" (p. 187).

Cyberspace as a mediating frame for psychotherapeutic work may enable the exploration of identity and intersubjective space under the guidance of the therapist. This relates to Winnicott's (1971) description of infants' play as being a symbolic and practical exploration of their limits in the facilitating environment controlled by their caretakers. Based on Winnicott's (1958) concept of the "transitional space," cyberspace can be considered to be composed of elements from both one's inner world and outward reality. In psychoanalytic terms, the virtual space can be thought of as an extension of the intrapsychic, a transitional space between the self and the other, between the inside and outside (Lemma, 2015; Suler, 2004). These parallels between virtual interaction and Winnicott's concept of the transitional space, have been pointed out by several authors (Bayles, 2012; Scharff, 2013; Lemma & Caparrotta, 2014) and are summarized by Lingiardi (2011) as follows:

"Computer-mediated communication allows the user to play with realities and identities. It can thus contain transitional elements as defined by Winnicott; the transitional object, in fact, lies halfway between Me and not-Me, between reality and fantasy, between near and far, between what we create and what we discover (p. 487)."

It appears that in online therapy the screen image can function as a transitional object, "allowing the patient to maintain the representation of the therapist and the functions of the potential room even after the therapy conversation has ended, enhancing the internalization of the therapist and his/her function" (Agar, 2019, p. 71). Based on this framework, we can consider the client as a self that experiences complex states of emotional pain and relationship dilemmas and seeks an "online third party" that will take on an engaging function and be "as close and as far as I wish." It is a self that, within a reflective and self-referential plan of life, continues to need the "other." In the online environment, this "other" can be available at any time and for any duration as long as he/she satisfies the individual's needs. In fact, this type of relationship characterizes the hypermodern subject who connects and disconnects online at any time. Using the shared online environment, the therapist can still help the patient experience states of transitional awareness and enable him/her to use this transitional space as the doorway to self-discovery and therapy.

Conclusion

Seeking support in an online environment (or following online therapy when traditional therapies are not available), highlights the common psychological need of individuals in their constant struggle to be contained by the "other" and at the same time to maintain individuality (Weinberg, 2014). Online therapy meets the needs of people who do not have access to physical, traditional psychotherapy. The search for online psychotherapeutic support reveals the coexistence of seemingly opposing needs: that of intimacy, security, and a bond through which emotional needs will be met while at the same time retaining the ability to remain at a distance and to control whether to connect or disconnect, to reveal oneself or resist and withdraw into an online cocoon. Although these processes also apply to in-person interactions, the challenge in the Internet environment arises from the paradox of the coexistence of proximity and distance forming a unique matrix of online transitional space that facilitates the expression of projections and of communication and relationships independent of time and distance (Weinberg, 2014). It has become apparent that the new "intimacy media encounter" can evoke a sense of integration or disconnection depending on whether the individual feels recognized or not. The need to belong raises critical questions and deeply conflicting emotions in the subject, reflecting the ambivalence of relatedness, i.e., the profound desire for autonomy together with a longing for the other (Marouda-Chatjoulis, 2014). In this context, new forms of intimacy emerge in response to the search for a way of communicating online that can also lead to inner self-actualization and the maintenance of personal identity.

Therapists should be aware that online communication may imply new features and rules for therapeutic interactions in an intersubjective space, where the therapeutic dyad has an active role regarding the therapeutic course. The therapist and the patient do not passively experience the new intimacy encounter. Instead, they actively process and reshape what it means to meet the "other" in an online therapeutic context. As we attempt to meet human needs with technology, we must innovate and adapt to optimally satisfy these needs. Thus, we should reevaluate the changes observed in the construction of identity and intimacy today, when experiencing this new therapeutic encounter in cyberspace.

Contemporary forms of digital expression have to meet our profoundly unconscious need to recognize, be recognized and relate to each other. Human needs for intimacy, holding, belonging, and the need to engage under conditions of possible relational rejection, loss, pain, and ambivalence have to be satisfied. The Internet seems to be able to take on this function to some extent attaining a social character, which "feeds" the sense of self. The need to connect has not changed. The need to recognize and be recognized remains the same. The need to seek the other and the need to be wanted remains constant over time. What has changed are the conditions under which both the analyst and the client attempt to meet these needs. Whether on or offline these needs are influenced by the temporal, spatial, and ontological components on the basis of which identity is constructed.

Practical Considerations

- The multiple changes in the rituals of communication brought about by the use of online therapy lead us to rethink the notion of "intimacy."
- Online communication may create the conditions enabling the client's self-expression considerably more quickly than in face-to-face therapy.
- In online psychotherapy, some dimensions of the therapeutic relationship are reinforced while others are impaired due to the new bodily presence. This implies a newly transformed form of interaction: the patient may oscillate between an "untouched-touched" position.
- Therapists should consider how technology-related issues can affect their presence or absence in therapy; they should recognize when this transition occurs so they can soften their expressions or resolve any misunderstandings.
- Within the context of online psychotherapy, we can describe the "intimacy media encounter" as experienced in an intermediate "private" space of the screen which is at a distance "away from me" but at the same time uniquely personal "in me."
- Therapists should consider that online communication may imply new features and rules in therapeutic interactions; however, the therapeutic dyad creates an intersubjective space holding an active role regarding the therapeutic course.

References

Agar, G. (2019). The clinic offers no advantage over the screen, for relationship is everything, video psychotherapy and its dynamics. In H. Weinberg, & A. Rolnick (1st Eds.), *Theory and Practice of Online Therapy* (pp. 66–78). Routledge. eBook ISBN9781315545530.

Aryan, A. (2013). Setting and transference-countertransference reconsidered on beginning teleanalysis. In J. Scharff (Ed.), *Psychoanalysis Online* (pp. 119–132). London: Karnac.

Attwood, F., Hakim, J., & Winch, A. (2017). Mediated intimacies: Bodies, technologies and relationships. *Journal of Gender Studies, 26*(3), 249–253. 10.1080/09589236.201 7.1297888

Battich, L., & Geurts, B. (2020). Joint attention and perceptual experience. *Synthese,* 1–14. 10.1007/s11229-020-02602-6

Bayles, M. (2012). Is physical proximity essential to the psychoanalytic process? An exploration through the lens of Skype? *Psychoanalytic Dialogues, 22*(5), 569–585. 10.1080/10481885.2012.717043

Baym, K. (2010). *Personal Connections in the Digital Age.* Cambridge, MA: Polity Press.

Benson, V., Saridakis, G., & Tennakoon, H. (2015). Information disclosure of social media users: Does control over personal information, user awareness and security notices matter? *Information Technology and People, 28*(3), 426e441. 10.1108/ITP-10-2 014-0232.

Campos-Castillo, C., & Hitlin, S. (2013). Copresence: Revisiting a building block for social interaction theories. *Sociological Theory, 31*(2), 168–192. 10.1177/07352751134 89811

Casale, S., Fiovaranti, G., & Caplan, S. (2015). Online disinhibition: Precursors and outcomes. *Journal of Media Psychology, 27,* 170–177. 10.1027/1864-1105/a000136

Castells, M. (2001). *The Internet galaxy: Reflections on the Internet, Business and Society.* New York: Oxford University Press.

Cheung, C. M., Wong, R. Y. M., & Chan, T. K. (2020). Online disinhibition: conceptualization, measurement, and implications for online deviant behavior. *Industrial Management & Data Systems.* 10.1108/IMDS-08-2020-0509

Corbella, V. (2020). From the couch to the screen: Psychoanalysis in times of virtuality. In F. Irtelli et al. (Eds.), *Psychoanalysis: A New Overview.* IntechOpen. 10.5772/intechopen. 95092.

Dowling, M., & Rickwood, D. (2013). Online counseling and therapy for mental health problems: A systematic review of individual synchronous interventions using chat. *Journal of Technology in Human Services, 31,* 1–21. 10.1080/15228835.2012.72 8508

Elliott, A., & Urry, J. (2010). *Mobile Lives.* London: Routledge

Fischbein, S. V. (2010). Psychoanalysis and virtual reality. *The International Journal of Psychoanalysis, 91*(4), 985–988. 10.1111/j.1745-8315.2010.00300.x

Gabbard, G. O. (2001). Cyberpassion: E-rotic transference on the internet. *The Psychoanalytic Quarterly, 70*(4), 719–737. 10.1002/j.2167-4086.2001.tb00618.x

Geller, S. (2020). Cultivating online therapeutic presence: Strengthening therapeutic relationships in teletherapy sessions. *Counselling Psychology Quarterly,* 1–17. 10.1080/ 09515070.2020.1787348

Geller, S. M. (2018). *A Practical Guide to Cultivating Therapeutic Presence.* Washington, DC: American Psychological Association.

Giddens, A. (1992). *The Transformation of Intimacy: Sexuality, Love and Eroticism in Modern Societies.* Oxford: Polity press.

Gutierrez, L. (2017). 'Silicon in "pure gold"? Theoretical contributions and observations on teleanalysis by videoconference'. *The International Journal of Psychoanalysis, 98*(4), 1097–1120. 10.1111/1745-8315.12612

Haythornthwaite, C. (2005). Social networks and Internet connectivity effects. *Information, Community & Society, 8*(2), 125–147. 10.1080/13691180500146185

Heath, S. (2004). Peer-shared households, quasi-communes and neo-tribes. *Current Sociology, 52*(2), 161–179. 10.1177/0011392104041799

Isaacs Russell, G. (2015). *Screen Relations: The Limits of Computer-Mediated Psychoanalysis and Psychotherapy.* London: Karnac Books.

Isaacs Russell, G. (2020). Remote working during the pandemic: a Q&A with Gillian Isaacs Russell: Questions from the editor and editorial board of the BJP. *British Journal of Psychotherapy, 36*(3), 364–374. 10.1111/bjp.12581

Jamieson, L. (1998) *Intimacy: Personal Relationships in Modern Societies.* Cambridge and Malden, MA: Polity Press.

Koch, R., & Miles, S. (2020). Inviting the stranger in: Intimacy, digital technology and new geographies of encounter. *Progress in Human Geography.* 10.1177/030913252 0961881

Kocsis, B. J., & Yellowlees, P. (2018). Telepsychotherapy and the therapeutic relationship: Principles, advantages, and case examples. *Telemedicine and e-Health, 24*(5), 329–334. 10.1089/tmj.2017.0088

Lemma, A. (2015). Psychoanalysis in times of technoculture: Some reflections on the fate of the body in virtual space. *The International Journal of Psychoanalysis, 96*(3), 569–582. 10.1111/1745-8315.12348

Lemma, A. (2020). The aesthetic link: The patient's use of the analyst's body and the body of the consulting room. *Psychoanalytic Perspectives, 17*(1), 57–73. 10.1080/1551 806X.2019.1685313

Lemma, A., & Caparrotta, L. (2014). *Psychoanalysis in the Technoculture Era.* London: Routledge.

Lingiardi, V. (2008). Playing with unreality: Transference and computer. *The International Journal of Psychoanalysis, 89*(1), 111–126. 10.1111/j.1745-8315.2007. 00014.x

Lingiardi, V. (2011). Realities in dialogue: Commentary on paper by Stephen Hartman. *Psychoanalytic Dialogues,* 21, 483–49510.1080/10481885.2011.595342.

Lobinger, K., Venema, R., Tarnutzer, S., & Lucchesi, F. (2021). What is visual intimacy? Mapping a complex phenomenon. *MedieKultur: Journal of Media and Communication Research, 37*(70), 151–176. 10.7146/mediekultur.v37i70.119750

Locke, J. L. (1998). *Why We Don't Talk to Each Other Anymore: The De-Voicing of Society.* New York, NY: Touchstone.

Marar, Z. (2012). *Intimacy.* London: Routledge.

Marouda - Chatjoulis, A. (2014). *The Need to Belong: Groupishness and Conflict Within Groups. A Psychodynamic Approach.* Athens: Papazisi eds.

Martin, J., McBride, T., Masterman, T., Pote, D. I., Mokhtar, D. N., Oprea, E., & Sorgenfrei, M. (2020). Covid-19 and early intervention: Evidence, challenges and risks relating to virtual and digital delivery. *Early Intervention Foundation, London.* https://www.eif.org.uk/files/pdf/covid19-early-intervention-virtual-digital-delivery.pdf

Miguel, C. (2018). *Personal Relationships and Intimacy in the Age of Social Media.* Springer.

Nebeling Petersen, M., Harrison, K., Raun, T., & Andreassen, R. (2018). Introduction: Mediated intimacies. In R. Andreassen, M. Nebeling Petersen, K. Harrison, & T. Raun (Eds.), *Mediated intimacies. Connectivities, Relationalities and Proximities* (pp. 1–16). New York: Routledge. 10.4324/9781315208589-1

Neumann, D. A. (2013). The frame for psychoanalysis in cyberspace. In J. Scharff (Ed.), *Psychoanalysis Online: Mental Health, Teletherapy, and Training* (pp. 171–181). London: Karnac Books.

Ogden, P., & Goldstein, B. (2019). Sensorimotor psychotherapy from a distance: Engaging the body, creating presence, and building relationship in videoconferencing. In H. Weinberg, & A. Rolnick (Eds.), *Theory and Practice of Online Therapy* (pp. 47–65). New York, NY: Routledge.

Oshni Alvandi, A. (2019). Cybertherapogy: A conceptual architecting of presence for counselling via technology. *International Journal of Psychology and Educational Studies, 6*(1), 30–45. 10.17220/ijpes.2019.01.004

Roesler, C. (2017). Tele-analysis: The use of media technology in psychotherapy and its impact on the therapeutic relationship. *Journal of Analytical Psychology, 62*(3), 372–394. 10.1111/1468-5922.12317

Roth, B. (2014). Mutual attention and joint gaze as developmental forerunners of the therapeutic alliance. *The Psychoanalytic Review, 101*(6), 847–869. 10.1521/prev.2014. 101.6.847

Sayers, J. (2021). Online psychotherapy: Transference and countertransference issues. *British Journal of Psychotherapy, 37*(2), 223–233. 10.1111/bjp.12624

Scharff, J. (2020). In response to Kristin White "Practicing as an analyst in Berlin in times of the coronavirus". *The International Journal of Psychoanalysis, 101*, 585–588.

Scharff, J. (Ed.) (2013). *Psychoanalysis Online: Mental Health, Teletherapy and Training*. London: Karnac Books.

Sfoggia, A., Kowacs, C., Gastaud, M. B., Laskoski, P. B., Bassols, A. M., Severo, C. T., Machado, D., Krieger, D. V., Torres, M. B., Teche, S. P., Wellausen, R. S., & Eizirik, C. L. (2014). Therapeutic relationship on the web: To face or not to face? *Trends in Psychiatry and Psychotherapy, 36*, 3–10. 10.1590/2237-6089-2013-0048

Simpson, S., Richardson, L., Pietrabissa, G., Castelnuovo, G., & Reid, C. (2020). Videotherapy and therapeutic alliance in the age of COVID-19. *Clinical Psychology and Psychotherapy, 28*(2), 409–421. 10.1002/cpp.2521

Singleton, A., Abeles, P., & Smith, I. C. (2016). Online social networking and psychological experiences: The perceptions of young people with mental health difficulties. *Computers in Human Behavior, 61*(August), 394–403. 10.1016/j.chb.201 6.03.011

Suler, J. (2004). The online disinhibition effect. *Cyberpsychology & Behavior, 7*(3), 321–326. 10.1002/aps.42

Svenson, K. (2020). Teleanalytic therapy in the era of Covid-19: Dissociation in the countertransference. *Journal of the American Psychoanalytic Association, 68*(3), 447–454. 10.1177/0003065120938772

Trub, L., & Magaldi, D. (2017). Left to our own devices. *Psychoanalytic Perspectives, 14*(2), 219–236. 10.1080/1551806X.2017.1304118

Turkle, S. (2011). *Alone Together: Why We Expect More from Technology and Less from Each Other*. New York: Basic Books.

Weinberg, H. (2014). The *Paradox of Internet Groups: Alone in the Presence of Virtual Others*. London: Karnac.

Weinberg, H. (2020). Online group psychotherapy: Challenges and possibilities during COVID-19—A practice review. *Group Dynamics: Theory, Research, and Practice, 24*(3), 201. 10.1037/gdn0000140

White, K. (2020). Practising as an analyst in Berlin in times of the coronavirus: The core components of psychoanalytic work and the problem of virtual reality. *The International Journal of Psychoanalysis*, *101*(3), 580–584. 10.1080/00207578.2020. 1761816

Winnicott, D. W. (1958). *Through Paediatrics to Psycho-Analysis*. London: Tavistock.

Winnicott, D. W. (1960). The theory of the parent–infant relationship. In D. W. Winnicott (Ed.), *The Maturational Process and the Facilitating Envorment* (pp. 37–55). New York: International Universities Press.

Winnicott, D. W. (1971). *Playing and Reality*. London: Tavistock.

Zelizer, V. A. (2009). *The Purchase of Intimacy*. Princeton: Princeton University Press.

5 Me and My "Otherness" or: Who is the Other on the Screen Who Looks Exactly Like Me?

Vered Bar

Introduction to the "Otherness"

The Cambridge Dictionary defines "otherness" as "being or feeling different in appearance or character from what is familiar, expected, or generally accepted."[1] Work in the virtual space has been emerging steadily over the past decade or so. However, until the outbreak of the recent global pandemic in 2020, for most mental health practitioners, it has not been the main therapeutic platform. Instead, classic face-to-face in-person sessions have been the prevailing treatment paradigm. Virtual work exposes us to self-states (Bromberg, 2001) which we may prefer to avoid in daily routine. The "otherness," which is usually embedded within the self and is invisible and inaccessible, is available for our examination in virtual work in a way that undermines our subjective self-perception and self-image. The intent is not only to our self-image and our perceived external appearance (good or not) but to an internal discourse that takes place in light of the visual encounter that sometimes reflects the gap between the internal emotional experience and the way it appears and is transmitted. In virtual space we are more aware of the gap between what is inside and how it is outwardly expressed. In addition, everything that is not familiar to us on the screen is eyed critically. Because this encounter occurs between ourselves and our "otherness," the visible on-screen image exacerbates the gap (or the adequacy) between what is happening inside us (what we really want to say or think and what we really feel) and how this desire visually appears on screen, and is "said," both verbally and non-verbally. The visual meeting between our inner reality and our outer reality brings us face-to-face with the discomfort created by this gap and thus takes us out of our comfort zones. Therefore, virtual space, being new and unfamiliar, may pose a threat.

Usually, we have a sense of self which has been constructed from our subjective inner experience. In the virtual space, our sense of self is informed by our subjective experience in addition to our "objective" experience – from outside in. We may experience a split between our "self" as a subject (how I experience myself) and as an object (a "not-me"). In this manner the "object self" represents our "otherness." In Levinas' view (Epstein, 2005) the "other"

DOI: 10.4324/9781003205029-7

penetrates the world of the self without asking for "permission," and without considering the ability and willingness of the self. Similarly, Freud (Kedar, 2013) writes that one of the characteristics of the unconscious system is the replacement of external reality (objective self) with psychic reality (subjective self). During virtual work we experience the opposite. We experience how our psychic reality appears when exposed to the external reality. The encounter with our inner reality that is reflected outwards is complex. There are gaps, differences, false and authentic self-states, which are particularly visible in the therapeutic work in the virtual space. The outer "mask," namely our "Persona" (Jung, 1966) that we put on ourselves every day and feel comfortable in, can and does visually confront us in the virtual on-screen encounter with ourselves.

When there is a large gap between the inner and outer state, the feeling is that of "estrangement." That is, the presence of the self on the screen is "I am a stranger" who responds and behaves differently from the "familiar me," that increases the awareness of the gaps and the presence of the "familiarity" and the "strangeness" within us. Thus, tension is created, which, on the one hand induces an automatic return to the familiar, and on the other, constitutes an opportunity for growth, development, and construction of accepting relationships between the "familiar" and the "stranger" within us. In this context "I am a stranger" is like our "otherness," since the intent is not necessarily to the difficulty in reference to how we look but rather to the visual gap between our inner self and its outward expression. The encounter between our inner public self and our inner experience can also produce a sense of defamiliarization.

Thus, an examination of the nature of the encounter between ourselves and our "otherness" that we stare at on the screen while we engage in virtual work might raise many questions, such as: How does a person perceive his/her/their self?[2] What is the nature of the difficulties of seeing ourselves? Are we able to maintain a subjective view of ourselves or do we become an object for ourselves? Is our experience of "otherness" related to our perception of ourselves as attractive people? Is the reflection we meet on the screen familiar to us and recognizable as our "inner self"? The intention here is to elucidate what in the meeting with our "otherness" is so powerful and at the same time, precisely because of this power, produces an experience of rejection. It shows how the encounter makes the self-states that we do not like in ourselves accessible, and thus has the potential to expand our self. Ultimately, this experience may enable us to accept some of our own "otherness" and contain what we refer to as our subjective self and our objective self.

The Virtual Space and Our Self-States

In virtual work everything is amplified, namely both positive and negative emotions. On the screen where the gaze is more focused on facial expressions and every movement, mimicry of the other and ours is heightened. The face appears sharper and there is nothing that the eye cannot see (Levinas, 1991). All this in the interaction between us and the other within us that will be revealed to us on screen. My clients and students, mostly female, complained that it was a very difficult experience to see themselves on screen. The reasons they reported varied. It often related to external appearance but also included an awareness of "flawed mimicry" when there is a gap between their internal experience and how they see their face/facial expressions on screen. They also reported incongruence when saying something that did not genuinely match what they felt inside. They were preoccupied with the gaps between the external perception of self as encountered on the screen and the internal experience. Some participants discovered the option of turning off the self-view in order to avoid seeing themselves. I see it as a missed opportunity for growth.

Most of the responses revolved around their hopes that at the end of the pandemic they would return to working face-to-face. Under this circumstance, they believed they could present themselves more authentically and fully in the therapeutic space.[3] They describe a prevailing discrepancy between one "me" and another "me." The one on the screen was neither authentic nor complete but the "me" brought to a face-to-face encounter was both. The emotional experience was similar to the defense mechanism of splitting. Several anecdotes serve to illustrate this point. For some of the participants the negative self-image was emphasized. Several found a "method" of placing a sticker on the screen to hide their "window," allowing them to block their self-view. They reported that not seeing themselves allowed them to feel more comfortable and relaxed in their virtual work. In an informal conversation with colleagues, there was a discussion of a feature that allows the lecturers not see themselves on screen while the students see the lecturer. One female colleague noted she welcomed this option and reported that her concentration improved, and her mind became less distracted ever since she began to use this feature. To summarize, the tension in working with myself "while I see myself" is created both due to the self-perception and self-image (how I look) and because of the inner discourse produced as a result of the gap between our "inner" and "external" reality when they are not congruent.

Bromberg (2001) argues that mental health is the understanding that we are all divided and maintain multiple self-states while simultaneously feeling a continuous and coherent self despite the multiplicity. According to this stance, we have the ability to "stand in the spaces" by accessing self-states from which we have disconnected and are no longer in contact, and nonetheless with which we are able to have a conflict or a dialog. Below I shall argue that on screen we encounter our other parts, specifically those disconnected aspects of ourselves that are less accessible to us or that we are less in touch with and therefore the "me" on the screen is the "not me" as my participants have asserted. Following Bromberg, the therapist's role is to facilitate the client's accessibility to their self-states and to guide them into a conflict or dialog with these aspects of the self so that the participants may meet the spaces or crevices between their split self-states. With this in mind, it is postulated that the virtual therapeutic space and work are the venue, the opportunity, and the possibility to befriend our less-liked self-states and form a more integrated whole. While participants experience a profound desire to avoid confronting themselves on the screen, as therapists, we should not give in to this desire, but instead encourage our participants to explore this desire as a part of the therapeutic content.[4]

The "Otherness" as a Symptom of the Cultural Mirror

Body Dysmorphic Disorder or BDD (DSM-V) is defined as an excessive preoccupation with imaginary or minor external defects and external appearance in a way that leads to distress or impaired functioning (American Psychiatric Association, 2013). Popular culture and media emphasize standardized ideals of beauty and often link "ugliness," or aesthetic unattractiveness to malice, and imperfections. Men and women suffer equally from body dysmorphic symptoms. They obsess over individual physical features, combinations of features, or even the entire body and appearance (Bienvenu et al., 2000). Features such as one's nose, hair, skin, weight, or body shape may represent the focus of obsession. This culturally mediated division invites intense preoccupation with appearance and may be significant for people who are highly vulnerable to their self-image. In most cases, the excessive fixation with external appearance begins in adolescence and tends to become fixed for years. Over time, the preoccupation can expand to other areas of the body in the absence of appropriate treatment (e.g., social, physical, neurological) (Gluck, 2013). Susan Bordo (1985) argues that the dominant preoccupation with the body has become a kind of self-regulating detachment mechanism. Since the relation to the physical aspect is alienated, as if it is something foreign, it is regarded as not part of the self, the "not- self."

For many of us (Pfund et al., 2020), the virtual encounter produces preoccupation with our appearance and our inwardness as it is expressed outwardly. Pfund et al. found a positive correlation between self-objectification and dissatisfaction with appearance. Consequently, in order to accept and assimilate our "otherness" we may need to bridge the gap between our "objective -self" (on screen) and our "subjective- self."

Apparently, many virtual participants have outwardly displayed behaviors or conduct similar to those suffering from dysmorphic body disorder. On the screen they may perceive themselves as much wider, thiner, smaller or larger than the actual circumference of their physical body. Because virtual work zooms in and frames certain aspects of our physical presence (and there are many parts that remain "invisible"), what appears is more prominent and amplified. Hence, reasonably it can be claimed that this is a "*temporary situational dysmorphic disorder"* resulting from the encounter with a new and unfamiliar space. The encounter returns most of us to regressive defenses and basic assumptions about ourselves and in relation to ourselves. That said, it is also realistic to assume that as most of us return to work face-to-face, *the "temporary situational disorder"* will lessen (something that does not transpire among people with body dysmorphic disorder for whom it expands and solidifies).

The Virtual Meeting: An Opportunity to Get Out of Our Comfort Zones

The "otherness" often has been perceived with negative connotations, as a state of being where something is defective and lacking. This may explain what happens when we meet our other parts on the screen. It is more comfortable for us to see these parts as "not me," instead of accepting them as part of our self, however foreign and irrelevant they may feel. Furthermore, societal communal and cultural explanations of "otherness" or support of our self-image see "otherness" as the expression of anomalies, loneliness, and lack of acceptance. In this inner dialog our other self-states are unworthy and therefore excluded. The "otherness" does not yield coherence with the perception of who we are; therefore, we deny it and develop a relationship of reluctance and avoidance towards it. Yet the virtual encounter, especially in this period when we are new to it and still "naive in it," can also serve as a fertile ground for development and learning.

Virtual space is perceived as threatening because it jeopardizes the integrity of the self. According to Bion (1965) there are thoughts without a thinker. Thoughts waiting for the thinker to think them. Failure of expectations can lead to thought and therefore also potentially to mental development. In Bion's view, although it might not be a pleasant experience, it nonetheless can lead to growth. Therefore, Bion asserts (2000, p. 115) that "when the painful experience is eliminated, there is a blockage of mental development. Rejecting a painful feeling is like blocking the development of thinking or thwarting growth." Precisely because virtual space is perceived as frustrating, alienating, and disappointing (Weinberg, 2020), we are afforded a broad cushion for mental development and growth. Some of the feelings of alienation we experience in virtual space are, of course, from the "otherness," that is, from the space perceived as cold and alienated from our experience and tasks. However, some feelings are the internal projections of alienation of which Bordo (1985) speaks. These projections are the parts of our bodies and of our self-states of which we are usually less aware. The virtual space reduces the ability to avoid dealing with the "otherness" we have split off within ourselves. This is a separation that is binary, convenient, and heuristic; it does not automatically lead to reflective processes. The reflection will allow participants to examine where their self-states that are expressed in the virtual space will meet them in life and how they are part of them ("I am both") and not their own private cases and representations that exist only in the virtual space. Befriending the "other" on the screen, which is also us, means, therefore, integrating the "otherness" within us – creating a broader conception of our self, laying the groundwork for deeper self-acceptance and building accepting relationships between the familiar me (the inner experience) and the strange me (that appears on the screen), for both the therapists and their clients and students.

Biases While Working in Virtual Space

It appears that those who define themselves as introverts feel more comfortable with virtual work and those who define themselves as extroverts – less so (McConnon, 2021). Weinberg (2020) argues that some participants, such as those with social anxiety, benefit more from online therapy. What has resurfaced and is prominent in virtual groups is that participants who experience themselves as extroverts have reported difficulty and even suffering in the virtual space while people who experience themselves as introverts have found that they can more easily take more dominant roles than usual, via virtual groups (Weinberg, 2020). Virtual space has enabled the "otherness" of both, since it is regressive and returns us to self-states that are not always under our control and make it possible to present our less socially accepted needs through the high emotional arousal that meets us when we are alone on screen.

In a group, what is perceived as the "otherness" splits the group in a way that disrupts group coherence. Expanding the range of group self-states allows additional self-states to become accessible. This continuum includes those self-states that symbolize the "otherness." It is also the space for the mental and developmental growth of each participant. The "otherness" is accessed when the self can recognize it. It does not just appear, it is revealed. It brings its renewal in its arrival or outburst into the self. Revelation is entirely the fruit of the other's initiative, and it requires the reaction and response of the self (Epstein, 2005). In other words, the movement is that we refuse to contain it within us. It is as if our shadow is floating upwards and defying our "otherness" in public.

Winnicott's article "Hate in the Counter-Transference" (1949) was a breakthrough in this regard, because for the first time he opened the door for therapists to hate their patients. Winnicott stated that the therapist must not deny the hatred that really exists within him. The analyst must be aware of his or her own fear and hatred. In the present context, hatred must be cultivated, contained, and available for comment. Respectively, a facilitator or counselor who refuses to acknowledge their hateful self-states will not be able to process them and have a dialogue with them (Bar, 2021). This implies that therapists should connect with their "otherness," namely with the same seemingly unacceptable or unprofessional self-states and emotions, so that the patient can recognize them within themselves, and so that the therapist can recognize them in the patient. The virtual work requires the therapist/counselor/facilitator to connect and acknowledge their "otherness," and in order to accept the "otherness" of others in the virtual space, to enable the self to expand and not eradicate it or cooperate with the distinction between the "me" and the "not-me."

Finally, I would like to point out two cognitive biases that I identify in virtual work. These biases can become an emotional barrier which might prevent reflection and work on both our "otherness" as professionals and our others, i.e., clients/groups/patients.

1   Actor-observer bias (Watson, 1982) is the tendency of people to attribute their actions to external circumstances, but the actions of others to their inner world and characteristics. This bias relates mainly to one's negative behaviors. In virtual space we tend to attribute the "otherness"; i.e., behaviors that we do not identify with, to the external (virtual) environment while the behavior of others to who they are. This effectively avoids the process of reunion and connection to the "otherness." The virtual space becomes another actor who has motives and intentions and has an effect on our behavior.

2   Loss aversion bias (Tversky & Kahneman, 1991) refers to the hatred of loss. What motivates people is the fear of losing what they have rather than the desire to win. The virtual environment creates an experience which we define as a loss because it challenges our former perceptions of ourselves. The loss aversion bias provokes a rejection, specifically the person who I seem to be in the virtual space is not who I really am. This experience takes away self-states that I had and loved, reduces me, and carries me away. Therefore, it is hard to perceive virtual space as an opportunity to grow.

As a therapist we need to be aware of these two biases in order to enable progress and change.

Working with Our "Otherness": Personal Reflections on "Otherness"

In this section, I provide two examples of working with the "otherness." The first example concerns my own self experience of my "otherness." The second example stresses the challenges in adopting what is perceived as "not me" as "me."

Example #1 As I watched the recordings of the lectures I gave in the first semester of 2021, I noticed that I often played with my hair. This was a behavior I was not aware of in face-to-face encounters with participants. The experience of the "stereotypical woman playing with her hair" created an uncomfortable feeling for me: primping, preoccupied with "her" outward appearance, not attentive, preoccupied with what "she" looks like and her (flirtatious/playful) effect on others. This created the potential for a possible refraction of my self-image in my own eyes as a professional invested in knowledge and reason. I wondered if my clients and students saw this gesture as an over-attempt to look good or a desire to be perceived as attractive. Did me, playing with my hair, bother them as it bothered me? Were they even aware of this, and why did it bother me so much? Was this effectively a kind of incoherence between who I think is on the outside as a lecturer and consultant and the self I met in the virtual meetings?

Example #2 During a group meeting, feedback was given to an on-screen participant who joined our virtual sessions with his microphone muted and his video turned off. He had been highly charismatic and en-gaged in face-to-face sessions. When this difference between his in-person demeanor and his participation in the virtual space was shared with him, the participant agreed with the group and said that on screen he felt in-effective due to the fact that his body was not visible. He explained that he has always relied on his appearance and in general he likes to present and lecture while standing. Now that he is sitting, and his body is not visible he feels absent and ineffective.

I challenged him and asked if the experience of lack of presence and lack of influence was familiar to him and whether the virtual space is the only venue that challenges him in this manner? He acknowledged being aware of other places where he experiences this, but in virtual work he encountered these feelings with great intensity. I suggested that the virtual encounter enables that which also exists outside the virtual space to be present in the virtual one. However, there is no doubt that feelings exist within him. Usually these are self-states which are less accessible to him and easy for him to ignore and repress, while the virtual space forces him to confront the feelings. I also told him that in my opinion this is an opportunity for him to deal with processes that he managed to bypass and avoid on a daily basis. In fact, I recommended that he not "disappear" or "lose his words" in the new and unfamiliar virtual space. I pointed out that this is an opportunity to grow and gain control of his presence and his degree of influence in a way that is independent of external conditions – such as virtual vs. face-to-face or what he defines – as "not me." I suggested reframing to define "you too." To my delight, he, as well as the group, agreed with me. I challenged ev-eryone to identify self-states they may have "lost" or of which they had less control over in the virtual space. Their responses included "lack of power," "difficulty connecting after," "empathic failure," "a feeling that I am not significant," "lack of authority," "charisma is not felt," "low motivation," and "lack of interest and curiosity."

Next, I suggested that we think about what was found, revealed, and dis-covered about ourselves during the virtual work. This time there was silence. I recognized that it was easier to discuss the loss and more difficult to talk about what had been gained. After a relatively long silence, participants began to answer, stating "I learned about myself that I was less sociable than I thought," "I was actually comfortable being in 'my cave' without mixing with others," "I love the ease with which I can be or not be present," "lack of responsibility for others," "an emotional disconnect that pleases me," "I enjoy being in my own company and not really needing others," "comfortable," and "I don't have to make an effort to please."

The common denominator is that many of the answers imply a lower social need than the participants initially thought and perhaps an enjoyment of solitude, distance, and alienation. Most of the group members agreed that they were more comfortable with the solitude of being alone in the virtual space than they initially thought. They expressed the need to be together, yet not as experienced before the virtual work. They discovered that both needs exist, namely the need for social engagement and the need for solitude. Furthermore, they learned that both can co-exist. Of course, it is possible that virtual work also exposes a strong social bias that stems from the fact that people are social creatures.

Summary

This chapter reviews and discusses how the challenging virtual space and our "otherness" can be used as an ongoing simulation and how the virtual dimension as well as the high emotional arousal that it brings to the surface can be used as an opportunity for growth. It presents a case study to demonstrate how to utilize and harness its potentially overwhelming power in order to enable the participants to accept their "otherness" and facilitate the growth and expansion of their self. Virtual work allows us to connect to our self-states that are not accessible on a daily basis. Often these are self-states that we do not automatically like. Though we can easily ignore these self-states in our daily routine or during face-to-face work, it is harder to do so in virtual work where they are embodied on the screen. As such, the virtual space is an opportunity to expand the self and accept the non-self as part of the self. In virtual work, for both the therapist and the client, the participating self is experienced as a subjective self, i.e., "me," while the on-screen self is newly experienced as an object and therefore as an alien and isolated, "not me." Though the automatic response is often to reject this splitting of the self into "me" and "not me," as detrimental or unhelpful, the author invites the readers to consider the potential growth that is inherent in this novel experience of the self. Additionally, as therapists we need to be aware of the cognitive biases and the "*temporarily virtual dysmorphia*" that may impede our ability to work within the novel space and encourage our participants to receive and benefit from the on-screen object experienced as "not me" as part of the subject experienced as "me"; in other words, accept our "otherness."

Accepting My "Otherness" – Personal Worksheet

- Draw: "who I am in the virtual space?" Share and explain? What do I bring to face-to-face setting that I do not bring to the virtual experience? Why?
- Suggest a name / title to the "other" who is you in the virtual space? Explain
- Tell the story of the "other" who is you considering who you perceive they are in the virtual space. in what way is their story different or similar to "your" story?
- Which self-states are less familiar to me which I met in the virtual experience?
- Everyone says what surprises them when they see themselves in a virtual setting. What will people see in person that they will not see virtually?
- Have I discovered something I love/appreciate about myself in the "virtual space" that is less expressed face -to -face?
- What did I learn about myself in the virtual space that I would want to have in face -to -face setting?

Notes

1 Cambridge dictionary ("otherness"): https://dictionary.cambridge.org/de/worterbuch/englisch/otherness (Retrieved on 2021, July 7)
2 With the aim of addressing assumed binary and gendered distinctions in referring to people in a general way, the pronouns they/there will be used in this chapter, unless specifically referencing a particular gender.
3 The participants are not allowed to join the virtual session without their camera turned on.
4 This approach is congruent to Schema therapy: "Schema Therapy in the Online Setting – from Challenges to Opportunities".

References

American Psychiatric Association. (2013). *Diagnostic and statistical manual of mental disorders* (5th ed.). Washington, DC: Author.

Bar, V. (2021). *Benign dissociation in groups and organizations*. Resling (Hebrew).

Bienvenu, O. J., Samuels, J. F., Riddle, M. A., Hoehn-Saric, R., Liang, K. Y., Cullen, B. A., Grados, M. A., & Nestadt, G. (2000). The relationship of obsessive-compulsive disorder to possible spectrum disorders: Results from a family study. *Biological Psychiatry*, *48*(4), 287–293. 10.1016/S0006-3223(00)00831-3.

Bion, W. R. (1965). *Transformations*. London: Heinemann.

Bion, W. R. (2000). *The clinical thinking of Wilfred Bion*. Bookworm (Hebrew).

Bordo, S. (1985). Anorexia nervosa: Psychopathology as the crystallization of nature. *Philosophical Forum*, *17*(2), 73.

Bromberg, M. P. (2001). *Standing in the space: Essays on clinical process, trauma, and dissociation*. Routledge.

Cambridge Dictionary. (n.d.). Otherness. In *Dictionary.Cambridge.org*. Retrieved on July 7, 2021. https://dictionary.cambridge.org/de/worterbuch/englisch/otherness

Epstein, D. (2005). *Near and far*. Ministry of Defense (Hebrew).

Gluck, S. (2013). What is Body Dysmorphic Disorder, BDD (DSM-5)?. In *HealthyPlace*. Retrieved on July 7, 2021. https://www.healthyplace.com/ocd-related-disorders/body-dysmorphic-disorder/what-is-body-dysmorphic-disorder-bdd-dsm-5

Jung, C. G. (1966). *Two essays on analytical psychology, collected works* (Vol. 7, 2 ed.). Routledge.

Kedar, M. (2013). The other and the responsibility to the other in Levinas and the unconscious and the responsibility for the unconscious content that became conscious in Freud. *Hebrew Psychology*. Available at: https://www.hebpsy.net/articles.asp?id=2911 (Hebrew).

Levinas, E. (1991). *Totality and infinity: An essay on exteriority*. Kluwer.

McConnon, A. (March 9, 2021). Zoom fatigue: The differing impact on Introverts and extroverts. *The Wallstreet Journal*. https://www.wsj.com/articles/zoom-fatigue-the-differing-impact-on-introverts-and-extroverts-11615291202

Pfund, G. N., Hill, P. L., & Harriger, J. (2020). Video chatting and appearance satisfaction during COVID-19: Appearance comparisons and self-objectification as moderators. *International Journal of Eating Disorders*, *53*(12), 2038–2043. 10.1002/eat.23393

Tversky, A., & Kahneman, D. (1991). Loss aversion in riskless choice: A reference-dependent model. *The Quarterly Journal of Economics*, *106*(4), 1039–1061. 10.2307/2937956

Watson, D. (1982). The actor and the observer: How are their perceptions of causality divergent? *Psychological Bulletin*, *92*(3), 682–700. 10.1037/0033-2909.92.3.682

Weinberg, H. (2020). Online group psychotherapy: Challenges and possibilities during COVID-19 – A practice review. *Group Dynamics: Theory, Research, and Practice*, *24*(3), 201–211. 10.1037/gdn0000140

Winnicott, D. W. (1949). Hate in the counter-transference. *The International Journal of Psychoanalysis*, *30*, 69–74.

6 Zooming in Zoom: Mental-Body-Brain Perspectives on Online Psychotherapy Sessions

Hadas Mor-Ofek

The COVID-19 pandemic influenced our lives tremendously. Massive changes in everyday life altogether with medical and financial threats led to increase in mental distress. The need to protect the physical health of therapists and patients and the frequent lockdowns raised the necessity to find "out of the box" solutions to the growing need for psychotherapy. Online psychotherapy seemed like a reasonable option. Prior to this worldwide crisis, online therapy had taken its first steps as a common practice in psychodynamic based therapies (Scharff, 2013) as well as cognitive-behavioral ones (Andersson, 2018). However, the current situation accelerated the use of online therapy for the majority of psychotherapists.

Interestingly, coinciding with the outbreak of the pandemic, a paper concerning ways to improve nonverbal interpersonal communication during online treatment was published by Rolnick and Ehrenreich (2020). The authors discussed the partial absence of the body and suggested few technological solutions that could assist "to bring the body back to the scene," such as using psychophysiological sensors as conduits of the patient's bodily expressions or choosing a unique type of camera that enables zooming in on the patient's face and concurrently seeing his or her full body. However, most therapists who had to move into online therapy did not have such equipment. This state of affairs enables us to take a look at online therapies under less favorable conditions, and to reflect on the challenges of online therapy from a mind-body-brain perspective.

In the following chapter, we survey online therapy from the point of view of patient-therapist relationships. We describe the Interpersonal Neurobiology and the Polyvagal's Theory perspectives on nonverbal communication and its role in psychotherapeutic alliance. We specify the patient-therapist synchronization process through updated models of brain functioning – the Free Energy Principle and the "common currency" of world-brain relations. On the basis of this theoretical background, we characterize patients who are more prone to influences of the compromised nonverbal communication during online therapy. In addition, we refer to certain aspects of online

DOI: 10.4324/9781003205029-8

sessions' nonverbal communication. We interpret the internet bandwidth interruptions as resembling the "sloppy" nature of interpersonal communication. We deal with the over presence of facial expressions at the expense of the whole body, and the lack of shared environment and shared attention. We suggest phenomenological inquiry as a means to overcome the aforementioned challenges. Finally, we present a scenario where online therapy might be beneficial to therapeutic progression.

Patient-Therapist Alliance and Nonverbal Communication

Allan Schore, an American psychologist and one of the leading theoreticians in the Interpersonal Neurobiology field (IPNB), was interviewed in March 2021. He was asked about the efficacy of online psychotherapy, which became prevalent during the COVID-19 pandemic. Schore pointed at two goals of psychological treatment. One is symptom reduction, and the other is mental growth prompting. He suggested that since essential elements for therapeutic change, e.g., nonverbal communication, is limited during online therapy, only symptom reduction may be achieved. True mental growth is questionable. Schore's presumption calls for a deeper look on the patient-therapist communication in general and during online sessions in particular.

Therapeutic alliance was already identified in a vast body of research as the best predictor of positive outcomes across a wide range of modalities (Martin et al., 2000; Norcross, 2014).

The therapist's presence promotes a positive therapeutic alliance (Geller et al., 2012), and in conjunction with affective involvement, they facilitate neuroplasticity required in the course of learning and repetition, i.e., working through, during therapy (Allison & Rossouw, 2013).

Patient-therapist nonverbal communication appears to be as central as the ideational-verbal aspect of the therapeutic dialogue. The therapeutic dyad creates experiential context that loads the cognitive content with personally negotiated meaning. Emotional experiences constitute brain states of vitality that facilitate mutual influences (Trevarthen, 1993), and that promote generation of renewed meanings and therapeutic change.

What is the mechanism of this mutual nonverbal influences between therapist and patient? Synchronization of rhythms, gestures, and behaviors are the basis for dyadic regulatory processes. The nonverbal aspects that convey information about the inner emotional state and establish the vital experience of being "feel felt" (Siegel, 2007) include body postures, movements, gestures, facial expressions, eye contact, as well as prosody, changes in breathing, skin color, and even smell. These vast range of expressions constitute what Stern (2010) calls "forms of vitality," that attune the patient-therapist intersubjective field and guide the course of the session.

Nonverbal Communication from IPNB's Lens

The research and the clinical perspectives of the patient-therapist relationship and its influence over mental-physiological processes are at the heart of the Interpersonal Neurobiology (IPNB) field, an interdisciplinary attitude that aims to integrate science and subjective domains. IPNB presents some relevant ideas regarding online therapy.

Siegel (2015) emphasizes the importance of integration as a basis of physical and mental health. Since brain and mind, as living systems, are open to the flow of sensory data from the environment, especially to information about other's emotional states (Cozolino, 2006), interpersonal integration serves as the main vehicle to achieve neural integration (Siegel, 2006). According to Siegel, interpersonal integration is the result of a relationship, where one person is present for another person. Presence and attunement create resonance between the bodies, brains, and mental experience of the two partners and build trust and resilience.

Therapeutic setting facilitates these interpersonal processes by establishing a physical realm, an appointment in a given place and time, that enables the therapeutic couple to align and resonate. Siegel (2007) claims that "resonance circuits" are at the heart of this alignment. By this term, he refers to a reciprocal stream of energy and information between two people. Moreover, this interbrain connectivity allows early detection and repair of ruptures of the alliance (Ray et al., 2017).

In the IPNB field, mental experiences of the self, the world, and relationships, are mainly associated with right hemisphere activation. This notion is a cornerstone in Schore's ideas (2019). Schore claims that therapeutic conversations are in fact a dynamic interplay between two right hemispheres of the therapeutic couple. It is a moment-to-moment state sharing, that acts as an interactive matrix in which patient and therapist match states. This dynamic facilitates neuroplastic changes in the patient's regulatory systems, which in turn allows for optimal treatment outcomes in both symptom-reducing and mental growth.

The IPNB ideas highlight the importance of the continuous transition of non-verbal vocal, bodily, and facial gestures between the patient and the therapist, for the psychotherapeutic change. That raises the question whether online therapy provides adequate conditions for the required patient-therapist nonverbal communication. Before we reflect on this issue, we present another aspect that might be relevant for the interpersonal experience during online therapy.

Safety and the Polyvagal Theory

A sense of safety provides optimal conditions to engage in effective psychotherapeutic work. Social circuits attenuate amygdala-based influences, and therefore increase a sense of safety (Badenoch, 2008). From this perspective, a strong patient-therapist relationship is crucial for feeling safe during therapy sessions.

Exploring the connections between safety and interpersonal relationships, is at the heart of the polyvagal theory, a model of the autonomic nervous system (ANS), that brings together risk evaluation processes and bodily regulation, at the service of physical and mental health.

The polyvagal theory (PVT) was introduced by Stephan Porges (2011), who claimed that in contrast to Cannon's (1929a) well-known model of the ANS as a bimodal system, ANS contains three parts, which are hierarchically phylogenetically ordered. The first two subsystems in PVT are similar to Cannon's model: the ventral parasympathetic subsystem (ventral-vagal complex – VVC, composed of myelinated vagal fibers), the most evolved part in the ANS, and the sympathetic subsystem. The third subsystem, according to the PVT, is the DVC (dorsal-vagal complex, composed of unmyelinated vagal pathways), the most primitive part of the system. Each part of the ANS provides an adequate subbase for the actions required to meet environmental demands, via its influences over the cardio-pulmonary (heart-lungs) functioning.

The VVC regulates the body in perceived safe environments, through inhibition of the spontaneous heart rate. This regulation is characterized by calmness and tranquility. It promotes physical growth and restoration, as well as mental activities such as learning and social engagement, processes associated with psychotherapeutic change. By contrast, under threats, the sympathetic system is recruited to support the defense actions of fight and flight. The sympathetic regulation resulted in high cardiac and metabolic output. Its typical experiential quality is alertness, anxiety, and irritation. In addition, the DVC regulates the body under extreme life-threatening states that are combined with helplessness. DVC regulation would be manifested in metabolic depression, hypoarousal, and defensive shutdown.

The coordination between the three parts of the ANS and the environmental demands is based on "neuroception" (Porges, 2011), a continuous automatic risk evaluation monitoring. Neuroception is supported by pre-frontal and temporal cortices with projections to the amygdala and the periaqueductal gray.

Neuroception is vital for interpersonal connection. The main source of information concerning safety is interaction with others. Via facial expressions, vocalizations and gestures, information about "what is going on out there," especially in the interpersonal field, is conveyed. Projections from neuroceptive process shift the autonomic regulation.

When indications of safety are detected, the ANS regulation shifts to VVC, i.e., parasympathetic regulation, that down-regulates defense strategies and enables social engagement behaviors and connectedness. This dynamic represents a bi-directional neural communication between the face and the heart. The VVC is linked to the striated muscles in the face, that control facial expressions, the middle ear muscles that extract human voice from background noise, the laryngeal and pharyngeal muscles that support prosody and head tilting, and turning muscles that are involved in social gestures and orientation. All the above form the social engagement system that underlies emotional communication. Its importance to the psychotherapeutic process is undoubted. In psychotherapy, safe interpersonal interactions encourage shift to VVC regulation. That helps to alleviate emotional dysregulation (Geller & Porges, 2014).

When threat is detected, sympathetic autonomic reactions enhance defensive reactions and decrease the awareness of others. In the therapeutic scene, this state drives the patient to perceive others in a negative direction, and may affect the therapist as well, through a bias to interpret the patient's responses in a more reactive and less reflective manner.

If "inescapable attacks" signals are detected, ANS shifts to DVC regulation. Physiological and mental state of the patient shifts toward behavioral and emotional shutdown. In therapy it may put therapist and patient at risk of disconnection and dissociation (Geller & Porges, 2014).

The elegant model of the polyvagal theory, and its straight forward implications, drove many clinicians and theoreticians to implement the theory into their work and has gained much popularity. However, the polyvagal theory is not without criticism, particularly regarding the lack of scientific evidence to support the theory (Grossman & Taylor, 2007). Despite the criticism, polyvagal theory provides a feasible metaphor for understanding the relationships between safe interpersonal relations and emotional growth in psychotherapy. Using it as a useful metaphor is conceivable, since its premises concerning the role of the parasympathetic regulation and neuroception, are supported by the neurovisceral integration theory, a more scientific-based model concerning autonomic functioning (Smith et al., 2017).

The polyvagal's premises concerning the neuroceptive-driven ANS regulation add the issues of safety to the question concerning the feasibility to provide good-enough interpersonal information transition during therapy meetings. However, in order to explore this issue, we take a closer look at the aforementioned interpersonal processes that are sketched in a rather metaphoric-general manner in the IPBN and the polyvagal theory.

Patient-Therapist Nonverbal Communication: Synchronization Processes through the Free Energy Principle Lens

Common denominator of the above perspectives, is the patient-therapist duet of movements and sounds, the "communicative musicality" (Trevarthen & Malloch, 2000) that synchronizes physiological/mental states. Thus, synchronization seems like a centerpiece of therapeutic alliance and change.

What is the mechanism of synchronization? We may answer it by conceptualizing nonverbal communication between patient and therapist as a particular expression of world-brain relations.

The relations between the person and the environment are based on mutual influences. These influences can be described as interactions between temporospatial dynamics of the environment and temporospatial dynamics of the brain. Temporospatial dynamics refer to changes in time and space in the person's external environment vs. the brain neuronal activity. Mental features are attributed to these interactions (Northoff, 2019). In order to understand it in depth and connect it to online psychotherapy challenges, let's take a look at the brain's functioning through the Free Energy Principle (FEP), an integrative model concerning the brain functioning.

The FEP was introduced by Karl Friston (2010, 2006). The FEP (a.k.a. the predictive coding/processing theory) is based on Helmholtz's (1866, in Friston et al., 2006) notion that the brain is an inference machine. According to FEP, the brain generates and uses internal statistical hierarchically organized models to infer the causes for its sensory input, in the service of survival and well-being. The models, i.e., predictions, are formed by extracting regularities from the environment, so in that manner, they assist the organism to adjust to its environment.

A mismatch between these predictions and the upcoming sensations (exteroceptive or interoceptive data) creates prediction-error and releases free energy. Free-energy is a measure of discrepancy between two systems, which in our case are the brain (prediction) and the world (sensations). This is not an abstract concept; it can be quantified and is used routinely in modelling empirical data (Friston et al., 2007). When the organism succeeds in anticipating the state of the environmental context, free energy is low. The free energy has also to do with the energy that was supposed to be directed to a prediction-based action (Friston et al., 2009) and remained redundant and unbound due to prediction error. The brain's job is to minimize its free energy since it jeopardizes the organism's survival.

Free energy minimization is aimed to recouple the organism/brain's internal dynamics and the world/environment's external dynamics. It is achieved by either changing the prediction, i.e., learning, or by changing the upcoming sensory data, "active inference," in the FEP terminology, that refers to resampling the environment or to acting upon it till the sensations fit the prediction (Hohwy, 2013). These bidirectional processes create synchronization between the world/environment and the brain/individual.

But how does synchronization exactly occur? How do the world's external dynamics and the brain's internal dynamics interact, and how is it connected to online therapy?

World-Brain Temporospatial Synchronization

Northoff (2018) claims that this interaction requires something like a shared code, "common currency." The temporospatial dynamic may be a good candidate to provide it (Northoff, 2019).

The spontaneous brain activity shows continuous changes over time and space that form statistical frequency distributions. These statistical distributions were named by Northoff (2014a) "neuronal statistics." Environmental stimuli show certain statistical frequency distributions as well, and were coined "natural statistics" (Barlow, 2001). The interaction between the brain's "neuronal statistics" and the environment's "natural statistics" results in stimulus-induced neuronal activity. This interaction can be experienced as mental activity, such as perceptions, affects, or other subjective experiences (Panksepp, 1998b; Solms, 2017, 2018).

According to Northoff (2019), the brain's neuronal statistics, reflect the prediction. Prediction is actually a temporospatial pattern, resulted from past interaction between environment and organism. This temporospatial pattern, interacts with the current upcoming sensory data, the "natural statistics." Discrepancy between the two creates the aforementioned prediction error that would create the change in the prediction or in the environment. This is the proposed process that serve as a substrate for the patient-therapist synchronization, in which each partner of the "therapeutic couple" provides the other the "natural statistics" that interact with the other's "neuronal statistics," and drive the mutual synchronization.

Following the above neuronal process that underly patient-therapist synchronization, we can refine our question concerning online therapy and ask **what may interrupt the patient/therapist's neuronal-natural statistics interaction during online therapy?**

The "Weak Link" Patient-Therapist Temporospatial Alignment

Temporospatial synchronization between two systems, patient and therapist in our case, requires a minimal internal temporospatial synchronization of different aspects in each system. When the brain's internal synchronization is reduced, the alignment to the environment is less efficient (Northoff, 2018). Reduced neuronal synchronization prevents integration of different mental functions including perceptual, cognitive, and affective aspects. This sort of dynamic was found in individuals who had experienced negative life events (Duncan et al., 2015). In that case, in order to establish patient-therapist synchronization, the "natural statistics," i.e., the nonverbal data from the therapist, should be clearer and less interrupted. Thus, we may hypothesize that online interruptions would be more problematic during online treatment of patients whose temporospatial synchronization is reduced, such as childhood-traumatized patients. This is supported by Holmes and Nolte (2019) that claim that the more disturbed the individual, the longer biobehavioral synchrony would take.

Sharon, a 50 years old woman, has been in therapy for several years. She applied for treatment because she couldn't bear criticism, and that affected her marital and professional relationships. During therapy, Sharon revealed distant and ambivalent relations with her mother. The therapeutic relations were intense. She was needy and demanding. Whenever I disappointed her, she became detached and hostile. When COVID-19 pandemic started, Sharon was trying to push me to meet her f2f. I offered her online sessions instead, and she accepted it reluctantly. In the first online session, things seemed alright. Two weeks later, I slightly moved my computer, so my background was changed a little, and my face seemed distant. During the following session, Sharon became quiet and hostile. She was furious at me for changing the whole picture. It took her a long time to calm down. She insisted I would promise I'd never change position again.

Some patients seem vulnerable to online interruptions; however, the majority of online therapies do seem beneficial (Fernandez et al., 2021). What enables online psychotherapeutic processes to work? In the due course of the chapter, we present the main characteristics of online meetings that could compromise the therapeutic experience, discuss their actual impact, and suggest ways to overcome it.

Synchronization, Interruptions, and "Sloppiness"

The essential task of establishing patient-therapist biobehavioral-mental synchrony is a challenge in f2f treatment, and it is doubly true in online therapy. The dependency on the internet bandwidth may cause interruptions to the fluency of video/audio transmissions. Delays, lags and freezes of face or voice characterize online sessions. Although these interruptions challenge synchronization, the majority of online treatments overcome it. How?

Let's begin with referring to one of the surprising findings concerning mother-child attunement. Tronick (2003), who studied mother-child interactions, found that mothers attune with their children only 33% of the time. This ratio characterized all mothers. It did not differentiate securely attaching mothers from insecure ones. Tronick (2003, p.5) concluded that all relationships are "sloppy." Adding FEP perspective, we conclude that the mechanism to generate predictions concerning secure attachment can be settled by extracting regularities from relatively noisy sample (Clark, 2019 p.174), "sloppy" dyadic relationships. Therefore, establishing and maintaining good-enough synchrony is still possible under "sloppy" communication during online sessions.

"You're in My Face"

Another aspect of online therapy is the overemphasis on the visibility of the participants' faces, at the expense of the entire body. The faces are in higher resolution. This feature of online treatment is different from the f2f setting, where the face is at distance and the whole body is visible. How does it affect psychotherapy, especially when we take into account the importance of bodily gestures in the patient-therapist "communicative musicality" and in neuroception?

Ramseyer and Tschacher (2014) conducted an analysis of the patient-therapist face vs. bodily movements synchronization and their association with treatment outcomes. Using motion energy analysis, they compared the influences of head movements synchrony compared to body movements synchrony on post session assessment (micro-outcomes) and post treatment achievements (macro-outcomes). Findings suggested that head synchrony predicted macro-outcomes, while body-synchrony predicted session outcomes.

They interpreted the differential influences of head/body synchrony as reflecting different processes. Body synchronization was associated with nonverbal signals that operate outside conscious awareness, and thus are more susceptible to being automatically triggered in resonating individuals and impact post-session emotional experience.

Head movements synchrony was connected to a more deliberate control. It was correlated with speech activity, a more consciously controlled activity. Thus, head movement synchrony is connected to more verbal-explicit aspects of communication and may serve as an indicator of agreement on treatment goals and relationship quality, that is linked to macro-outcomes of therapy.

Thus, we may infer that although online psychotherapy enables mainly head movement synchrony, patient-therapist alliance can be still achieved and maintained since head movement synchrony carries more integrative and long-scale impacts. It may reflect formation of an integrative prediction (FEP) on the basis of these long-scale impacts, that enables patient and therapist to "stay in sync" despite lack of body movements. This conclusion is consistent with the notion that the face is where presence is communicated (Geller & Greenberg, 2012).

Yael, is a 32 year old woman, married, and mother of four. She started therapy a year before the COVID-19 outbreak. She suffered from free-floating anxiety and health anxiety.

Yael and I started to meet on a weekly basis. Her relationship with her mother was brought up. She described ambivalent feelings towards her mother, who was available and helpful, but at the same time, emotionally detached and demanding. At that stage, Yael was becoming attached to me. She was over occupied with my opinions and feelings, and longed for my presence. She was very attentive to my physical presence, my clothing, my hair style.

When the lockdown started, we moved to online sessions. During the first meetings Yael neither spoke, nor looked at me. She seemed overwhelmed. After a few weeks she said: "I can't feel that's you. You're too close. I see eyes, mouth, hair, but I don't see you."

Shared Attention

In his critique of psychoanalysis, Levenson (1989) mentioned that the question that therapists should ask is "what's going on around here?" rather than the usual psychoanalytic inquiry "What does it mean?". This remark emphasizes the importance of state sharing between patient and therapist. Thus, sharing states during the session allows patient and therapist to share their mental landscapes.

Shared attention might be a real challenge in online therapies. Patient and therapist do not share the same space as in f2f meetings. They experience different environmental events during the hour. This way, important data concerning the context for various reactions is not shared, and does not serve in mental processing.

Human beings have a specific drive to share emotions, experiences, and activities with others (Gergely, 2007). What underlies this motivation? Shared-attention is a cognitive-emotional-interpersonal tool. Faced with limited processing resources, the human mind must prioritize some of the environmental aspects. A main prioritizing means is to focus on the aspects that were signaled by others' attention. Research suggests that shared attention can amplify memories, goals, evaluations, emotions, and behavioral learning (Shteynberg, 2015). Stronger shared-attention states are likely when close others are more synchronously attending to the object of one's attention.

According to Shteynberg (2007), shared attention increases the focus of emotional scenes only when it is thought to be synchronized. That creates a shift from first-person singular to first-person plural.

The importance of shared attention is demonstrated position in another study that measured synchronization of physiological and emotional states among individuals in physical proximity but without direct interaction (Golland et al., 2015). The participants watched emotional movies together while seated side by side. The researchers found that autonomic signals of subjects were synchronized and correlated with their emotional responses. This finding suggests that the shared state, i.e., the emotional movie, was the common factor in the subjects' synchronization.

The conclusion is that online therapies challenge the generation of both synchronization and shared attention, thus compromise the creation of "we" experience which is so vital to the therapeutic alliance. In the process of world-brain temporospatial synchronization, the presence of separate events, e.g., sources of external data, for each of the therapeutic partners interrupts the alignment.

The online sessions with Eve, continued long after lockdowns ended, since she just moved to another city. The following vignette took place in May 2021, during the security crisis in Israel. From my clinic I could hear distant bombings, although I was not at risk. Eve's place was far from the war zone. During one session, while talking about her job, I heard bombings. A minute later Eve stopped talking, and seemed hurt. I asked her about that. She said: "I guess I bore you. I know my job is not that interesting." I was surprised, since I didn't feel uninterested. Then I realized that hearing the bombing evoked my worries and despair, and that was probably what my face expressed. I hypothesized she interpreted my facial expression as a reaction to her, instead of the actual reaction to bombing. She and I did not share the same state.

Phenomenology, Markedness, and Re-Constructed Synchronization

How can we overcome the lack of shared attention? We propose that Levenson's inquiry "What's going on around here?" may help us here.

Phenomenological inquiry, that aims to obtain knowledge about the person's mental experience directly, as it is experienced by the person herself, may serve as a means to establish synchronized shared attention. Following Daniel Stern's ideas about the importance of the present moment in psychotherapy, Ramberg (2006) suggests that the therapist should ask the patient probing questions with regard to what is taking place. He recommends using questions like when, where and how, instead of why.

What is the hypothesized process that underlies the use of phenomenological stance to overcome the lack of synchronized shared attention? According to studies in this domain (Shteynberg, 2007), the **experience** of shared attention, and not the actual act of both participants attending to the same object is the critical component to generate shared attention. Therefore, shared attention experience can arise in different ways, such as informing the other about what you attend to. Phenomenological stance may provide a suitable way to create this kind of perception.

Phenomenological inquiry and the shared state it may invoke, can be conceptualized as a kind of markedness between the therapist and the patient. Markedness is an interpersonal process, where affect mirroring display is modulated in several ways, so the presented affect would be referentially being anchored as belonging to the other, and not to the displayer's state (Fonagy et al., 2004). This selective imitation reflects a match of internal feeling states, and signals that a sense of mutual understanding has been established (Stern, 2010).

The possibility to infer emotional states through gathering information about the patient's external environment during online therapy may serve as a kind of markedness process. The when, where, and how questions oblige the therapist to infer the patient's affect not by a simple imitation and resonance, rather through using verbal bypass. This may supply the required data for the predictions concerning the patient-therapist alliance.

"Don't Stand So Close To Me" – Benefits of Online Therapy

Weeks after returning to f2f meetings, Yoav, a man in his thirties, asked whether we could return to online meetings. Prior to the pandemic, Yoav was tense, and felt the therapy was stuck. Between the meetings he had many thoughts concerning the therapy, but whenever he sat in front of me, he was blocked. During the online sessions, he was more free and emotionally present, compared to the previous stage. While talking about his request, he said: "Do you know this song 'don't stand so close to me'? it's not exactly the same, but I feel that sitting in front of you makes me feel so needy. That's terrifying. I need you to be present, but not so intensively. Zoom, where I felt you're there, not here, was safer."

This paper mainly dealt with the challenges of online therapy. However, I was surprised to realize that after the lockdown was over, a few of my patients asked to continue with online sessions. The flexibility and accessibility of online sessions were some of the reasons for that wish. But as the above clinical vignettes demonstrates, other motivations were presented as well.

The challenge in creating patient-therapist resonance, seemed like an advantage in a few cases. Some patients, who were hypervigilant to my emotional expressions or were concerned about feeling exposed during f2f meetings, found the online sessions relieving. Their possibility to attenuate or to have some control over the stream of nonverbal signals, helped to strengthen a sense of safety. Issues that were not revealed till then, have suddenly emerged. "It is much easier for me to share it with you when I know that you are not sitting right in front of me" was one of the remarks that a patient has made after sharing some traumatic episodes from his early childhood. I hypothesize that sometimes the option to leave some blur in the patient-therapists interaction through the online communication was beneficial in cases in which creating a clearer prediction about the therapist's emotional experience and synchronizing with the therapist reactions was overwhelming for the patient.

Closing Remarks and Recommendations

Schore's hypothesis, concerning the partial therapeutic outcomes of online therapy, can be readdressed now. Understanding of the mechanisms that underlie patient-therapist synchronization, enables us to offer a spectrum on which the efficacy of online therapy can be spread.

It seems that there is a connection between the patient's intrinsic brain synchronization, and the ability to sustain the obstacles and partiality of online nonverbal communication. Patients with less synchronized temporospatial brain patterns may gain less from online sessions. This state is often correlated with past history of negative life events.

However, using phenomenological inquiry, i.e., being more interested in the "where," "when," and "how" and less of the "why'" may serve as a bypass for the challenges of online psychotherapy.

References

Allison, K. L., & Rossouw, P. J. (2013). The therapeutic alliance: Exploring the concept of "safety" from a neuropsychotherapeutic perspective. *International Journal of Neuropsychotherapy, 1*, 21–29.

Andersson, G. (2018). Internet interventions: Past, present and future. *Internet Interventions, 12*, 181–188.

Badenoch, B. (2008). *Being a brain-wise therapist: A practical guide to interpersonal neurobiology*. New York: WW Norton.

Barlow, H. (2001). The exploitation of regularities in the environment by the brain. *Behavioral and Brain Sciences, 24*(4), 602–607.

Cannon, W. B. (1929a). *Bodily changes in pain, hunger, fear and rage. An account of recent researches into the function of emotional excitement*. New York: Appleton.

Clark, A. (2019). *Surfing uncertainty: Prediction, action and the embodied mind*. NY: Oxford University Press.

Cozolino, L. J. (2006). *The neuroscience of relationships: Attachment and the developing social brain*. New York: Norton.

Duncan, N. W., Hayes, D. J., Wiebking, C., Tiret, B., Pietruska, K., Chen, D. Q., Rainville P., & Northoff, G. (2015). Negative childhood experiences alter a prefrontal-insular-motor cortical network in healthy adults: A preliminary multi-modal rsfMRI-fMRI-MRS-dMRI study. *Human Brain Mapping, 36*(11), 4622–4637.

Fernandez, E., Woldgabreal, Y., Day, A., Pham, T., Gleich, B., & Aboujaoude, E. (2021). Live psychotherapy by video versus in-person: A meta-analysis of efficacy and its relationship to types and targets of treatment. *Clinical Psychology & Psychotherapy, 28*(6), 1535–1549.

Fonagy, P., Gergely, G., Jurist, E., & Target, M. (2004). The social bio-feedback theory of affect -mirroring: The development of emotional self-awareness and self-control in infancy. In *Affect regulation, mentalization, and the development of the self*. London: Karnac.

Friston, K. (2010). The free-energy principle: A unified brain theory? *Nature Reviews Neuroscience, 11*(2), 127–138.

Friston, K. J., Daunizeau, J., & Kiebel, S. J. (2009). Reinforcement learning or active inference? *PLoS ONE, 4*, e6421.

Friston, K., Kilner, J., & Harrison, L. (2006). A free energy principle for the brain. *Journal of Physiology, 100*, 70–87.

Friston, K., Mattout, J., Trujillo-Barreto, N., Ashburner, J., & Penny, W. (2007). Variational free energy and the Laplace approximation. *Neuroimage, 34*, 220–234.

Geller, S. M., & Greenberg, L. S. (2012). *Therapeutic presence: A mindful approach to effective therapy*. Washington, DC: American Psychological Association.

Geller, S. M., & Porges, S. W. (2014). Therapeutic presence: Neurophysiological mechanisms mediating feeling safe in therapeutic relationships. *Journal of Psychotherapy Integration, 24*, 178–192.

Geller, S. M., Pos, A. W., & Colosimo, K. (2012). Therapeutic presence: A common factor in the provision of effective psychotherapy. *Society for Psychotherapy Integration, 47*, 6–13.

Gergely, G. (2007). The social construction of the subjective self: The role of affect-mirroring, markedness, and ostensive communication in self-development. In L. Mayes, P. Fonagy, & M. Target (Eds.), *Developments in psychoanalysis. Developmental science and psychoanalysis: Integration and innovation*. Karnac.

Golland, Y., Arzouan, Y., & Levit-Binnun, N. (2015). The mere copresence: Synchronization of autonomic signals and emotional responses across co-present individuals not engaged in direct interaction. *PLoS One, 10*(5).

Grossman, P., & Taylor, E. W. (2007). Toward understanding respiratory sinus arrhythmia: Relations to cardiac vagal tone, evolution and biobehavioral functions. *Biological Psychology, 74*(2007), 263–285.

Hohwy, J. (2013). *The predictive mind*. NY: Oxford University Press.

Holmes, J., & Nolte, T. (2019). Surprise and the bayesian brain: Implications for psychotherapy theory and practice. *Frontiers in Psychology, 10*, 592.

Levenson, E. A. (1989). Whatever happened to the cat? *Contemporary Psychoanalysis, 25*, 537–553.

Martin, D. J., Garske, J. P., & Davis, M. K. (2000). Relation of the therapeutic alliance with outcome and other variables: A meta-analytic review. *Journal of Consulting and Clinical Psychology, 68*, 438–450.

Norcross, J. C., & Lambert, M. J. (2014). Relationship science and practice in psychotherapy: Closing commentary. *Psychotherapy*, *51*(3), 398–403.

Northoff, G. (2014a). *Unlocking the brain. Volume I: Coding.* New York, NY: Oxford University Press.

Northoff, G. (2018). The brain's spontaneous activity and its psychopathological symptoms - "Temporo-spatial binding and integration". *Progress in Neuro-Psychopharmacology & Biological Psychiatry*, *80*(Pt B), 81–90.

Northoff, G. (2018). *The spontaneous brain: From the mind–body to the world–brain Problem.* Cambridge: The MIT Press.

Northoff, G. (2019). Lessons from astronomy and biology for the mind—copernican revolution in neuroscience. *Frontiers in Human Neuroscience*, *13*, 319.

Panksepp, J. (1998b). The periconscious substrates of consciousness: affective states and the evolutionary origins of the SELF. *Journal of Consciousness Studies*, *5*, 566–582.

Porges, S. W. (2011). *The polyvagal theory: Neurophysiological foundations of emotions, attachment, communication, self-regulation.* New York: Norton & Company.

Ramberg, L. (2006). In dialogue with Daniel Stern: A review and discussion of the present moment in psychotherapy and everyday life. *International Forum of Psychoanalysis*, *15*(1), 19–33.

Ramseyer, F., & Tschacher, W. (2014). Nonverbal synchrony of head- and body-movement in psychotherapy: Different signals have different associations with outcome. *Frontiers in Psychology*, *5*, 979.

Ray, D., Roy, D., Sindhu, B., Sharan, P., & Banerjee, A. (2017). Neural substrate of group mental health: Insights from multi-brain reference frame in functional neuroimaging. *Frontiers in Psychology*, *8*, 1627.

Rolnick, A., & Ehrenreich, Y. (2020). Can you feel my heart (via your camera and sensors)? The role of the body, its absence, and its measurement in online video psychotherapy. *Biofeedback*, *48*(1), 1–5.

Scharff, J. S. (Ed.). (2013). *Psychoanalysis online: Mental health, teletherapy, and training.* London, UK: Karnac.

Schore, A. N. (2019). *Right brain psychotherapy (Norton Series on Interpersonal Neurobiology).* New York: WW Norton & Company.

Shteynberg, G. (2015). Shared attention. *Perspectives on Psychological Science*, *10*(5), 579–590.

Siegel, D. (2006). An interpersonal neurobiology approach to psychotherapy. *Psychiatric Annals*, *36*(4), 248–256.

Siegel, D. (2007). *The mindful brain.* New York: W.W. Norton.

Siegel, D. (2015). Interpersonal neurobiology as a lens into the development of well-being and resilience. *Children Australia*, *40*(2), 160–164.

Smith, R., Thayer, J., Khalsa, S., & Lane, R. (2017). The hierarchical basis of neurovisceral integration. *Neuroscience & Biobehavioral Reviews*, *75*, 274–296.

Solms, M. (2017). What is "the unconscious," and where is it located in the brain? A neuropsychoanalytic perspective. *Annals of the New York Academy of Sciences*, *1406*, 90–97.

Solms, M. (2018). The neurobiological underpinnings of psychoanalytic theory and therapy. *Frontiers in Behavioral Neuroscience*, *12*, 294.

Stern, D. (2010). Forms of vitality: Exploring dynamic experience in psychology, the arts, psychotherapy, and development. UK: Oxford University Press.

Trevarthen, C. (1993). The self born in intersubjectivity: The psychology of an infant communicating. In U. Neisser (Ed.), *The perceived self: Ecological and interpersonal sources of self-knowledge* (pp. 121–173). New York: Cambridge University Press.

Trevarthen, C. and Malloch, S. (2000). The dance of wellbeing: Defining the musical therapeutic effect. *Nordic Journal of Music Therapy*, 9(2), 3–17.

Tronick, E. (2003). Of course all relationships are unique: How co-creative processes generate unique mother–infant and patient-therapist relationships and change other relationships. *Psychoanalytic Inquiry*, 23(3), 473–491.

Section II

Individual Therapies – Specific Modalities

7 Telehealth Delivery of Dialectical Behavior Therapy

Chelsey R. Wilks and Kyrill Gurtovenko

Dialectical Behavior Therapy

Dialectical Behavior Therapy (DBT; Linehan, 1993) is a third wave behavioral treatment that was originally designed for clinically complex patients at high risk for suicide (see Linehan & Wilks, 2015 for more historical background on DBT). DBT is a leading evidence-based treatment for borderline personality disorder (BPD) in adults. It is also the leading treatment for adolescent self-injurious thoughts and behaviors (Glenn et al., 2019), and has growing evidence for its efficacy with preadolescent youth (Perepletchikova et al., 2017).

DBT consists of four modes of treatment: individual psychotherapy, group skills training, between session phone coaching, and therapist consultation team. Each mode of treatment serves a vital treatment function. For example, individual therapy primarily functions to build and maintain motivation for change, and to work towards reaching individual therapy goals (i.e., "building a life worth living"). DBT skills training was developed because patients enrolled in DBT had considerable skills deficits, which inhibited their therapeutic progress. Thus skills training, most commonly delivered in a group format, serves the primary function of skills acquisition (Linehan, 2014). The phone coaching mode is also included in DBT as high-risk complex patients often need help implementing and generalizing nascent skills into relevant contexts, particularly during periods of elevated distress. The primary function of phone coaching is to support and strengthen skills generalization, as well as provide additional flexibility for between session therapeutic contact for crisis management and repairing the client-therapist relationship when needed. Finally, weekly therapist consultation team was developed to mitigate the potential of therapist burn out when treating highly suicidal and complex patients. The function of the consultation team is to enhance therapist motivation and for therapists to utilize DBT skills and principles with one another as needed to ensure they are doing DBT in an adherent and effective manner.

Telehealth for Complex Behavioral Dysfunction

Telehealth or telemedicine refers to the provision of healthcare services, including psychotherapy, delivered via telecommunication or digital technologies

DOI: 10.4324/9781003205029-10

(i.e., internet, web, or telephone-based applications). Coronavirus 2019 (COVID-19) greatly accelerated the transition to this more flexibly accessible mode, and as a result, many of the structural barriers to accessing treatment (e.g., transportation, lack of providers in close proximity) have changed as patients can access a therapist in the comfort of their homes. There is a rapidly growing research evidence base supporting the effectiveness of telehealth for a wide range of mental health problems (Fernandez et al., 2021; Hubley et al., 2016). Unfortunately, in many of these studies, patients with current suicidal ideation are often excluded (Rojas et al., 2020). Only recently has there been emerging research and professional guidelines for the telehealth delivery of mental health care to patients at high risk of suicide (e.g., Holland et al., 2021; McGinn et al., 2019), and such guidelines have been developed in the absence of clinical trial data. Another challenge of implementing teletherapy for high-risk patients is low willingness among clinicians. For example, Gilmore & Ward-Ciesielski (2019) surveyed therapists who treat suicidal patients about their likelihood and experience of treating suicidal patients via telehealth. Most respondents indicated that they were unwilling to implement telehealth with suicidal patients, citing discomfort with the lack of control in managing high-risk clients. The combination of limited research and lower motivation on the part of clinicians has resulted in a lack of disseminated telehealth protocols for complex suicidal patients. This is particularly problematic as individuals who are most likely to benefit from teletherapy are those with limited access to health services, including those living in rural communities, who are approximately 60% more likely to die by suicide than their urban counterparts (Ivey-Stephenson et al., 2017). However, since COVID-19, the bulk of DBT therapists have been pushed to quickly adapt to telehealth with high-risk patients, regardless of their prior willingness, comfort, or therapeutic skills in this mode.

Rapid Implementation of Telehealth-DBT

The complexity of the patient population and the multifaceted nature of the treatment make delivery of DBT via telehealth complicated for patients and providers (Zalewski et al., 2021). Each mode of DBT presents unique challenges when conducted over telehealth. Below we discuss some of these challenges, and describe how each mode requires unique flexibility, adaptations, and solutions to maintain its effectiveness via telehealth.

Individual Therapy

Challenges

Topics covered in DBT tend to be highly stressful and personal (e.g., suicide, substance use, trauma) and simply finding private accommodations for both patients and therapists proves complicated (Zalewski et al., 2021).

Stage one patients at high risk for suicide require frequent and thorough risk assessment, and DBT clinicians report that conducting assessments and crisis interventions via telehealth is challenging (Zalewski et al., 2021). The content and structure of DBT individual sessions is also heavily guided by the use of the DBT diary card (Linehan, 1993). The diary card is a worksheet that is routinely completed by DBT patients on a daily or weekly basis and is used to monitor clinical variables such as suicide and self-harm urges, behaviors, emotions, skills use, as well as other relevant idiographic variables. Zalewski and colleagues (2021) surveyed DBT clinicians during the transition to tele-DBT, and most noted frustration with integrating the diary card into treatment. There are limited streamlined options and guidelines for how to transfer identifiable diary card information easily and privately over telehealth. Although there are a small handful of technological tools designed to augment tele-DBT (i.e., mobile apps), they vary widely in cost, scope, utility, and quality (Wilks et al., 2021). Another complicating factor for individual therapy is that clinicians are unable to observe the entirety of the patient's non-verbal behavior (outside of where the camera is positioned). This may contribute to attenuated rapport in teletherapy compared to in-person treatment (Wood et al., 2021), as therapists may be unable to observe and respond to subtle shifts in a patient's demeanor. This is particularly crucial in DBT, where therapists are regularly expected to flexibly respond to a patient's changes in emotion via "movement, speed, and flow," and respond appropriately via validation, irreverence, or problem solving (Linehan, 1993).

Solutions and Adaptations

Related to conducting suicide risk assessment, it is recommended that telehealth DBT therapists are aware of a patient's location throughout clinical interactions, utilizing multiple modes of risk assessment (i.e., observational, brief screening measures administered securely via shared computer screen, collateral reports from family and friends), and being ready to work with other persons in the patient's environment to assist with assessment and intervention if needed (McGinn et al., 2019). Being able to observe a patient's home environment can give teletherapy a distinct advantage. Observing the patient's home environment can contextualize cues and triggers for crises. Clinicians can instruct *and observe* the removal of instruments of self-harm, for example, flushing medications down the toilet or locking up firearms. Relatedly, with regard to skills practice and generalization, these new behaviors are being implemented in a highly relevant context for the patient-their home, potentially increasing the skills' generalizability (Harvey et al., 2020). Clinicians can exploit this benefit by having clients walk through a skill in the area they were most likely to need it, as opposed to the clinician's office (Hyland et al., 2021). DBT therapists have implemented a variety of novel solutions to improve the delivery of individual treatment. One cohort of therapists utilized a Qualtrics survey, which included questions from the diary card and was easily accessible during sessions (O'Hayer, 2021). Other solutions included using mobile apps, a shared Google sheet, and verbally reporting diary cards (Lakeman & Crighton, 2021). With regard to stylistic strategies, validation is especially important in DBT, and requires therapists to be mindful to patient cues conveyed over telehealth. Therapist's expressions of validation and empathy may also need to be more overt, visible, or amplified, for instance relying on more non-verbal forms of validation and communication (e.g., facial gestures, thumbs up/thumbs down, applauding, etc.).

Skills Training

Challenges

DBT skills training is a didactic process in which patients acquire new behavioral skills to apply to their daily lives. Group therapy delivered via telehealth has considerably less research than individual teletherapy, with only six randomized clinical trials as of 2019 (Gentry et al., 2019). Preliminary research has indicated that, although DBT group teletherapy is comparable to in person DBT groups with regard to connection to skills leaders and overall satisfaction, patients experience less cohesion in teletherapy groups compared to in-person groups (Lopez et al., 2020). When a skills group is delivered in person, there are two therapists: a group leader whose job is to teach the skills and manage the group, and a co-leader whose job is to manage group interfering behaviors, respond to in the moment crises, and manage logistics. An obvious logistical issue when delivering telehealth is technological problems, which can suddenly thrust DBT co-leaders into a position of IT professional. Another challenge is defining and identifying group interfering behaviors. While in-person group interfering behavior can include outbursts or talking to other group members during teaching, in the telehealth format group interfering behaviors can present in a variety of new ways. Patients can be keeping the camera off, not muting their microphone, over or underutilizing the "chat" function, or not being in a private location-potentially violating other group members' privacy. The group leader's responsibility is to clearly define the group rules and expectations, while the co-leader's is to attend to and respond appropriately to dysfunctional group behaviors; however, these may not be readily apparent to group leaders with limited experience on the telehealth medium (Zalewski et al., 2021). Some clinicians reported that the teleconferencing format prompted unique challenges for group members. Specifically, O'Hayer (2021) stated that DBT group members experienced elevated distress from the persistent notifications, and patients with body dysmorphia reported distress associated with having their image on screen within a telehealth platform. Finally, the many exercises, role plays, examples, and activities designed to enhance skills training were designed to be delivered in-person (Linehan, 2014), and translating these practices to an online format may have limited the teaching repertoire of clinicians (particularly for those with lower computer literacy).

Solutions and Adaptations

Telecommunication software has improved drastically over the past several years allowing for relative ease in delivering group therapy via telehealth. There are now several platforms that enable users to easily log on, interact with group members, enable and disable various features, all with negligible lag or diminished picture quality. One critical element of running a successful DBT telehealth skills group is fluidity and ease in use of telehealth technology. Lopez et al., (2020) recommend that both patients and clinicians consider "practice sessions" with telehealth software prior to joining or leading a DBT skills group. This way, DBT leaders could solve any technological problems that emerge prior to skills teaching. Puspitasari and colleagues (2021) recommend a system level set of guidelines to be determined prior to rolling out group treatment that can be rapidly disseminated to clinicians. In DBT, this can be developed at the team level; however, empirically derived DBT-specific guidelines are needed to reduce redundancy. This can include telehealth specific guidelines such as: (1) logging onto group in a secure and private location, (2) keeping microphone muted unless speaking, (3) keeping the camera on, (4) ensuring members are in a well-lit location, and (5) practicing the skill of "one-mindfully" by closing web browsers and disabling computer notifications. Finally, video conferencing software enables clinicians to implement creative solutions to enhance engagement in skills training. Zalewski et al. (2021) recommend implementing features within telecommunication platforms (e.g., Zoom) such as quizzes, breakout rooms, and annotation in order to improve participation, as well as offer participants to enter conference rooms 15 minutes early in order to enable group cohesion. Relatedly, some telecommunication platforms allow users to customize their video conferencing experience, such as disabling their own camera so that it is visible to others, but invisible to the user, or adjust how speakers are presented. Users can also customize other features such as disabling notifications, which may be distracting as group members enter and exit the group.

Phone Coaching

Challenges

Phone coaching is one of the unique aspects of DBT, and also presents many challenges as well as heightened risk of burnout for therapists (Ruork et al., 2021). The psychological impact of the pandemic on patients has been significant (Lakeman & Crighton, 2021; Liu et al., 2020), and many DBT clinicians may have experienced increased phone coaching demands since then. O'Hayer (2021) reported that their DBT team noticed an increase in casual conversations during the pandemic, which they attributed to lockdowns and associated loneliness. However, of all the DBT modes, phone coaching had minimal adaptations for telehealth because phone coaching has always shared many similarities with telemedicine.

Solutions and Adaptations

Despite the elevated number of crises, clinicians reported the highest level of satisfaction with phone coaching compared to the other three modes during the pandemic (Zalewski et al., 2021). This is likely due to the fact that very little adaptation is necessary in implementing phone coaching. Indeed, phone calls, texts, and email communication has been and will likely continue to be implemented by DBT therapists (Rizvi & Roman, 2019), and phone coaching was least susceptible to disruptions in care during the shift to tele-DBT. As is noted in the DBT treatment manual (e.g., Linehan, 1993), if patients are contacting the therapists too frequently or during inopportune times, therapists should utilize contingency management strategies to continually orient and shape effective phone coaching use.

Consultation Team

Challenges

The consultation team provides an opportunity where clinicians can seek problem solving and validation and express grievances in a structured consultation setting. The challenges inherent in telehealth consultation teams are similar to those entailed in group skills training, with technological problems, undefined guidelines, etc. One of the functions of the DBT consultation team is to acknowledge and problem solve potential burn out. During an era of persistent teleconferencing use, clinicians experienced increased "Zoom fatigue" (Hyland et al., 2021). Similar to DBT skills group, DBT clinicians reported moderate frustration about not being able to respond spontaneously to colleagues over telehealth, which interfered with group cohesion (Hyland et al., 2021). In addition, similar to group DBT, clinicians in consultation teams were presented with a variety of other stimuli such as incoming emails, temptation to complete unfinished notes, or private sidebar chat conversations vying for a clinician's attention during consult team sessions. The potential consequences of this phenomenon can include limited accountability, collaboration, cohesion, and a compromise in DBT adherence and quality.

Solutions and Adaptations

Consultation team is an opportune time to brainstorm creative solutions for adapting skill delivery, solving technology problems, and increasing engagement. As all therapy is being delivered via computer software, it is easier than ever to record and review sessions during team, allowing for more precise and effective problem solving and adherence. Structured time should be allotted for technology related problems including managing suicide risk via telehealth, burn out, technical difficulties, and skill adaptations. Similar to DBT skills groups, DBT teams should be creative and flexible, and lean into using technology to strengthen engagement, cohesion, and support for one another. DBT teams may benefit from collaboratively developing and committing to a set of agreements around what it means to be fully engaged and mindfully present during team sessions. Such guidelines can non-judgmentally identify the potential pitfalls of remote consult teams, and proactively prevent the serious challenges that can arise.

DBT for Adolescents

DBT has been adapted for a wide range of populations, with DBT for adolescents (Miller, Rathus, & Linehan, 2007) being one of the most widely implemented and effective variations of the treatment. There are many unique considerations relevant for delivering quality adolescent DBT via telehealth, a few of which we discuss here.

Adolescents living at home with parents, siblings, and other family members may find it especially difficult to find a quiet and confidential space from which to engage in teletherapy. This may be particularly true for teenagers from lower income households where living spaces are smaller, and these patients and families may experience difficulties with access to robust internet connections and well-functioning devices for engaging in teletherapy. The DBT-A therapist must remain flexible and aware of each patient and family's needs, and be ready to troubleshoot such treatment interfering factors, which may not be 100% in the patient's control. DBT case management strategies, among other approaches, should be applied to helping clients overcome and solve such barriers.

During risk assessment and management via telehealth for adolescents, DBT clinicians should ensure that both audio and video is used to maximize observational cues about the patient's emotional state and environment. Along with guidelines for adult DBT discussed earlier, managing risk for adolescents should also involve contact, orientation, and obtaining consent from caregivers early on, conducting interviews with caregivers to assist with determining risk levels, and orienting and involving caregivers in the development of crisis interventions and safety plans (Holland et al., 2021; O'Brien et al., 2020).

Adolescents may also be particularly anxious and avoidant when it comes to verbally sharing clinically sensitive information over telehealth, particularly in a group setting. Thus, DBT-A clinicians should be especially adept at incorporating the use of common video teleconferencing features such as white boards for drawing/writing, screen sharing, the chat function, and breakout rooms, for eliciting and strengthening participation in an effective and inclusive manner (Lopez et al., 2020). Principles of shaping and contingency management are essential for eliciting and strengthening treatment engagement for adolescents over telehealth.

Adolescent patients may also be more prone to engaging in therapy interfering behaviors over telehealth compared to adult DBT patients. This may be due to several factors – for example, youth are more likely to find themselves in treatment due to parental influence rather than their own intrinsic motivation. They may also be more distractible or find it harder to engage with treatment via telehealth due to variability in cognitive and developmental factors. Treatment interfering behaviors may be more accessible or normalized for youth over telehealth, for example, muting and tuning out a therapist, turning off their camera and feigning technical issues, shutting off their device and ending a session prematurely, or never logging on to the session in the first place. Thus, there may be more need for parental involvement to ensure strong attendance and engagement in telehealth DBT, particularly during early stages of treatment. In the same way that parents may drive youth to their in-person appointments, caregivers may need to facilitate and assist youth with logging on to telehealth sessions. DBT-A multi-family skills groups may benefit from guidelines that require all youth to log on from the same device and room as their caregivers, which in our experience, significantly mitigates a variety of otherwise tempting treatment interfering behaviors for adolescents. Orientation to additional telehealth guidelines and expectations which can help to define what it means to attend DBT sessions may be essential (e.g., camera on, able to see your face, answering questions and speaking so that leaders know client is listening).

Strong rapport and therapeutic alliance are essential for effective youth mental health treatment (Karver et al., 2018). Establishing and maintaining alliance in DBT via telehealth may require particular attention to the effects of technology, patient and family culture, and the teletherapist's characteristics. Goldstein and Glueck (2016) provide several recommendations with this goal in mind, including increased use of non-verbal and interactive approaches to communication (videos, images, slideshows, polls, virtual white board drawings, etc.) as well as taking breaks to "explore the virtual world together" (looking up images/videos of the adolescent's favorite shows/games/hobbies, looking up interesting facts on the internet, watching funny videos, etc.).

Although we have described a few guiding principles above, it is notable that there is currently little to no research on the implementation of DBT over telehealth for adolescents and families. Studies are needed to determine whether this mode of delivery is effective for this population and to develop more specific guidelines and strategies to ensure positive DBT outcomes for adolescents and their families engaging in DBT via telehealth.

Summary and Future Directions

Evidence to date suggests that although various forms of technologically as-sisted DBT show promise, more research is needed to inform guidelines in this area of practice (van Leeuwen et al., 2021). There is a lack of clinical trial data comparing the effectiveness of tele-DBT to standard delivery. While some clinicians and clients have reported a moderate level of ease in implementing the treatment virtually, it does not come without unique problems and challenges to overcome. In this chapter, we have described some of the specific challenges, potential solutions, and strengths of delivering DBT via telehealth, and this area of study calls for considerably more work moving forward. Given that a higher percentage of patients and clinicians will enroll in telehealth post-pandemic (Bakken, 2020), more research is needed to un-derstand the strengths and limitations of tele-DBT.

Practical Considerations and Tips

- Have contact information for family, friends, roommates, and other supports readily available in case more in-person supports are needed for risk assessment and crisis management.
- Make use of other resources to facilitate treatment such as mobile applications, secure Google Drive, and/or survey soft-ware for diary card review and homework.
- Lean in to the unique opportunities of telehealth to support engagement. Use polls, streaming audio/video, and other crea-tive ways to practice, demonstrate, and engage patients in the tasks of DBT individual therapy and skills acquisition.
- Ensure that patients are logging onto therapy in a private and secure location, particularly in group formats in order to maintain confidentiality for group members.
- Incorporate teleconferencing practice sessions for both clinicians and patients, to ensure smooth navigation of technology during therapeutic interactions.

References

Bakken, S. (2020). Telehealth: Simply a pandemic response or here to stay? *Journal of the American Medical Informatics Association*, 27(7), 989–990, 10.1093/jamia/ocaa132

Crowell, S. E., Beauchaine, T. P., & Linehan, M. M. (2009). A biosocial develop-mental model of borderline personality: Elaborating and extending linehan's theory. *Psychological Bulletin*, *135*(3), 495.

Fernandez, E., Woldgabreal, Y., Day, A., Pham, T., Gleich, B., & Aboujaoude, E. (2021). Live psychotherapy by video versus in-person: A meta-analysis of efficacy and its relationship to types and targets of treatment. *Clinical Psychology & Psychotherapy*, 28(6), 1535–1549. 10.1002/cpp.2594

Gentry, M. T., Lapid, M. I., Clark, M. M., & Rummans, T. A. (2019). Evidence for telehealth group-based treatment: A systematic review. *Journal of Telemedicine and Telecare*, 25(6), 327–342.

Gilmore, A. K., & Ward-Ciesielski, E. F. (2019). Perceived risks and use of psychotherapy via telemedicine for patients at risk for suicide. *Journal of Telemedicine and Telecare*, 25(1), 59–63.

Glenn, C. R., Esposito, E. C., Porter, A. C., Robinson, D. J. (2019). Evidence base update of psychosocial treatments for self-injurious thoughts and behaviors in youth. *Journal of Clinical Child and Adolescent Psychology*. 48(3), 357–392. doi: 10.1080/153 74416.2019.1591281

Goldstein, F., & Glueck, D. (2016). Developing rapport and therapeutic alliance during telemental health sessions with children and adolescents. *Journal of Child and Adolescent Psychopharmacology*, 26(3), 204–211.

Harvey, A., Callaway, C. A., Zieve, G. G., Gumport, N. B., & Armstrong, C. C. (2020). Applying the Science of Habit Formation to Evidence-Based Psychological Treatment: Improving Outcomes for Mental Illness. *Perspectives on Psychological Science*, 17(2), 572–589.

Holland, M., Hawks, J., Morelli, L. C., & Khan, Z. (2021). Risk assessment and crisis intervention for youth in a time of telehealth. *Contemporary School Psychology*, 25, 12–26. 10.1007/s40688-020-00341-6

Hubley, S., Lynch, S. B., Schneck, C., Thomas, M., & Shore, J. (2016). Review of key telepsychiatry outcomes. *World Journal of Psychiatry*, 6(2), 269.

Hyland, K. A., McDonald, J. B., Verzijl, C. L., Faraci, D. C., Calixte-Civil, P. F., Gorey, C. M., & Verona, E. (2021). Telehealth for dialectical behavioral therapy: A commentary on the experience of a rapid transition to virtual delivery of DBT. *Cognitive and Behavioral Practice*. 10.1016/j.cbpra.2021.02.006

Ivey-Stephenson, A. Z., Crosby, A. E., Jack, S. P., Haileyesus, T., & Kresnow-Sedacca, M. (2017). Suicide trends among and within urbanization levels by sex, race/ethnicity, age group, and mechanism of death—United States, 2001–2015. *MMWR Surveillance Summaries*, 66(18), 1.

Karver, M. S., De Nadai, A. S., Monahan, M., & Shirk, S. R. (2018). Meta-analysis of the prospective relation between alliance and outcome in child and adolescent psychotherapy. *Psychotherapy*, 55(4), 341.

Lakeman, R., & Crighton, J. (2021). The impact of social distancing on people with borderline personality disorder: The views of dialectical behavioural therapists. *Issues in Mental Health Nursing*, 42(5), 410–416.

Lenz, A. S., Del Conte, G., Hollenbaugh, K. M., & Callendar, K. (2016). Emotional regulation and interpersonal effectiveness as mechanisms of change for treatment outcomes within a DBT program for adolescents. *Counseling Outcome Research and Evaluation*, 7(2), 73–85.

Linehan, M. (1993). *Skills Training Manual for Treating Borderline Personality Disorder* (Vol. 29). New York: Guilford Press.

Linehan, M. (2014). *DBT? Skills Training Manual*. Guilford Publications.

Linehan, M. M., Korslund, K. E., Harned, M. S., Gallop, R. J., Lungu, A., Neacsiu, A. D., McDavid, J., Comtois, K. A., & Murray-Gregory, A. M. (2015). Dialectical behavior therapy for high suicide risk in individuals with borderline personality disorder: A randomized clinical trial and component analysis. *JAMA Psychiatry*, *72*(5), 475–482.

Linehan, M. M., & Wilks, C. R. (2015). The course and evolution of dialectical behavior therapy. *American Journal of Psychotherapy*, *69*(2), 97–110.

Liu, C. H., Stevens, C., Conrad, R. C., & Hahm, H. C. (2020). Evidence for elevated psychiatric distress, poor sleep, and quality of life concerns during the COVID-19 pandemic among US young adults with suspected and reported psychiatric diagnoses. *Psychiatry Research*, *292*, 113345.

Lopez, A., Rothberg, B., Reaser, E., Schwenk, S., & Griffin, R. (2020). Therapeutic groups via video teleconferencing and the impact on group cohesion. *MHealth*, *6*(0), Article 0. 10.21037/mhealth.2019.11.04

Lynch, T. R., Chapman, A. L., Rosenthal, M. Z., Kuo, J. R., & Linehan, M. M. (2006). Mechanisms of change in dialectical behavior therapy: Theoretical and empirical observations. *Journal of Clinical Psychology*, *62*(4), 459–480.

McGinn, M. M., Roussev, M. S., Shearer, E. M., McCann, R. A., Rojas, S. M., & Felker, B. L. (2019). Recommendations for using clinical video telehealth with patients at high risk for suicide. *Psychiatr Clin*, *42*(4), 587–595.

Miller, A. L., Rathus, J. H., & Linehan, M. M. (2007). *Dialectical Behavior Therapy with Suicidal Adolescents*. Guilford Press.

Neacsiu, A. D., Rizvi, S. L., & Linehan, M. M. (2010). Dialectical behavior therapy skills use as a mediator and outcome of treatment for borderline personality disorder. *Behaviour Research and Therapy*, *48*(9), 832–839. 10.1016/j.brat.2010.05.017

O'Brien, K. H. M., ALmeida, J., View, L., Schofield, M., Hall, W., Aguinaldo, L., Ryan, C. A., & Maneta, E. (2020). A safety and coping planning intervention for suicidal adolescents in acute psychiatric care. *Cognitive and Behavioral Practice*, *28*(1), 22–39 10.1016/j.cbpra.2019.08.003

O'Hayer, C. V. (2021). Building a life worth living during a pandemic and beyond: Adaptations of comprehensive DBT to COVID-19. *Cognitive and Behavioral Practice*. 10.1016/j.cbpra.2020.12.005

Perepletchikova, F., Nathanson, D., Axelrod, S. R., Merrill, C., Walker, A., Grossman, M., Rebeta, J., Scahill, L., Kaufman, J., Flye, B., Mauer, E., & Walkup, J. (2017). Randomized clinical trial of dialectical behavior therapy for preadolescent children with disruptive mood dysregulation disorder: Feasibility and outcomes. *Journal of the American Academy of Child and Adolescent Psychiatry*, *56*(10), 832–840. 10.1016/j.jaac.2017.07.789

Puspitasari, A. J., Heredia, D., Gentry, M., Sawchuk, C., Theobald, B., Moore, W., Tiede, M., Galardy, C., Schak, K., & Clinic, M. (2021). Rapid adoption and implementation of telehealth group psychotherapy during COVID 19: Practical strategies and recommendations. *Cognitive and Behavioral Practice*.

Rizvi, S. L., & Roman, K. M. (2019). *Generalization Modalities: Taking the Treatment Out of the Consulting Room—Using Telephone, Text, and Email*.

Rojas, S. M., Carter, S. P., McGinn, M. M., & Reger, M. A. (2020). A review of telemental health as a modality to deliver suicide-specific interventions for rural populations. *Telemedicine and E-Health*, *26*(6), 700–709.

Rudge, S., Feigenbaum, J. D., & Fonagy, P. (2020). Mechanisms of change in dialectical behaviour therapy and cognitive behaviour therapy for borderline personality disorder: A critical review of the literature. *Journal of Mental Health, 29*(1), 92–102.

Ruork, A. K., Yin, Q., & Fruzzetti, A. E. (2021). Phone consultation and burnout among providers of dialectical behaviour therapy. *Clinical Psychology & Psychotherapy*, 1–10. 10.1002/cpp.2668

Sampaio, M., Navarro Haro, M. V., Wilks, C., De Sousa, B., Garcia-Palacios, A., & Hoffman, H. G. (2021). Spanish-speaking therapists increasingly switch to telepsychology during COVID-19: Networked virtual reality may be next. *Telemedicine and E-Health, 27*(8), 919–928.

van Leeuwen, H., Sinnaeve, R., Witteveen, U., Van Daele, T., Ossewaarde, Egger J.I.M., van den Bosch, L.M.C. (2021). Reviewing the availability, efficacy and clinical utility of Telepsychology in dialectical behavior therapy (Tele-DBT). *Borderline Personal Disord Emot Dysregul, 8*(1), 26. 10.1186/s40479-021-00165-7

Wilks, C. R., Gurtovenko, K., Williamson, J., Rebmann, K., & Lovell, J. (2021). A systematic review of mobile apps for dialectical behavior therapy for content and usability. *Journal of Emotion Dysregulation and Borderline Personality Disorder*, 8 (1), 29. 10.1186/s40479-021-00167-5

Wood, M. J., Wilson, H. M., & Parry, S. L. (2021). Exploring the development and maintenance of therapeutic relationships through e-Health support: A narrative analysis of therapist experiences. *Medicine Access@ Point of Care, 5*, 23992026211018090.

Zalewski, M., Walton, C. J., Rizvi, S. L., White, A. W., Gamache Martin, C., O'Brien, J. R., & Dimeff, L. (2021). Lessons learned conducting dialectical behavior therapy via telehealth in the age of COVID-19. *Cognitive and Behavioral Practice*. 10.1016/j.cbpra.2021.02.005

8 Schema Therapy in the Online Setting – from Challenges to Opportunities

Hagara Feldman

Introduction to Schema Therapy

Schema therapy (ST) is an integrative psychotherapy model developed from Cognitive Behavioral Therapy (CBT), with the intention of helping hard-to-treat cases, especially clients with chronic Axis I or personality disorders. The model combines theories and intervention techniques from different approaches, including CBT, Attachment, Gestalt, Object relations, constructivist theories, and psychoanalytic schools (Rafaeli et al., 2011; Flanagan et al., 2020).

ST was first introduced by Young (1990) and then elaborated by Young and his colleagues (Young et al., 2003) who presented the full model and its implementations for borderline and narcissistic PD. During the following years, numerous specific versions of the model were put to use: protocols for other personality disorders (Bernstein et al., 2021; Arntz & Jacobs, 2012; Arntz & Jacobs, 2013; Arntz, 2012); implementations for groups setting (Farrell et al., 2009); suggestions for integrating ST with contextual and "third wave" concepts (Roediger et al., 2018); and even ST self-practice/self-reflection for therapists (Farrell & Shaw, 2018).

The original ST model (Young, 2003) postulates a set of five universal **childhood core emotional needs**, for example, secure attachment to others, a clear sense of identity, and realistic limits. The model asserts that difficulties in adult life are explained by the extent to which such needs went unmet in childhood. Adequate satisfaction of these needs facilitates healthy emotional development, whereas chronic frustration of needs leads to the development of early maladaptive schemas (EMS). Naturally, individual differences in temperament also play a role in the development of EMS, since temperament determines the dominance of each need and provokes different responses from the environment.

Each **EMS** is "a broad, pervasive theme or pattern; Comprised of memories, emotions, cognitions and bodily sensations; regarding oneself and one's relationships with others; developed through childhood or adolescence; elaborated throughout one's lifetime and dysfunctional to a significant degree" (Young et al., 2003, p.7). When an EMS is activated in the present, the

DOI: 10.4324/9781003205029-11

individual feels, senses, and thinks as they did in the original childhood situations linked to the schema. Therefore, schemas maintain and perpetuate themselves, creating vicious circles. Young and his colleagues (2003) identified eighteen schemas, e.g., abandonment, defectiveness/shame, failure, mistrust and abuse, and undeveloped self. They sorted them under five schema domains of early environment characteristics, like disconnection and rejection (unmet need for safe attachment), or impaired autonomy and performance (unmet need for autonomy, competence, and sense of identity). In response to schema activation, individuals tend to behave in one of three **coping styles,** which are variations of the three basic responses to threat. In **schema overcompensation** (fight), individuals believe, feel, and behave as if the truth is the opposite of the EMS. For example, an adult who felt like a failure as a child will do everything they can to constantly feel successful. In **schema avoidance** (flight), individuals use behavioral or mental avoidance to prevent EMS activation. For example, the same adult described above will avoid any challenges to circumvent even the slightest chance of failure. Finally, in **schema surrender** (freeze), individuals accept the EMS as true and feel its pain, but make life choices that maintain it. For example, the same adult described above continues making life choices that maintain and "prove" the feeling of failure. Each coping style may be manifested in various coping behaviors that, for the most part, lead to frustration of needs and to schema maintenance. They are automatic and can be unconscious.

As ST evolved, it became clearer that the model based on needs, EMSs, and coping styles cannot fully explain or treat the problems in more complex cases. Such patients – often ones with borderline or other personality disorders and with extensive comorbidity – presented a multitude of schemas, alongside extreme and quick fluctuations between different cognitive, emotional, and functional states. That led Young to develop the concept of **Schema Modes** (Modes). Modes are temporary (adaptive or maladaptive) emotional-cognitive-behavioral-neurobiological states, in which the individual is at any particular time. A maladaptive mode usually occurs when multiple EMS and coping behaviors are activated. Young described four types of modes: (1) **Child Modes**: experienced as extreme emotional states, in which the individual is reliving the pain of having their core needs unmet in childhood. These are thought to be innate, and are typically triggered when we feel rejected, under pressure, or left alone. Young described three subtypes of child modes: vulnerable, angry, and impulsive. The most dominant component of child modes is emotions. (2) **Dysfunctional Introjected Modes** (also called "**Inner Critics**"): the internalization/introjection of the negative elements of attachment figures or other influential others during childhood. Young identified two subtypes of introjected critic modes – punitive and demanding. These modes are experienced as internal voices (self-talk) or images, putting pressure ("you need to work harder!") or criticizing ("you are so worthless!"). These modes usually trigger or intensify the pain within the vulnerable child mode. The most dominant component of introjected/critical modes is negative cognition. (3) **Maladaptive Coping modes:** Versions of the child's attempt to have their needs met by an early environment which was emotionally depriving or abusive. These behaviors were usually helpful during childhood, providing protection or a sense of love and worth, but became dysfunctional in adult life, as they are broadly "overused" in the present environment – therefore perpetuating the pain of unmet needs. Young suggested three groups of coping modes (each has few sub-types), corresponding with the aforementioned basic responses to threat: Surrendering Coping modes, Avoidant/Detached Coping modes, and Overcompensating Coping modes. The most dominant component of dysfunctional coping modes is behavior. (4) **Healthy Modes:** The **Healthy Adult mode** – the integrative, reflective, and self-compassionate part of us. During therapy, this part is "trained" to deal with the inner dynamics between the different modes, so that current life problems will be more adaptively handled. Another type of healthy mode is **Happy/Contented Child** mode – usually occurs when our emotional needs are met, so we can feel close to other people, safe, satisfied, playful, and joyful.

During the following years, with accumulating research and clinical insight, the list of modes' sub-types grew longer (Flanagan et al., 2020).

ST begins with creating a strong bond with the client and a clear **case conceptualization**. The conceptualization, alongside with **psychoeducation** regarding needs, schemas, and modes, is shared with the client as a "road map" for the therapy process. Throughout the course of therapy, schema therapists use **emotional/experiential**, **cognitive**, **behavioral**, and **interpersonal** interventions. They focus on both schema healing and growing the healthy adult mode to help meet the needs in adult life. Schema therapists involve two fundamental therapeutic stances – **Limited Reparenting** and **Empathic Confrontation**. These stances stand by themselves but also provide the ground and the frame for the other strategies that are used during therapy. This chapter highlights and expand only on the aspects that seem more challenging or unique to the online setting.

Online Schema Therapy

Schemas, Modes, and Limited Reparenting in the Online Setting

The online environment may be intimidating, both for the therapist and the client. It brings up technological challenges as well as clinical challenges, such as keeping the therapeutic frame, dealing with the implications of physical distance on creating a sense of real connection, and applying specific therapeutic interventions that seem easier to deliver when the client is in the same room. Since EMS might be triggered due to any situation that is implicitly or explicitly linked to the content of the schema, the online setting might also be a fruitful ground for EMS activation. Clients' responses to the challenges derived from the online setting itself, can provide useful clinical information for schema therapists, as they provide opportunities to identify schemas and modes. Therefore, the therapists will be more likely to respond beyond the technical solution, from a **limited reparenting** stance already at an early stage of therapy. **Limited Reparenting (LR)** is the central therapeutic stance in ST and it directs and defines the therapeutic relationship. It derives from the theoretical basic assumption about the role of unmet needs in current life problems (Flanagan et al., 2020). Practically, it means identifying the specific emotional need that comes up at a certain moment and responding by fulfilling it, within the professional limits. This stance encourages the therapist to be "a real person," and to provide a warm, close, authentic relationship that serves as an antidote to the EMS and the origins of them. The triggers that are related to the online setting itself, provide early opportunities for LR.

A common trigger for schemas and modes activation in the online setting is internet instability, which is quite frequent in online work. When internet connection slows down or is lost, clients with **abandonment schema** may readily expect their therapist to get tired of them, to blame them, or to get frustrated and terminate therapy. This may lead to intense anxiety (i.e., to the experience of both their **punitive parent mode** and their **vulnerable child**). In response, some clients may take full responsibility whenever technical problems appear and may apologize profusely (entering the **compliant surrender mode**), whereas other clients may respond in rage, refusing to pay for "lost time" (entering an **overcompensating mode**). From a **LR** stance, this would be a good opportunity to provide safety and stability in the relationship – "I know it's frustrating, I am sorry. This is no one's fault, I am here and not going anywhere." It is also important to offer a contingency plan for such situations, like changing to a different app or using a phone call instead. These verbal and practical responses meet the client's need for stability and safety underlying the abandonment schema, is a LR response.

Facing the same erratic internet connection, a client with a **defectiveness schema** may expect the therapist to see them as stupid or clumsy, therefore feel shame (**vulnerable child**). To cope with such shame, the client might stop therapy (**avoidant protector**), or instead blame or try to humiliate the therapist (**overcompensating**). Meeting the needs underlying defectiveness schema (i.e., **LR**) includes providing a sense of being "ok" and accepted. It can be done through self-disclosure, normalizing technology challenges, providing gentle guiding and calming messages – "Technology can be hard, isn't it? I felt the same when I started, and I still do sometimes … But hey, no worry, I am here and will help you through it step by step!".

Another common trigger in the online setting is "The Limited Perspective" (Feldman & Liu, 2020), meaning that information that is available in the face-to-face setting, such as the office decoration or the therapist's body language is missing. The missing information might activate a **mistrust/abuse schema**, giving rise to concerns regarding what is happening outside of the camera frame. The most dominant need underlying the mistrust/abuse schema is the need to feel safe and trustful. From a **LR** stance, it might be helpful giving an audiovisual tour of the therapy room at the start of therapy.

The therapist can walk around the room with the laptop, as if the client were walking into the room. By getting closer to small details like the bookshelves or an art piece, even paying sensorial attention to details like the texture of a sofa or cushion – the sense of closeness and trust may increase (Feldman & Liu, 2020).

Adapting Experiential Techniques to the Online Environment

ST applies cognitive, behavioral, experiential, and relational interventions in the course of therapy. The aim of experiential interventions is to experience and express emotions and needs that are related to one's EMS. Once the relevant emotions are triggered, the therapist can partially meet unmet childhood needs and heal the schemas. These interventions are meant to trigger high levels of emotional reaction, therefore therapists might feel insecure to apply them when the client is not physically in the same room with them. The most central and widely used emotional interventions in ST are Imagery Rescripting (IR) and Chair-Work (CW). This section describes the challenges and the adaptations needed when providing them online.

Imagery Rescripting (IR)

IR in ST means providing, through imagery, a corrective emotional experience in negative or traumatic childhood situations that are linked to the origins of the schemas. Practically, the client is asked to close their eyes or gaze at a specific point, bring to life a painful or unpleasant childhood memory, using a "here-and-now" language when describing the situation from the perspective of the child. To amplify the sense of realness and to activate the emotional connection to the memory, the client is asked to pay attention to senses (what do you see? hear?), to emotional and cognitive reactions (what do you think and feel when looking at dad right now?) and to bodily sensations (where do you feel it in your body?). After "setting the scene" in the most vivid way possible, the therapist will ask for permission to join the child in the situation, to help them fulfil the needs that come up and were unmet at the time. They may encourage the client to express feelings and needs, or to play and "just be a child," or they may provide warmth or protection from an abusive figure or situation. Before embarking on full rescripting episodes, it is usually recommended to practice a "safe place" in imagery and to gain some grounding techniques if necessary. Delivering IR in the online setting is not largely different from the traditional face to face setting, considering the intervention is done in the non-physical "imagery space." However, IR might trigger extremely strong emotions and it might be more difficult to stabilize the client while they are not physically nearby. It is therefore recommended to carefully assess any risk factors like impulsivity or suicidality, and to proceed with the intervention more gradually than one would in a traditional face to face setting. Remember to stay within the "window of tolerance" (Siegel, 1999) while gently and gradually expanding it, to allow deeper emotional interventions. Start with "training" your client to feel comfortable with closing their eyes, and then use their senses to "bring to life" a pleasant image/situation in the present or in the past. Focus on creating a safe place in imagery. At that stage it is helpful to also practice some grounding techniques, like bare foot on the cold floor or scanning the room. You may suggest to your client to hold a "soothing object," like a favorite soft toy or a blanket. After a safe bond is created and the client can cooperate with grounding or self-soothing guidance from the therapist, you can start with full rescripting. Start with short rescripting interventions with no antagonist, just focusing on connecting with the child and meeting their needs (also serves as a by-pass to the detached protector). Then gradually move to more painful or traumatic memories with an antagonist. The time spent on every stage differs from one client to another, depending on the size of their healthy adult mode and the scope of the poisoning experiences in childhood.

Although it might seem more cumbersome to provide IR online, it also provides a benefit. The gradual use of imagery to prepare for full IR, can meanwhile enhance the connection with the child modes. Also, the client's growing ability to visualize and feel connected in imagery, can be used to decrease the sense of physical absence by imagining being together in the same space. It can be an imaginary place or even the therapist's office, whether it is familiar to the client or presented to them by the audio-video tour (Feldman & Liu, 2020).

Another benefit of the online setting for conducting imagery interventions, is the activation of schemas due to the setting itself (as described above). These can be used as a starting point for an "affect bridge" – an imagery tool usually used in the assessment phase, aiming at linking a current emotional activation to a childhood situation.

Chair-Work (CW)

Another experiential technique widely used in ST is CW. The root of CW is planted in Psychodrama and Gestalt, with later developments by Lesley Greenberg, Kellogg and others (Kellogg, 2012; Greenberg & Pascual-Leone, 2006). CW in ST serves mainly to externalize different modes by placing each mode onto a different chair. Practically, the client moves between different chairs, each representing a different mode. CW increases modes awareness, enabling dialogue between different modes as well as targeting a specific one. It can be used in a variety of ways and for different purposes (Roediger et al., 2018). Unlike IR, CW requires physical space and movement, therefore applying it online raises different concerns for therapists. Moving between chairs is important since it helps the client to step in and out of the modes. When the client is not in the therapist's space, which is pre-arranged for this kind of work, the therapist will have to be creative and work within the limits of the client's space: Ask your client to bring more chairs or cushions or even use the floor. Help them arrange the different seats according to the planned intervention, using verbal instructions or demonstration. If the space is small and it is impossible to add more chairs, you can offer to gently move the same chair to different angles or sides of the room; or using different areas on a wide sofa or a bed. Also possible to use a different room in the client's house, if it suits them, like a dining room or a living room, to enable more movement. If needed, guide the client to move the laptop/mobile to enable sufficient sound and frame of the specific chair/mode which we are currently talking with. After setting the stage, the interventions and instructions are no different from a traditional setting. We can even guide the client to literally remove an "unwelcome mode" – "Please take that chair of the inner critic out of the room, it is damaging you! Let's stop him together!"; or when dealing with a strong coping mode that blocks contact with the vulnerable child – "I know that part is trying to protect you, but you are safe here and it doesn't let us reach out to 'little you'. Maybe the protector can move aside, at least for a while?". When speaking to an empty chair which represents a specific mode, adjust your body posture and eye contact and direct it to the empty chair on the client's side. Make sure the client knows that you are talking to the mode and not to him as a whole – "I am talking to the inner critic now, telling him to stop bullying you!".

Another way of enhancing mode awareness and externalizing mode dialogues online, is the use of objects (like mode cards or soft toys) to represent modes. It is preferable that clients choose representations that have meaning for them, also keeping in mind size and material. for instance, choosing a large and stiff object to represent an inner critic, and a small, soft cute toy to represent the child. Still, allow yourself to improvise with objects that are available around you, or draw a modes map on the whiteboard or share photos on share-screen. When using representations as a substitute to the traditional chair work, it is important to remember that the movement is missing. It is therefore essential to slow down even more, encouraging the client to take the time to connect to each mode when shifting between them.

Chair work and imagery work are very central interventions in ST, but there are many other experiential tools therapists use creatively to raise emotions and to leverage the therapeutic relationship. For some of these, the online setting and the related technology can be a benefit. **Childhood photos**, for example, are usually used to by-pass a strong detached protector and to enhance the connection to the child. In the traditional face to face setting, we use the physical photo that is usually quite small. In the online setting we use the "share screen" option to look at the photo together, and we can enlarge it or focus on specific areas like the eyes or the little hands. This amplifies the emotional response and therefore the effectiveness of the tool.

Other emotionally focused interventions, like writing letters or using associative cards, can be easily delivered online.

From Challenges to Opportunities – Conclusions and Further Implications

ST can be successfully delivered in an online setting with only a few
adaptations and precautions when applying experiential interventions.
Furthermore, combining the lens of the model, with the therapeutic stance
and the experiential tools, may in fact increase the sense of connection
when delivering therapy online. LR directs the therapist to be warm,
creative, natural and act as "a real person." That stance combined with the
space for playfulness, invites therapists to naturally use physical gestures
towards the camera (combined with verbal description), e.g., "here's my
hand," "give me five," or "let's take 'a warm hug moment'." Even what is
usually seen as "disturbances" in the client's setting, for example a child or a
pet trying to enter the room during a session – can be used to enhance the
therapeutic relationship and bond while addressing it with warmth and
curiosity. The use of imagery can also be a platform for "sitting together
side by side," and the warm therapist's approach may provoke stronger
emotions when even just saying things like "I would have helped you if
I were there." In summary, addressing schemas and modes, alongside the
use of varied experiential techniques and a limited reparenting stance, can
help bypass the barrier of physical absence. Most of these can be implemented into other therapeutic approaches as well, to increase the sense
of closeness and warmth when delivering online therapy.

Practical Considerations and Tips

- Limited reparenting: use the opportunities that the setting
  provides by activating schemas and modes; use imagery,
  physical gestures towards the camera, a virtual tour of the office
  and other creative ways to create a sense of closeness and
  "being together."
- Imagery rescripting: teach grounding and stabilization techniques; practice "safe place," establish a safe relationship
  before rescripting and work gradually within the window of
  tolerance.
- Chair Work: help in "setting the stage" on the client's side; work
  creatively with what the space allows; use representations.

References

Arntz, A. (2012). *Schema therapy for Cluster C personality disorders*. In M. van Vreeswijk, J. Broersen, & M. Nadort (Eds.), *The Wiley-Blackwell Handbook of Schema Therapy: Theory, Research, and Practice* (pp. 397–414). Wiley-Blackwell.

Arntz, A., & Jacob, G. (2012). *Schema Therapy in Practice: An Introductory Guide to the Schema Mode Approach*. Chichester: Wiley.

Arntz, A., & Jacob, G. (2013). Schema therapy for personality disorders. A review. *International Journal of Cognitive Therapy*, *6*(2), 171–185.

Bernstein, D., Keulen-de Vos, M., Clercx, M., De Vogel, V., Kersten, G., Lancel, M., & Arntz, A. (2021). Schema therapy for violent PD offenders: A randomized clinical trial. *Psychological Medicine*, 1–15. https://www.cambridge.org/core/journals/psychological-medicine/article/schema-therapy-for-violent-pd-offenders-a-randomized-clinical-trial/A6A8E0C8E512EFF14D50B98A798A3C71

Farrell, M. J., & Shaw, A. I. (2018). *Experiencing Schema Therapy from the Inside Out: A Self-Practice/Self-Reflection Workbook for Therapists. Self-Practice/Self-Reflection Guides for Psychotherapists*. Guilford Press.

Farrell, M.J., Shaw, A.I., & Webber, M. (2009). A schema-focused approach to group psychotherapy for outpatients with borderline personality disorder: A randomized controlled trial. *Journal of Behavior Therapy and Experimental Psychiatry*, *40*, 317–328.

Feldman, H., & Liu, X. (2020). Schema anywhere: The opportunities and pitfalls of delivering schema therapy online. *Schema Therapy Bulletin*, March 17, 2020. https://schemasociety.wildapricot.org/Schema-anywhere-The-opportunities-and-pitfalls-of-delivering-Schema-Therapy-online

Flanagan, C., Atkinson, T., & Young, J. (2020). An introduction to schema therapy. Origins, overview, research status and future directions. In G. Heath, & H. Startup (Eds.), *Creative Methods in Schema Therapy Advances and Innovation in Clinical Practice* (pp. 1–16). Taylor and Francis Inc.

Greenberg, L. S., & Pascual-Leone, A. (2006). Emotion in psychotherapy: A practice-friendly research review. *Journal of Clinical Psychology*, *62*, 611–630.

Kellogg, S. (2012). On speaking one's mind: Using chairwork dialogues in schema therapy. *The Wiley-Blackwell Handbook of Schema Therapy: Theory, Research and Practice*, 197–208.

Rafaeli, E., Bernstein, D. P., & Young, J. (2011). *Schema Therapy: Distinctive Features*. New York: Routledge.

Roediger, E, Stevens, A. B., & Brockman, R. (2018). *Contextual Schema Therapy. An Integrative Approach to Personality Disorders, Emotional Dysregulation, and Interpersonal Functioning*. Context Press.

Siegel, D. J. (1999). *The Developing Mind*. New York: Guilford.

Young, J.E. (1990).Cognitive therapy for personality disorders: A schema-focused approach. Professional Resource Exchange, Inc.

Young, J. E., Klosko, J. S., & Weishaar, M. E. (2003). *Schema Therapy: A Practitioner's Guide*. New York: Guilford Press.

9 Implementing the Unified Protocol Online: Adaptations and Considerations

Andrew J. Curreri, Molly E. Fitzpatrick, David H. Barlow, and Elizabeth H. Eustis

Introduction

In recent years, the popularity of "telehealth" (i.e., delivering healthcare using internet-based videoconferencing platforms) has grown substantially in the field of psychology (Gros et al., 2013). This trend was spurred in part by the global COVID-19 pandemic, during which governments around the world implemented policies intended to limit the spread of the virus, including physical distancing. For many mental health practitioners, telehealth offered a solution whereby psychotherapy could be provided over synchronous video-conferencing platforms, largely meant to approximate in-person psy-chotherapy while therapists and patients participated from separate locations.

Telehealth offers clear advantages, including broadening the accessibility of mental health services for individuals who otherwise may experience barriers to accessing care. For example, telehealth can improve accessibility for people who live far from providers and can address barriers related to childcare and work schedules. For individuals with mobility limitations, telehealth may provide a more physically accommodating option for treatment. Additionally, attending sessions from the privacy of one's home can be helpful when stigma prevents individuals from seeking in-person treatment.

Telehealth also poses a number of challenges. For example, not all thera-pists or patients have access to fully private space in which they can com-fortably conduct sessions, nor to optimal technology (e.g., internet access, webcam). Additionally, many therapists who provide evidence-based care utilize manuals to guide treatment, which are largely written under the as-sumption that therapy is being conducted in-person. Therefore, there is a need for guidance on how to adapt in-person manuals to telehealth delivery.

The Unified Protocol for Transdiagnostic Treatment of Emotional Disorders (UP; Barlow et al., 2018) is a transdiagnostic, emotion-focused cognitive-behavioral therapy (CBT). In contrast with single-diagnosis CBT protocols, which largely target surface-level symptoms of specific disorders, the UP targets neuroticism, a personality dimension that represents the pri-mary shared process underlying all emotional disorders (e.g., anxiety, de-pression, and related disorders; Bullis et al., 2019). Individuals who are high in

DOI: 10.4324/9781003205029-12

neuroticism tend to feel emotions intensely and/or frequently, react to negative emotions with a sense of aversion, and engage in behaviors to reduce or avoid emotions (Sauer-Zavala & Barlow, 2021). This short-term avoidance tends to backfire in the long-term, leading to an increase in emotion and interference in accomplishing meaningful goals. By targeting neuroticism, the UP can be applied flexibly with individuals who report a range of emotional difficulties, fostering change by altering individuals' relationships with their own emotional experiences.

Over the years, studies have demonstrated the UP's efficacy across a range of disorders. One large randomized controlled equivalence trial found that the UP improved symptom severity to the same degree as gold-standard single-diagnosis CBT protocols for several anxiety disorders (Barlow et al., 2017). Further evidence supports the UP as an efficacious treatment for a wide variety of disorders marked by difficulty with emotions (e.g., Cassiello-Robbins et al., 2020).

The UP consists of eight modules, each introducing a specific skill aimed at promoting more flexible, adaptive responses to emotions in the service of helping patients accomplish their goals. This chapter provides a brief overview of all eight modules, highlighting specific ways that therapists may deliver them via telehealth. All adaptations are meant to maintain close adherence to the principles of effective CBT within the constraints of this modality. For additional considerations for administering the UP via telehealth, see Cassiello-Robbins et al. (2021).

Implementing the UP Online

Basic Considerations and Introductory Session

The first session of the UP is used to perform an initial functional analysis of patients' difficulties, set expectations for what treatment will involve, and build rapport. The functional analysis is largely discussion-based, as therapists attempt to understand their patients' presenting concerns through the lens of the transdiagnostic model of emotional disorders and within the context of their patients' daily lives, including their cultural background and identities. As with all therapy, the UP should be delivered in a way that is culturally responsive.

There are several unique considerations that warrant discussion when setting expectations for telehealth. Before beginning a session, therapists are encouraged to ensure that their patient is in a private space. As noted above, privacy at home is not always feasible; in this case, therapists may provide suggestions such as using headphones. Additionally, therapists should make a plan with patients at the start of a session regarding how they will proceed in the event of technological difficulties, including rescheduling or using the telephone instead. Similarly, it is helpful to identify emergency contacts in the event of any safety risks, including a family member in the home, if possible, and local emergency services.

Another logistical consideration for using a virtual format is how to transfer materials. Similar to other treatments, the UP utilizes worksheets and handouts to help explain concepts and facilitate skill practice; electronic versions can be emailed to patients before or immediately after the session. Moreover, the UP incorporates brief self-report questionnaires to track progress throughout therapy. These forms can be sent via email each week, completed together at the start of each session, or entered into a third-party system to which patients and therapists both have access. Although these adaptations may require additional preparation, such considerations are necessary to ensure that the treatment maintains its efficacy when being delivered online.

Module 1: Setting Goals and Enhancing Motivation

Module 1, which focuses on setting concrete treatment goals and discussing motivation for engaging in treatment, offers the first opportunity for therapists and patients to practice collaboratively completing worksheets in session. Based on the factors discussed earlier, either therapists or patients may share their screen during the session, and therapists are encouraged to ask their patients to share their thoughts about the logistics of completing worksheets online. It is worth noting that motivation for teletherapy may look different than motivation for in-person therapy, particularly if patients are choosing teletherapy because in-person therapy is not available to them; thus, Module 1 should involve a discussion of how participating in therapy remotely might impact engagement.

Module 2: Understanding Emotions

As a foundation for the skills presented in subsequent modules, Module 2 involves psychoeducation on the nature of emotions. First, therapists explain that emotions are adaptive cues that are meant to motivate helpful behavior despite potential discomfort. Next, therapists introduce the Three Component Model, a tool to help patients understand their emotional experiences by breaking them down into thoughts, physical sensations, and behaviors using worksheets. Finally, patients learn to place their emotional experiences into context using the Antecedents-Response-Consequences (ARC) form, which provides a framework through which patients and therapists can begin to examine the situations that trigger common emotions as well as the short- and long-term consequences of emotional responses.

Similarly to Module 1, therapists are encouraged to utilize the screen-share feature to complete these worksheets collaboratively. Preferences for whether therapists or patients enter text into the worksheet may have changed since the previous module; it is important to continually assess whether the logistics are working to best suit patients' needs and to modify accordingly.

Module 3: Mindful Emotion Awareness

Moving into Module 3, patients continue to build emotional awareness by learning the mindful emotion awareness skill, aimed at cultivating a non-judgmental, present-focused perspective toward emotions through several practice exercises. First, therapists lead a mindful meditation that is meant to promote mindful awareness of the three components of emotion: thoughts, physical sensations, and behavioral urges. Patients are asked to practice this meditation for homework. They may choose to audio record the meditation during the session on their phone or computer, or therapists may provide them with a premade recording via email.

The next activity is the mood induction, which involves practicing mindful emotion awareness in the context of an emotion that is intentionally elicited in-session. During the mood induction, patients select and then watch or listen to an emotionally evocative video or audio clip. Many patients choose a song that stirs up emotional memories; if they have trouble thinking of a song, therapists could select a video clip of an emotional film scene. The logistics of conducting the mood induction online differ based on the stimulus; if patients choose to play a song, they can do so on their own computer, whereas if therapists opt to play a video clip, they can find the video in a web browser and display it over screenshare.

It is helpful if patients and therapists can watch or listen to the stimulus together, as therapists may monitor patients' reactions during certain sections and gently draw attention to those reactions while debriefing the exercise. Thus, it is important to test out the connection in advance to be aware of and troubleshoot any issues that could hinder engagement. It is also helpful for therapists to be able to see patients' reactions during the exercise, which may require adjusting camera angle and lighting.

The final exercise in Module 3 is called anchoring in the present, which involves practicing mindful emotion awareness by cultivating nonjudgmental and present-focused awareness of emotional experiences as they unfold in daily life. Patients select an internal cue, such as their own breath, that they can use when they feel a strong emotion as a reminder to pause, reflect on the three components, and consider how to respond. Anchoring in the present is meant to be a skill that patients practice "off the page" in their day-to-day lives. As such, learning this skill in the context of their own home, rather than in a therapy room, could facilitate practicing this skill more easily and effectively in their daily life. In fact, this easier generalization of skill use to everyday life likely holds true for all UP skills.

Module 4: Cognitive Flexibility

The next three modules focus on each of the three components of emotion, starting with thoughts. In Module 4, patients learn cognitive flexibility, a skill that involves strengthening the ability to see situations from different perspectives. To illustrate this, therapists present patients with an illustration via screenshare depicting an ambiguous scene and ask patients to generate multiple interpretations. Therapists should elicit patients' first impression and then give patients space to take in more details and consider alternative interpretations, potentially using their cursor to draw attention to different details.

Patients then learn to apply cognitive flexibility to automatic thoughts about situations in their own lives using a worksheet completed via screenshare. The worksheet contains space for patients to record automatic thoughts, as well as alternative thoughts that represent different interpretations or perspectives. This process is guided by a list of questions that prompts consideration of alternative perspectives. Patients may find it helpful to keep a copy of these questions handy, such as in a note on their phone, to facilitate regular practice. It may also be helpful to write down alternative thoughts somewhere accessible, especially if the same negative thoughts are likely to recur (e.g., if someone ruminates about a particular situation before bed, they may keep an alternative thought on their nightstand). One advantage to conducting Module 4 online is that therapists can encourage patients to write down these reminders and place them somewhere accessible during the session.

Module 5: Countering Emotional Behaviors

As patients move into Module 5, the focus shifts from thoughts to behaviors. First, therapists and patients identify the function and consequences of behavioral components of emotions. In general, these components are "emotion-driven behaviors," such as the fight or flight component of fear, that function to avoid or suppress emotional discomfort or intensity. In addition, a strong tendency to avoid intense emotions is typically present. Both emotion-driven behaviors and avoidance are negatively reinforcing in the short-term; however, in the long-term, they can interfere with goals and confirm negative beliefs about emotions.

Patients are then encouraged to consider alternative actions, or behaviors that are different from, and potentially more helpful than, emotion-driven behaviors or emotion avoidance behavior. Alternative actions are likely to increase emotional discomfort in the short-term, but offer the long-term benefit of improving emotional tolerance. As in previous modules, patients plan and track their use of alternative actions, as well as the associated consequences, using worksheets that are completed via screenshare and assigned for homework.

Module 6: Interoceptive Exposures

Module 6 targets physical sensations through interoceptive exposures, or exposures to uncomfortable physiological sensations that are experienced in the context of strong emotions. For example, many people report muscle tension when they feel anxious or feeling weighed down when they feel depressed. In Module 6, therapists provide psychoeducation about the sensations that tend to accompany various emotions and the role that they play in the emotional response (e.g., shortness of breath while anxious may increase the likelihood a person avoids an uncomfortable situation).

Next, therapists lead patients through a symptom induction exercise that involves engaging in a series of physical exercises, such as hyperventilating, designed to bring on strong physical sensations. The goal is to find a few exercises that generate at least moderately distressing sensations that are similar to those experienced in the context of strong emotions. Due to the active and experiential nature of interoceptive exposures, adapting Module 6 to telehealth requires more creativity than previous modules, including planning logistics with patients in advance. There are three broad areas to consider: concerns about safety, the logistics of conducting the exercises, and identifying and addressing avoidance.

Although interoceptive exposures are not physically dangerous to patients who do not have medical or physical activity restrictions when performed correctly, safety should be considered given that patients will be conducting them on their own. For example, for exercises designed to elicit feelings of dizziness, such as repeatedly turning around, it would be important for therapists to ensure that patients have enough space before starting. If patients have access to a spinning chair, this may be the safest option. Each separate exercise might require unique safety considerations; therapists are therefore encouraged to contemplate potential safety concerns unique to each exercise and discuss them with patients ahead of time.

Whereas in person, therapists may be able to provide items to facilitate certain exercises (e.g., a thin straw to moderately restrict breathing), conducting these exercises remotely requires working within the constraints of whatever items patients have at their disposal, which may preclude certain exercises or necessitate modifications. This may also be an advantage in that patients may be able to practice exercises with therapist oversight that wouldn't have been as accessible in-person, such as wearing several layers of coats to feel overheated. Therapists are encouraged to participate in the symptom induction exercises along with patients to model safety and willingness to engage; thus, therapists should ensure that they are also prepared to engage in the exercises in their own space.

Finally, therapists and patients must identify potential avoidance intended to lessen discomfort during exercises. For example, if a patient is clenching their fists during an interoceptive exercise to soothe or distract themselves, a therapist would easily be able to notice this in-person. On the contrary, therapists might miss avoidant strategies over telehealth due to camera angle or video quality. To account for this, prior to each exercise, therapists and patients can brainstorm potential anticipated safety behaviors, and then after each exercise they can identify and process any avoidance.

Module 7: Emotion Exposures

The protocol culminates in Module 7, during which patients participate in emotion exposures. Exposures are a cornerstone of CBT and are effective in treating a variety of diagnoses (Hofmann & Smits, 2008). Traditional exposures emphasize extinguishing anxiety and distress to particular situations (e.g., contamination) or objects (e.g., needles). In contrast, emotion exposures emphasize developing new learning around *emotions* rather than specific stimuli. The goal is to promote emotional tolerance in service of one's goals: whereas in the past, patients may have engaged in self-limiting avoidance, emotion exposures offer the opportunity to build a broader repertoire for responding to emotional discomfort by fully experiencing uncomfortable emotions and responding in new ways.

The first step to conducting effective emotion exposures is creating a hierarchy, or a list of activities that can be used to intentionally evoke uncomfortable emotions. A good place to start is by revisiting the goals patients set in Module 1; if any have yet to be achieved, these may make good exposure opportunities. Patients can also consider the ways in which they are still avoiding emotions (e.g., avoiding specific situations). Ultimately, the UP's emotion-focused approach to exposure allows for creativity in designing exposures, as the emphasis is on evoking *emotions* rather than on recreating specific *situations*. Thus, many patients' hierarchies include activities like talking about an emotionally charged topic (e.g., a loved one who has passed away), looking at old photographs, or imaginal exposures (e.g., imagining an aversive future scenario using a written script). Additional examples of online exposures include displaying emotionally provoking media over screenshare (e.g., asking a patient with a rodent phobia to mindfully watch a clip of scurrying rodents) or utilizing virtual reality platforms (e.g., to simulate driving or flying). Therapists might also consider inviting a third-party (e.g., a colleague) to join the video session to assist with exposures. For example, a patient with social anxiety might give a presentation to a volunteer.

Exposures are then selected to be conducted in-session or independently for homework. Using screenshare, therapists and patients collaboratively complete worksheets before and after each exposure. The preparation worksheet asks patients to consider how the previous treatment skills could be helpful in conducting the exposure and experiencing their emotions fully. The debriefing worksheet provides space for processing the exposure by reflecting on how it went and what was learned.

Exposure planning should involve discussion about feasibility to conduct these exercises via telehealth. In-person, therapists are often able to directly observe as patients engage in the exposure activity, such as standing in a crowd. Remotely, however, it may not be feasible for these activities to be performed over video with therapists due to concerns about privacy and internet access while in public. Instead, these exposures can be assigned as homework, with preparation and review happening in session, and session time then also dedicated to conducting other exposures. In some cases, it may make sense for the therapist to offer phone support during initial exposures to increase buy-in and demonstrate support. For example, patients with trauma-related presentations may benefit from more support upfront to further establish and solidify a framework of trust with the therapist. However, it is not generally recommended that phone support be offered on a continual basis, as this could inadvertently function as a safety behavior, limiting the exposure's effectiveness.

During in-session exposures, therapists should be mindful of challenges and opportunities offered by technology. For example, certain avoidance behaviors may arise that are specific to the telehealth platform or that are more difficult to notice over video. This can include patients turning off their video so that they cannot see their own face, angling their camera in a specific direction, or engaging in a distracting or self-soothing activity off-screen (e.g., fidgeting beneath their desk).

Conversely, certain features of the telehealth platform may offer advantages. For example, in the context of a social anxiety exposure, a patient may benefit from being able to see their own face, either as a means to engage more fully with their anxiety or to test negative predictions (e.g., testing how red their face becomes). Furthermore, research suggests that the new learning that occurs during exposures may not always generalize easily across contexts (Mystkowski et al., 2002); thus, holding exposures virtually from patients' own everyday environment may help their new learning to better "stick," as this may be the environment in which strong emotions arise most often.

Module 8: Recognizing Accomplishments / Looking to the Future

The final module of the UP is focused on reviewing the gains made in therapy and planning for continued skill practice. This involves completing two worksheets via screenshare: one that summarizes the progress made throughout therapy and another that provides space to create a plan for continuing to practice skills. Patients often make plans for exposures that could not be completed during treatment; when treatment is conducted remotely due to temporary limitations (e.g., COVID-19 restrictions), this may involve planning for exposures that can be safely completed once restrictions have been lifted.

Conclusion

Increasing demand for online-delivered therapy has prompted interest in developing best practices for this modality. Effective treatments can be delivered over telehealth as long as therapists adhere to the evidence-based principles underlying these treatments. The UP offers a flexible, widely applicable treatment with strong support for its effectiveness. Considerations for delivering the UP online include thoughtfully managing logistics (e.g., completing worksheets over screenshare) and attending to telehealth-specific features that may undermine treatment effectiveness (e.g., the impact of the videoconference format on engagement or avoidance) or enhance it (e.g., promoting therapeutic learning directly in patients' home environments), as reducing avoidance and promoting new learning are central to the long-term management of emotional disorders.

References

Barlow, D. H., Farchione, J., Sauer-Zavala, S., Latin, H. M., Ellard, K. K., Bullis, J. R., Bentley, K. H., Boettcher, H. T., & Cassiello-Robbins, C. (2018). *Unified Protocol for Transdiagnostic Treatment of Emotional Disorders: Therapist Guide.* Oxford University Press.

Barlow, D. H., Farchione, T. J., Bullis, J. R., Gallagher, M. W., Murray-Latin, H., Sauer-Zavala, S., & Cassiello-Robbins, C. (2017). The Unified Protocol for Transdiagnostic Treatment of Emotional Disorders compared with diagnosis-specific protocols for anxiety disorders: A randomized clinical trial. *JAMA Psychiatry, 74*(9), 875–884.

Bullis, J. R., Boettcher, H., Sauer-Zavala, S., Farchione, T. J., & Barlow, D. H. (2019). What is an emotional disorder? A transdiagnostic mechanistic definition with implications for assessment, treatment, and prevention. *Clinical Psychology: Science and Practice, 26*(2), e12278.

Cassiello-Robbins, C., Rosenthal, M. Z., & Ammirati, R. J. (2021). Delivering trans-diagnostic treatment over telehealth during the COVID-19 pandemic: Application of the Unified Protocol. *Cognitive and Behavioral Practice, 28*(4), 555–572.

Cassiello-Robbins, C., Southward, M. W., Tirpak, J. W., & Sauer-Zavala, S. (2020). A systematic review of Unified Protocol applications with adult populations: Facilitating widespread dissemination via adaptability. *Clinical Psychology Review, 78*, 101852.

Gros, D. F., Morland, L. A., Greene, C. J., Acierno, R., Strachan, M., Egede, L. E., & Frueh, B. C. (2013). Delivery of evidence-based psychotherapy via video telehealth. *Journal of Psychopathology and Behavioral Assessment, 35*(4), 506–521.

Hofmann, S. G., & Smits, J. A. J. (2008). Cognitive-behavioral therapy for adult anxiety disorders: A meta-analysis of randomized placebo-controlled trials. *The Journal of Clinical Psychiatry, 69*(4), 621–632.

Mystkowski, J. L., Craske, M. G., & Echiverri, A. M. (2002). Treatment context and return of fear in spider phobia. *Behavior Therapy, 33*(3), 399–416.

Sauer-Zavala, S., & Barlow, D. H. (2021). *Neuroticism: A New Framework for Emotional Disorders and Their Treatment.* Guilford Press.

10 Remote Art Therapy: Engaging in a Shared Experience

Galit Mor

Introduction

This chapter covers the challenges facing therapists in their transition to remote art therapy (AT), illustrates creative online AT concepts and suggests an approach to advance remote processes while creatively utilizing the unique qualities of the media.

The insights and examples in the chapter are taken from my work with adolescents during the COVID-19 pandemic. However, I believe that the methods demonstrated in this chapter are suitable for patients of all ages, from childhood to the third age.

AT includes the use of expressive arts in the therapeutic process, integrated with psychotherapy approaches (Malchiodi, 2014). Arts therapies can be in the form of visual art, media, music, movement, drama and psychodrama, and bibliotherapy. Each of these disciplines can either stand alone or can be combined with tools from other fields as in intermodal expressive therapy (Berger, 2015). AT is suitable for all stages of life: childhood, adolescence, adulthood, and the third age.

During the COVID-19 pandemic, remote therapy became especially relevant, allowing ongoing therapy, as well as supervision and peer learning. Continued support and therapy are invaluable, especially in a difficult, isolating, complex, and anxiety-ridden period. Remote therapy can be offered through various media, including Zoom, WhatsApp video, cellphone conversations, text messaging, and sending photographs of artwork via cellphone or email, either synchronously or asynchronously.

For many therapists, this means daring to open-up, to leave their comfort zone, and to contemplate and err during the learning process, while coping with frustrating moments and with change in attitudes and perceptions. The transition demands adjustment from patients, as well. They, too, do not know in advance whether remote therapy will allow an ongoing beneficial process or which platform will suit them in particular: A phone call? Zoom meeting? WhatsApp call? Patients must experience the impact of the change on the therapeutic process, and their adjustment to change cannot be taken for granted (Mor, 2020).[1]

DOI: 10.4324/9781003205029-13

The COVID-19 pandemic invites us, as therapists, to train two mental muscles: first, the creativity muscle and thinking out of the box, and second, the ability to be present in an unknown situation, to contain the unknown until the space is filled with knowledge, and then to let go and be open, once again, to something new. To adjust to working remotely, art therapists are currently required to discover new models and creative interventions.

Even though, at first sight, the transition to remote therapy appears to invite less art-based intervention, it offers an opportunity for more creativity that enriches and rejuvenates the therapy.

The Challenge of the Setting: How Can We Form a Virtual Analytical Space?

The traditional approach attributes great importance to establishing and maintaining the physical boundaries of the therapeutic setting as a protected space that is separate from the outside world. In this space, transformation can occur in a process whereby unconscious elements can surface safely in the conscious sphere, using symbols that carry a message (Jung, 1997). In light of the absence of these boundaries in the virtual space (see Weinberg & Rolnick, 2019), how can we shape the online session as a "sacred space," in which the inside is separated from the outside – as a safe space where patients will dare to expose their vulnerability and connect to forgotten strengths, and where the therapist will succeed in being present and analytically attentive?

French and Simpson (1999) claim that learning depends largely on the ability to linger on the threshold of knowing and not knowing. Two things are necessary for this: having a considerable amount of knowledge and the willingness to engage with not knowing.

Between knowing and not knowing, therapists would do well to release the fear of erring vis-à-vis their patients and to contain being in the experience of not knowing.

If therapists synchronously hold the place that they know and the place that they do not know, they enable their patients and themselves to find a relative balance between the fear of the unfamiliar and responsiveness – in hope of opening a door to the analytical space. Something new can be found only by being open to the unknown (Bion, 1970; Ogden, 2003). Under conditions of uncertainty, a potential space is created; there, creativity is born. May (1975) mentions art-making processes as facilitating engagement with the not knowing stage: Creative people "knock on silence for an answering music; they pursue meaninglessness until they can force it to mean" (p. 93). I suggest, though, that art-based interventions enhance the ability to cope with and benefit from this stage.

What is the safe foundation in remote therapy that can allow us to set out to explore the balance that is called for vis-à-vis the unknown? Some therapeutic aspects that are mainstays of therapy in the physical space can also be part of remote therapy: the therapeutic figure, the therapist's focus on establishing his/her analytical attentiveness, the therapist's knowledge and experience, the therapist's commitment to the patient, and the therapeutic relationship as the most important layer of the therapeutic process (Aron, 1996; Bromberg, 1998; Ogden, 2009; Mitchell, 2000). These principles are a platform on which therapists can offer dynamic therapeutic interventions, while remaining open to what is happening from moment to moment. They are the safe base where implicit content may be embodied, where rigid defense mechanisms can be softened, fists can be un-clenched, fluid experiences can be gathered, and meaningful therapeutic processes can flourish. When the communicational space serves as a base in which the clear, familiar, and known is balanced with the unknown, the therapist and patient, like in a sturdy boat, can sail, and make discoveries outside familiar territory.

Unique Challenges for Remote Art Therapists

Art therapists, in their work, use creative means and nonverbal interventions because they recognize these tools' potential to set therapeutic processes in motion, to enhance the therapist–patient relationship, and to advance awareness and change. Creation is a resource for development and healing, facilitating sublimation processes (Malchiodi, 2002; Kramer, 2000; McNiff, 2004). The image is a container for the projection of elements of the inner world, offers the opportunity to give meaning to those elements, and advances processing of nonverbal and implicit content (Jung, 1997; Schaverien, 2000).

In AT, patients have an emotional encounter with implicit mental contents through processing with the creative, intuitive right hemisphere of the brain, while the conceptualization and meaning-making stage occurs in the left hemisphere that is associated with logic and rationality (Schore, 2012). The Creativity generates a transitional space that locates new channels for coping with troublesome issues (Winnicott, 1971). Artwork is a means of evaluation and intervention (Lahad, 1992).

What can help art therapists to advance remote AT processes while coping with the challenges of the transition to remote AT and utilizing the unique qualities of the media?

As I will illustrate further on, AT has unique qualities that can contribute to patient–therapist engagement and communication, as well as creating a shared experience from a distance.

Symbolic Portrayal of Psychological States on an Online Platform

Digital remote therapy offers art therapists an extension of their creative language and toolbox (Malchiodi, 2018; Zubala et al., 2021). In remote AT, themes in patients' lives can be portrayed in new ways with the help of technology. For example, when using creative means remotely, the way in which patients seek the therapist's presence reflects their individual needs or different stages in the process. Through making a joint drawing on the shared screen, patients may express the need to experience togetherness. They may ask the therapist to draw like them on the shared screen, out of the desire for a twinship experience or because of the need to echo content or for overt or covert mirroring. Other patients may prefer the therapist to watch them as they create, so that the content expressed through the artwork will be held in the gaze of the therapist, who serves as a witness and an audience. Some patients may express the wish to create in a space of their own, free of the therapist's gaze, to experience the capacity to be alone in the presence of another or may request a dialogue of creative images of which the therapist is a partner as a creative subject.

When therapists are analytically attentive and present, they are focused on an experience aimed to sense and understand occurrences in the therapeutic space in the context of the patient's psychological world. The context can emphasize either the interpersonal and/or the intrapersonal, depending on each case. Therapists will choose the interventions they believe to be most suited to the patient, according to their appraisal and understanding of the patient's needs.

Portrayal of Selfobject Needs

Fourteen-year-old Nir began therapy about a year before the COVID-19 outbreak. He is a sensitive, motherless boy, and was adopted by his aunt at his early childhood.

Nir's therapy in the physical space during the pre-pandemic period, focused on building a trusting relationships and primary relational needs. Moving to remote therapy during the pandemic, we met via Zoom. Nir needed me to be attuned and to respond to him empathically, with warmth and affection, and he expressed his primary needs in the therapy framework assisted by the means that this media offers. For example, in one of the Zoom sessions, Nir used graphic technology to scribble on my face. He seemed to be amused doing so, and I experienced his act as a way to create a rapport and an invitation to play. In another session, he used a different name in an attempt to deceive me. Using charm and a playful atmosphere, he was testing whether I would guess that it was him. I viewed this act as an expression of primary object relations or the pre-oedipal phase, which, in the physical space, could have been portrayed through playing hide and seek or peekaboo. Sometimes, he shared with me video clips and showed me dancing figures that he had created in an animation game, as I reacted with interest and enthusiasm.

I could identify his need for my presence as an admiring selfobject, in the sense defined by Kohut (1984) as an external figure who supports his psychological functions and helps him to internalize positive experiences; a figure who enables the patient to develop and sustain a sense of self-esteem. Nir did not require my interpretations, but the satisfaction of his selfobject needs through empathy, an audience (witnessing), admiration, and mirroring.

Remote Intersubjectivity

Manguel (2018) suggests that the bonding between the therapist and the patient in remote AT is not necessarily based on physical distance, but on emotional closeness. In the next examples, I will use the prism of the intersubjective approach to illuminate aspects of the therapeutic relationship. The intersubjective approach is based on the perception of the therapeutic relationship as an encounter between two subjects and on understanding the therapeutic occurrence as a process shared by two people. This is distinct from one-person psychology that focuses on one person's intrapsychic life (Aron, 1996; Bromberg, 1998; Mitchell, 2000). The approach emphasizes the healing role of the therapeutic relationship. Therapist–patient relations are perceived as equal yet asymmetrical, and the therapist and patient create an "analytic third" in the therapeutic setting (Ogden, 1994).

Schaverien (2000) mentions the artwork as a transference-object for the therapist–patient relationship. In this sense, the artwork reflects the shared therapist–patient experience, similar to the analytic third, as a shared creation of the therapist and patient and as a reflection of their interpersonal relationship. During the therapeutic process, the art therapist is often active and involved, sometimes even creating with the patient. These aspects reinforce the therapist's presence as a subject in the interaction and express the therapist's authenticity (Gerlitz et al., 2020). In addition, in AT, the art materials have therapeutic significance as a means of advancing processes and a bridge between therapist and patient (Orbach & Galkin, 2016).

With the passage of time, I was able to discern that my way of working remotely appears to be mostly through an intersubjective approach: placing the therapeutic relationship and the shared experience in the center as an engine for change and development in therapy, using self-exposure, being more active, sharing emotions, and using joint creation.

There are several reasons why this approach was particularly suitable for remote AT, especially during the COVID-19 pandemic: In the absence of traditional components, working on a different platform and in a physically distanced setting placed the therapeutic relationship as the focus. The main aim was to reach patients emotionally and to create a shared space and shared experience with them. Furthermore, in remote therapy, the exposure of the therapist as a subject is unavoidable when the patient can see the therapist's home environment on the screen, and additional aspects of the therapist as a subject are present in the interaction.

Another reason for the prominence of intersubjective relationships in remote therapy, during the COVID-19 period, is related to the shared elements of coping experienced by both therapist and patient. My personal exposure was on the table and positioned me as a subject. I found that instead of resisting and fighting against this exposure, I could use it to benefit the therapy. Additionally, I found that greater involvement was required of me, especially when reaching out to those patients who had withdrawn into their shells during the social distancing imposed by the pandemic.

Each of the patients in the following examples presented below had been in therapy for at least one year before the pandemic and had each come a long way in therapy; or more accurately, the therapeutic relationship had come a long way. In these therapies, I was present as a subject.

Walking Remotely, Together – A Clinical Example

Thirteen-year-old Liat had not left her home for several months – since the beginning of the first lockdown – for fear of infection with coronavirus. I suggested that we walk out "together," at the same time, during a WhatsApp video call. We each walked out into the public domain outside our homes, while creating a shared space for the two of us via the smartphone screen. We each experienced the other's perspective and the scenes that the other one saw through the phone screen. During this session, I was attuned and active until a flowing experience of togetherness was created. The session included use of the physical senses in the encounter with the outdoors, an experience of being present in the "here and now," as well as of movement, using photography as a creative means, sending photos, with dialogue in between, and remote verbal conversation. Our "walk together" allowed Liat to go outside after months of not having stepped out the door, as well as meeting her need for contact.

Establishing a Shared Experience

Seventeen-year-old Sari and I had remote therapy sessions for almost a year during the COVID-19 pandemic. Prior to the pandemic, we had met in the physical setting once a week over 2 years. During that time, the therapeutic relationship underwent a transition from a situation in which I experienced her as a difficult patient, whose attacks I must survive, to a patient who was able to see me as a separate subject and even to show empathy. As we created a foundation of trust and a safe space, Sari gradually became willing to encounter her vulnerabilities in the room, and to express them and herself authentically. At that point, we started to work remotely. Throughout that period, schools were closed, classes were online, and the pandemic constraints enforced social distancing. Sari appeared to withdraw into herself, in the absence of a daily routine, and was detached from her Zoom classroom learning. At that period we had remote therapy sessions via cellphone as her chosen means of communication since she preferred not to be seen during any remote communication with me and others. I sought ways to reach her remotely and to communicate with her. During one of our cellphone conversations, as an attempt to stimulate communication, I photographed and sent her a picture of a tree from my garden. I think this act was motivated partly by not wanting to do more of the same and partly by my despair and exhaustion with our halting communication. We discovered that we both live in houses with yards, which led to a discussion about plants, gardening, and our own gardens. Sari was aroused by our discussion and showed interest in cultivating her family's garden. In subsequent sessions, we exchanged and responded to photographs, taken simultaneously, of each other's gardens. This dialogue of images contributed a sense of presence and authentic expressions to our communication (Figures 10.1 and 10.2).

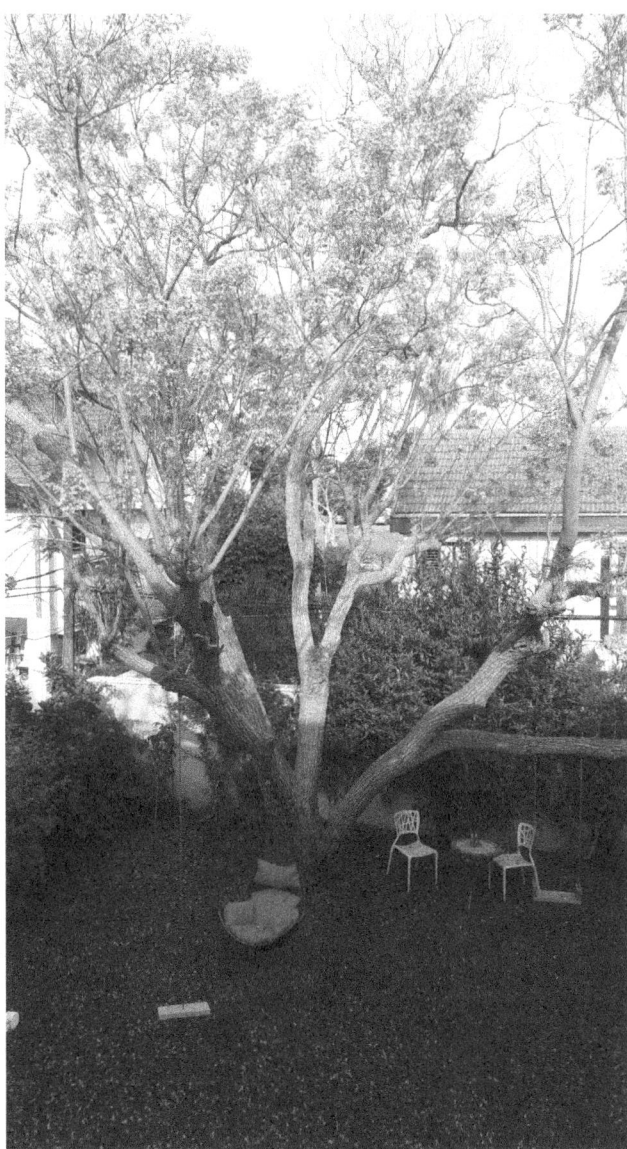

Figure 10.1 Photo of a tree in my garden.

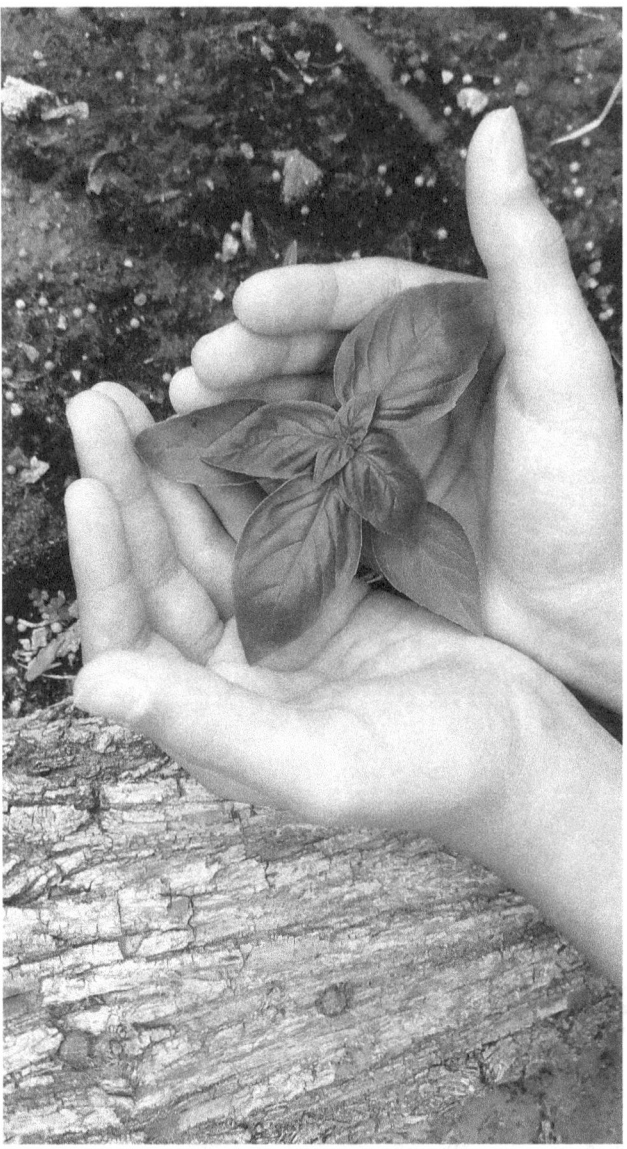

Figure 10.2 Planting a sapling.

Our sessions were filled with content. Sari shared about how she was nurturing her family garden. She seemed to experience herself as capable of cultivating and creating something at a time when the whole family was in lockdown and practicing social distancing. At this stage, I found that she discovered gentleness in herself and self-compassion.

A Voyage in New Directions Toward the Future

Rolnick and Ehrenreich (2020) note the absence of bodily presence as a fundamental challenge in remote therapy and propose ways to imbue physical presence in the therapy. They add that the experience of the concrete therapist–patient encounter can be reinforced through eye contact and positioning the camera so that the participants' bodies are visible. From my experience of remote therapy with 16-year-old Tomer (see below), I found that techniques involving the body in the therapeutic encounter contribute to the bodily presence of therapist and patient. Artwork that activates sensory motor channels can create physical presence by working with tactile art materials that stimulate the senses. In parallel, sensory channels may be integrated into the therapist–patient encounter; e.g., when therapist and patient are creating together while listening to music, combining the physical, emotional, creative, and social channels in an experience that is both separate and shared. The mindfulness concept represents the quality of an experience characterized by attentive presence. In certain therapies, particularly with patients who suffered from anxiety during the pandemic, I made use of interventions combining mindfulness and creativity with somatic experience techniques, such as breathing, grounding, and body scan, which the patient and I performed simultaneously under my guidance. These interventions contributed to the experience of shared presence in the session – of closeness despite the physical distance.

Tomer has CP. He has a rational temperament, is particularly bright, and suffers from stress. We began our remote therapy without a background of frontal sessions. Despite his initial hesitation as to whether he was interested in therapy, I persuaded him by explaining that we would combine mindfulness with artwork and that I would try to help him with balanced use of the creative brain hemisphere, since he acts from a very rational, task-focused, and self-demanding position. I explained that I would teach him relaxation techniques that can have added value during the pandemic. I was happy when he agreed to leave his comfort zone and to give it a try. In remote therapy, he responded to my guidance: to release control, to draw with eyes closed with his nondominant hand while listening to music; to roam across the page. Later, he described this as a relaxing, sensory experience, a release of judgmentalism, flowing, connecting to emotion (Figure 10.3).

I was especially moved by one of his drawings produced while listening to relaxing music, alongside the sound of waves and water. Tomer drew a boat and a figure with the caption: To the end and beyond. During lockdown and social distancing, at home, opposite the computer during the pandemic, he appeared to succeed in encountering new internal spaces, to sail in his imagination, to connect, through creative strengths, to an experience of space and a horizon, moving and advancing toward the future. He appeared to be expressing a positive experience of connection to resources of strength and hope (Figure 10.4).

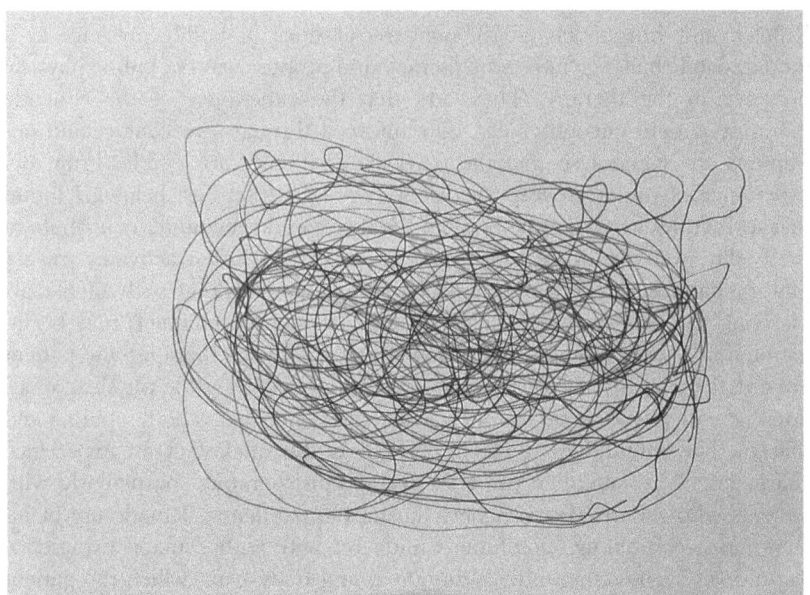

Figure 10.3 Tomer's creation through mindfulness (illustration).

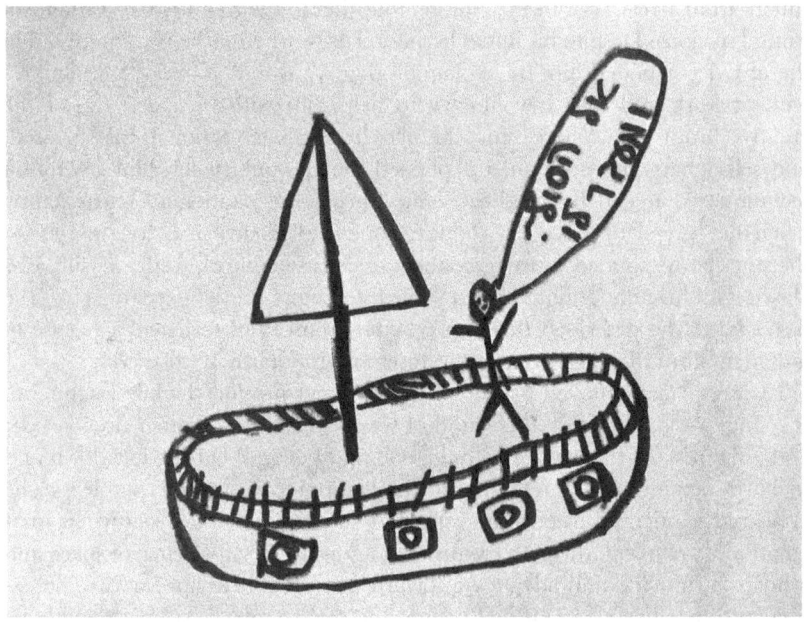

Figure 10.4 Tomer's drawing: "To the end and beyond".

Conclusion

I have pointed to challenges facing therapists in the transition to remote therapy during the COVID-19 pandemic and to factors that support this transition's success.

My remote therapy experiences during the COVID-19 pandemic showed me the centrality of the therapeutic relationship in the process of therapy. I found a variety of Art-based Interventions that enhance the patient-therapist engagement and establish a shared experience while promoting the therapy process.

Finding solutions in unexpected ways through the joy of discovery is a satisfying experience. If therapists are relatively competent in the technical side, they are able to draw tools from their professional toolbag by being dynamically attentive and emotionally available. What do we have in our professional toolbag? All of our therapeutic knowledge, our experience, and our creativity. When I open my toolbag, I discover a vast container; a space in itself in which I discover abundant options, far more than I imagined. I appreciate that the bag holds everlasting treasures and a diverse arsenal. The bag will always have space for new material, with the ability to create its own capacity. I am currently enjoying what this toolbag has to offer, but there were certainly times during the learning process when I broke my teeth on "Zoomish" to cope with the technology. Often, I overcame the difficulties thanks to my motivation. At other times, I stumbled, but kept on trying. Like with any new challenge, we need to be prepared to take the plunge.

Practical Considerations and Tips

- A creative, innovative approach advances discovery of new interventions, sustains interest, and opens new horizons.
- Varied, creative remote therapy interventions can revitalize the therapeutic encounter.
- The therapist's activism and a directive approach can help the patient, especially while adjusting to the new setting.
- Therapists can use their subjectivity to enhance the patient's engagement remotely.
- The therapist's use of dynamic, alive intonation alongside pronounced gestures and facial expressions can help pave the way to the patient.
- Parallel work by therapist and patient can establish a shared space as a platform for emotional work, as well as working synchronously with identical materials, developing a dialogue between images. Music can also be used as a shared acoustic space during the joint creative process.

- Patients can express their emotional world and embodied mental contents via technological means through creative applications, screen sharing, selecting online images, and YouTube clips and songs.
- Remote therapy opens the possibility for therapy outdoors, expanding options for intervention.
- The patient can send the therapist photos of the creation, to observe and relate to the art product together.
- In online therapy, we are exposed to the patient's real world via the screen. We can use this exposure to learn about the patient's life rather than trying to ignore the home space.
- The digital technology of remote therapy serves as a resonating chamber for transference–countertransference processes.

Note

1 This chapter is based on parts of a previous article: Mor, G. (2020). Remote art therapy: A call for initiative. *The Academic Journal of Creative Arts Therapies*, *10*(2), 1157–1165 (Hebrew).

References

Aron, L. (1996). *A meeting of minds: Mutuality in psychoanalysis*. Analytic Press, Inc.

Berger, R. (2015). Back to ritual. In V. Buchanan (Ed.), *Art therapy: Programs, uses and benefits* (pp. 51–66). New York, NY: Nova Science.

Bion, W. R. (1970). *Attention and Interpretation*. London: Tavistock Publications.

Bromberg, P. M. (1998). *Standing in the spaces: Essays on clinical process, trauma, and dissociation*. New Jersey: Analytic Press.

French, R., & Simpson, P. (1999). "Our best work happens when we don't know what we're doing": Discuss. *Socio-Analysis*, *1*(2), 216–230.

Gerlitz, Y., Regev, D., & Snir, S. (2020). A Relational Approach to Art Therapy. *The Arts in Psychotherapy*, 101644.

Jung, C. G. (1997). *Encountering Jung: Jung on active imagination* (J. Chodorow, Ed.). Princeton University Press.

Kohut, H. (1984). *How does analysis cure?* The University of Chicago Press.

Kramer, E. (2000). *Art as therapy: Collected papers*. Jessica Kingsley.

Lahad, M. (1992). Story-making in assessment method for coping with stress: Six-piece story- making and BASIC Ph. In S. Jennings (Ed.), *Drama therapy: Theory and practice 2* (pp. 192–208). Routledge.

Malchiodi, C.A. (2002). *The soul's palette: Drawing on art's transformative powers for health and well-being*. Boston: Shambhala/Random House.

Malchiodi, C. A. (2014). Creative arts therapy approaches to attachment issues. In C. A. Malchiodi & D. A. Crenshaw (Eds.), *Creative arts and play therapy for attachment problems* (pp. 3–18). New York: Guilford Press.

Malchiodi, C. A. (2018). *The handbook of art therapy and digital technology.* Jessica Kingsley.

Manguel, L. (2018). Proximity and distance in teletherapy. In J. Savege Scharff (Ed.), *Psychoanalysis Online 4* (pp. 91–108). Routledge.

May, R. (1975). *The courage to create.* W. W. Norton.

McNiff, S. (2004). *Art heals: How creativity cures the soul.* Shambhala.

Mitchell, S. A. (2000). Intersubjectivity: Between expressiveness and restraint in the analytic relationship. In *Relationality: From attachment to intersubjectivity* (pp. 125–146). Hillsdale, NJ: The Analytic Press.

Mor, G. (2020). Remote art therapy: A call for initiative. *The Academic Journal of Creative Arts Therapies, 10*(2), 1157–1165. (Hebrew).

Ogden, T. H. (1994). The analytic third: Working with intersubjective clinical facts. *The International Journal of Psychoanalysis, 75*(1), 3–19.

Ogden, T. H. (2003). On not being able to dream. *Int. J. Psycho-Anal., 84*(1), 17–30.

Ogden, T. H. (2009).*Rediscovering psychoanalysis: Thinking and dreaming, learning and forgetting.* Routledge/Taylor & Francis Group.

Orbach, N., & Galkin, L. (2016). *The spirit of matter: A database handbook for therapists, artists and educators* (Kindle edition).

Rolnick, A., & Ehrenreich, Y. (2020). Can you feel my heart (via your camera and sensors)? The role of the body, its absence, and its measurement in online video psychotherapy. *Biofeedback, 48*(1). 10.5298/1081-5937-48.1.1

Schaverien, J. (1989). The picture within the frame. In A. Gilroy & T. Dalley (Eds.), *Pictures at an exhibition: Selected essays on art and art therapy.* Routledge.

Schaverien, J. (2000). The triangular relationship and the aesthetic counter-transference in analytical art psychotherapy. In A. Gilroy & G. McNeilly. *The changing shape of art therapy: New developments in theory and practice* (pp. 55–83). Jessica Kingsley.

Schore, A. N. (2012). *The science of the art of psychotherapy.* W. W. Norton & Company.

Winnicott, D. W. (1971). *Playing and reality.* Tavistock.

Weinberg, H., & R., Arnon (2019). *Theory and Practice of Online Therapy: Internet-delivered Interventions for Individuals, Groups, Families, and Organizations.* 1st ed.Routledge.

Zubala, A., Kennell, N., & Hackett, S. (2021). Art Therapy in the Digital World: An Integrative Review of Current Practice and Future Directions. *Frontiers in Psychology, 12*, 595536.10.3389/fpsyg.2021.600070.

11 Zooming in on Experiential Dynamic Therapies

Joop Meijers

What is EDT?

EDT is an abbreviation of Experiential Dynamic Therapy. EDT is the collective name for a group of psychotherapies that have the following characteristics in common:

1 they share a few basic psychodynamic principles, the main ones being:

    a   the existence of a psychodynamic unconscious

    b   the importance of transference and countertransference, albeit differently from the classic psychodynamic meanings of the terms

    c   unconscious defenses against anxiety

2 they emphasize the role and importance of fully and consciously experiencing and expressing emotions

3 they integrate to some degree principles of other forms of psychotherapy that have proven to be effective in changing emotions, thoughts and behavior:

    a   from Cognitive-Behavior Therapy the principle and technique of Systematic Desensitization of the Fear of Affects (Affect phobia) or Exposure to stimuli that trigger 'authentic' emotions like: sadness, anger, joy, sexual longings and Response prevention i.e., preventing the use of defenses or 'avoidance behaviors' (McCullough, 1997).

    b   from Non-directive (Rogerian) Therapy the principle and technique of mirroring, even though in EDT the mirroring not only refers to what the client says and feels but also to what the therapist observes about the non-verbal behavior of the client

4 they attach great importance to the 'real relationship' and the 'real person' in therapy and not only or mainly to the so-called 'transference relationship'. The therapist does not hide behind a 'blank screen' on which the client projects his or her feelings, thoughts etc. An example: the author of this article was in many respects, computer illiterate at the beginning of the COVID-Zoom era. Not a few embarrassing things

DOI: 10.4324/9781003205029-14

happened during earlier Zoom meetings (such as accidently exposing personal material on my home screen when I wanted to screen-share a relevant diagram about the basics of EDT. This became an occasion to express my feelings of embarrassment as well as self-compassion on my part.

5   EDT is a focused, directive, active and therefore short-term or shorter-term therapy than most other psychodynamic therapies.

Clinical experience and empirical research have shown that EDT is an effective therapy for people who suffer from (originally called) axis 1 and axis 2 (personality disorders) problems. The therapy can be delivered as individual therapy, in couples and groups and to children and adolescents (Lilliengren et al., 2016, Derdikman Eiron, 2021).

Since its origins, starting with the pioneering work of Habib Davanloo in Canada (cf. Davanloo, 1995) in the late sixties of the previous century and the work of David Malan in England beginning in the seventies (c.f. Malan, 1995), EDT has proliferated and given birth to a variety of therapies that each has a different 'brand-name' to make it easier to differentiate the different kinds or 'tastes' of EDT. The better-known names: ISTDP (Intensive Short Term Dynamic Psychotherapy), IE-DP (Intensive Experiential Dynamic Psychotherapy), APT (Affect Phobia Therapy), AEDP (Accelerated Experiential Dynamic Psychotherapy). The originators of the different branches of EDT seem to agree that they stand on the shoulders of two giants: Habib Davanloo (a Canadian psychiatrist, born 1927) and David Malan (English psychiatrist 1922–2020), who developed the core model of EDT, then called ISTDP, in the last decade of the 20th century.

There are many books and articles about EDT and its derivatives and this is not the place to review or summarize them (for an excellent review see Osimo & Stein, 2018).

However, for the purpose of this chapter, it is important to understand the core theory of the model and the main techniques derived from the theory.

The main working assumption of EDT is that many psychological problems and symptoms with which people present to therapy, are the result of an acquired, learned fear of experiencing and/or expressing normal, authentic, adaptive emotions like anger, sadness, joy, and other emotions. This learning process happens, partly, 'unconsciously', i.e., without the patient being aware how and that it happened. Often this happens in childhood when a traumatic or aversive event threatens the crucial, life-saving attachment bond with a parent.

An example: A child with a depressive mother is either ignored or even scolded when he/she expresses anger towards his/her depressive mom. The child, who does not want to endanger the attachment bond or lose the mother's attention and care, over time 'learns', first to suppress the expression of his anger and later to suppress even the feeling itself, in order not to antagonize mom and be ignored or scolded. Since it is very difficult if not impossible to selectively suppress only specific feelings, the child gradually comes to suppress any feeling. When this mechanism lasts long enough it will become automatic and unconscious and may become a source of problems and symptoms.

The symptoms that bring people to therapy can be seen as the way or ways in which the client 'copes' with, or 'defends against' or 'avoids/escapes from the anxiety or extreme discomfort the patient felt or feels when exposed to the frightening and threatening feelings or situations, triggers, stimuli that give rise to the feelings.

Thus the goal of EDT, broadly defined, is to help people overcome their fear of experiencing and/or expressing normal authentic emotions. This is done by helping clients first see how their symptoms or problems are ways of coping with or defending against threatening but normal emotions, then giving up their defenses so that they can experience their emotions without experiencing anxiety or other inhibiting feelings. This happens first, in the safe environment of an accepting and understanding real person = therapist and later, hopefully, generalizes to the real-life situation of the client outside of therapy. As a sideline, it may be important to raise the issue of the possible 'cultural sensitivity' or 'bias' of a therapy that sets as its goal to help people freely experiencing and expressing their emotions. There are cultures and sub-groups within existing Western culture where the experiencing or ex-pressing of emotions is regulated by cultural norms. For example, in many ultra-orthodox Jewish circles the experiencing and expressing of anger is equated with idolatry and strictly forbidden. The cultural-religious norm is that one has to suppress the emotion of anger. For an EDT therapist working with this population this poses a huge challenge.

From a psychodynamic perspective, one might say that the therapy unfolds in and through a specific form of transference from the client to the therapist. Within the EDT context 'transference' means that the client expresses his feelings towards the therapist as a real present person and not as a stand-in for a person from the past. Alternatively, from a CBT point of view, one could say that EDT is a form of systematic desensitization of fear of feelings or a gradual exposure to experiencing and expressing emotions without needing to avoid or escape from the emotions. From an EDT point of view, the therapy is a new, unique experience for the client who will learn to overcome his fear of emotions in the context of a safe attachment relationship with the therapist as a real person (Osimo, 2003).

Since the focus of this chapter is the exploration of online therapy for EDT, the main questions to ask are:

> How will online, internet-based therapy, affect the crucial processes of overcoming the fear of experiencing and expressing emotions? Is experiencing and expressing emotions online fundamentally different from the same processes happening in the therapy room where client and therapist sit closely together (at least till COVID-19 forced 'social

distancing')? If there is a difference, does this difference significantly affect the outcome of therapy? How do clients and therapists experience this? And what can we learn from the relevant research?

Is Internet-based EDT Effective?

Compared to the quantity and quality of research of internet-based CBT (e.g., see Carlbring et al., 2018), there are very few studies on the efficacy or effectiveness of psychodynamic internet-based therapy in general and EDT in particular. As in the area of CBT, all relevant studies focus on the ***outcome*** of therapy and none (as far as we know) on the ***mechanisms*** of change.

Most high-quality research studies of the last 20 years support the so-called Dodo Bird -effect, after the famous character of 'Alice in Wonderland'. At the end of a competition between adversaries, the Dodo bird declares 'Everybody has won and all must have prizes'. When one only looks at the outcomes of different forms of therapy, assessed with empirically validated and agreed upon instruments, one will find few significant differences between the therapies (with notable exceptions, such as the treatment of OCD). A good example is a study by Lilliengren et al. (2016). The authors reported on a meta-analysis of 28 randomized controlled studies with almost 1800 patients who suffered from depression, anxiety, personality disorders and mixed problems. Both at the end of therapy and at a later follow-up, all EDT treated patients did significantly better than the patients in the inactive control groups. But compared with patients who were treated with drugs or CBT, there were no significant differences. As far as the different problem areas are concerned, the best outcomes happened in the depression group. The Lilliengren et al. study is representative. Most studies on the effect of EDT have similar results.

The same applies to internet-based therapies. Most studies on internet-based psychotherapy find the Dodo Bird effect. In their 2019 study, Berryhill et al. systematically reviewed 1253 articles about the effect of internet-based video-conferencing therapy versus therapy as usual on anxiety problems. After eliminating studies that did not meet stringent methodologic criteria, they based their review on 21 studies, 6 of whom were randomized controlled studies. The main finding of the review, not a meta-analysis, is that internet-based therapies, comprising a range of approaches, but no psychodynamic ones, do as well as face-to-face therapy as usual.

Since this chapter focuses on EDT, and not on psychodynamic therapies in general, we will only write a few words about the efficacy and effectiveness of internet-based psychodynamic therapies.

Almost all studies on the effects of internet-based psychodynamic therapy, IPDT, study a version of therapy based on text-based modules, homework assignment, and very limited therapist guidance, by mail or by video-conferencing. In this respect they are similar to the internet-based CBT studies, but with a different theoretical conceptualization. One of the more comprehensive studies is by Lindegaard et al. (2020). After having found 73 studies, they were eventually left with seven randomized controlled studies that fulfilled stringent methodological criteria. The research looked at the effect of therapist guided, verbal-text based IPDT on depression and anxiety in approximately 500 experimental and 500 control subjects. The control condition was a so-called 'inactive' control, meaning general support by a therapist but without specific tasks or instructions. The overall outcome of the study is disappointing. There were very small differences between the two conditions, not supporting the thesis that IPDT is efficacious or effective at all. Due to the design, nothing can be said about the efficacy as compared with psychodynamic treatment 'as usual'.

For our purposes it is important to ask how internet-based EDT compares with EDT administered as usual (i.e., in the therapy room in the physical presence of the therapist). If it turns out that the outcomes are similar, this may have important implications for the future of EDT in general and internet-based EDT in particular.

Given the crucial role of experiencing and expressing emotions, it is important not only to look at outcomes but also to understand the working mechanisms of EDT. How, if at all, is experiencing and expressing feelings different online versus in the reality of the therapist's physical presence? This applies to clients as well as to therapists.

A few available studies present some ***preliminary*** evidence that internet-based EDTs are effective. A good example would be a study by Johansson et al. (2013) on 100 people with problems of anxiety and depression. On a random basis, they were divided into an EDT self-help treatment with therapist guidance or another active therapist guided self-help supportive therapy. There were significant differences in favor of the EDT group and these remained at a follow-up of seven months. Whether the results are representative for internet-delivered EDT by a therapist, is to be seen. The study has several methodological limitations that make it difficult to derive conclusions. The term 'preliminary' has to be remembered in relation to almost all studies so far.

In the literature, there is some more evidence for the efficacy of psychodynamic internet-based therapy but those studies relate to classic psychodynamic therapy and not to the specific subgroup of EDT or EDT's.

An intermediate conclusion so far is that there is some preliminary support for the efficacy of internet-based EDT versus EDT in the clinic. But by far not enough to base the use of internet-based EDT on robust research evidence.

Therapist's Experiences in the Land of Skype and Zoom

This section is written from the perspective of 10 experienced and licensed EDT therapists in Israel, the first country to be almost COVID-free, in the summer of 2021 when it looked as if life would return to almost 'normal'.

These therapists (today there are still relatively few EDT therapists in Israel) were in a good position to reflect on their Zoom-experience, after many of them, but not all, had returned to face-to-face therapy in the clinic (since then, the Delta variant sent many of them back online). All of them worked in private practices since most public mental health settings of the government-managed health clinics did not permit or enable videoconferencing therapy.

On the basis of my personal communications with the Israeli EDT therapists, their experiences share several impressions and observations.

Non-Verbal Cues and the Expression of Emotions

Almost all therapists used to observe non-verbal expressions of emotions and feelings through seeing the whole body of the person in the therapy room. So when doing therapy by Zoom or Skype there was an initial difficulty of only having available a partial view of the body (head, shoulders). All of the therapists needed time to get used to this new situation. After the initial 'cut-off body shock' most of the therapists got used to the new situation and reported being able to notice tension, relaxation, different feelings (sadness, anger, fear, restlessness) on the basis of what they saw in and on the faces of their patients. Some therapists said that thanks to the very closeness of the face to the screen, they even had a better view of the face and so a close-up they never had in the clinic. They were able to notice tiny, small, changes in facial muscles they had not picked up in the therapy room.

Different therapists coped differently with the absence of the total body view. Some asked clients, more than they had done before, what and how they felt and where in the body they felt what they felt. Some therapists found this easier than doing the same in the face-to-face encounters in the clinic since now, on Zoom or Skype, they had a 'good excuse' to ask this several times in a session. They added that maybe, from the perspective of the client, now that the client is even more the 'eye and ear' of the therapist, s/he feels more motivation to notice his or her feelings and emotions and report on them, since the therapist cannot see part of the body.

Other therapists coped by asking the client to move away from the camera so that the therapist still could have a total body view, but then they had to pay the price of having a less clear view of the face area.

All therapists said that over time, they had learned to adjust to the new situation and none of the therapists felt that doing the therapy over Zoom or Skype had negatively affected the work of helping clients experiencing and expressing emotions.

Most therapists reported that observing bodily expressions of tension, feelings and emotions in this way, demanded more of their concentration than before and after each Zoom and Skype session, they had felt much more tired than before. The phenomenon of 'Zoom fatigue' has been described by different authors in different fields of expertise (c.f. Murphy, 2020).

Opening-Up of Clients

The degree to which clients were open and felt sufficiently comfortable to share their emotions and feelings was a function of several variables. For clients who had started therapy in the clinic or consulting room before the outbreak of COVID-19 and then continued on Zoom or Skype (or in a few cases other platforms) the passage from the clinic to teleconference was relatively easy, at least for those clients who were willing and interested to move to videoconferencing. Some clients stopped therapy once the therapist could not see them anymore in the clinic. A few other clients were willing to continue therapy, not by Zoom or Skype but by phone, without being seen or seeing the therapist. Most clients had no problem whatsoever being open and honest about their life, their feelings and emotions, and intimate details of their life. To the surprise of some therapists, a few clients said that they found it even easier to be open and honest about themselves than when they had been in the therapist's office. Also, some therapists said they had found it easier to face feelings of the client (like expressions of anger towards the therapist) than when they saw the client in the office clinic. The overall impression of the therapists was that Zoom and Skype therapy was as efficient and effective as the regular face-to-face therapy in the clinic. Yet, not surprisingly, most still preferred the direct personal contact they were used to before COVID-19.

Although the Israeli therapists interviewed for this article are not a representative sample, it is interesting to compare their impressions with 145 European and American therapists, whose attitudes and experiences were surveyed by Bekes and Aafjes van Doorn (2020). In the 2020 survey, psychodynamic therapists were less positive than CBT therapists about videoconferencing therapy. Overall, the therapists surveyed were somewhat insecure about the therapy and especially psychodynamic therapists questioned the effectiveness of the Zoom therapy compared to regular face-to-face therapy. They had doubts about the transference, therapeutic relationship, and emotional empathy; important factors in more psychodynamic-oriented therapies. The Israeli therapists were more enthusiastic. This could be explained by the fact that the Israeli therapists interviewed are EDT therapists. Videotaping plays a very important role in the training and supervision of EDT therapists. An integral part of their so called 'core training' is video recording their therapy session and getting supervision based upon watching the recorded session. Also watching the recorded session by themselves, with the guidance of checklists of variables to notice in the recorded therapy, is part of the training. This so-called 'deliberate practice' has become almost a standard of training in EDT and has proven to be a very effective form of supervision that improves the effectiveness of the therapist and therapy (see for example Rousmaniere, 2016).

An important research question is how ***clients*** experience videoconference-based therapy. Especially those clients who started therapy face-to-face and then because of COVID-19 had or wanted to continue therapy on Zoom or Skype. So far, we have not been able to find relevant published research on this issue.

Opening-Up of Therapists

For (us) therapists, the movement from in person sessions in our clinic to Zoom-sessions can maybe compared to a movement from three dimensions to two dimensions. Or from talking to someone while sitting opposite each other, face to face, with nothing in between us and talking with the other through a glass plate with the voice coming in through a microphone (sorry for the 'prison' association). Yes, the feeling is that something essential is lacking. The 'depth' of the interaction, which is very difficult to put into words. But there also are important gains. It is easier to carefully and closely observe what is going on in the client's non-verbal life, without embarrassing him or her too much. It is easier to make notes during a session. One can videotape the session, without having to use an external camera, which so often is experienced by clients as disturbing and an intrusion in the privacy of the session. And as mentioned before, for less internet and Zoom experienced therapists, sessions often offer a unique opportunity to model situations in which the therapist experiences difficult emotions, proving the famous expression that 'therapy is an interpersonal meeting of two souls who both have problems and experience complex emotions' (a variation on the words of Harry Stack Sullivan).

Zooming in on Post-COVID EDT: Conclusions

Based on research and experience so far, there is no reason to assume that internet-based EDT therapy is less effective than face-to-face, life therapy in the clinic or consulting room. That is, on the condition that both client and therapist feel comfortable enough with and agree to this setup and that both have good enough equipment for a smooth internet connection without disturbances in sound or sight.

The 'gut-feeling' of many therapists, and especially more psychodynamic-oriented therapists, is that in person-sessions are more effective than virtual sessions via Zoom or Skype, but the data and experiences of many therapists so far do not support the gut feelings. This is not to say that there is no difference in how one experiences a real life session versus a Zoom session. This is and will remain true, even if the 'objective data' show that there might be no significant differences between the outcome of therapy as measured by more objective and subjective data or even the 'acceptability' of internet-based therapy.

Maybe the difference between in person and internet-based EDT can be compared to the difference between a tasty meal at home or at a fancy restaurant. The meal and the food may be the same. They have the same caloric and health value. The food will be processed and prepared more or less in the same way and will have the same effect on the consumer's health. Still, depending on the preferences and economic status of the 'consumers', one may prefer home, the other the fancy restaurant.

The more the general public, clients, and therapists get used to internet-based therapy and the more comfortable they will feel with this medium, the more they will probably be willing to have and do therapy over Zoom or Skype, given external circumstances and logistics that will make this choice more and more probable and attractive. Many clients (and therapists!) have discovered the advantages of internet-based therapy in terms of time and distance. Where before COVID-19 they had to travel long distances and spent hours on the roads, now they can stay home and have therapy there. Of course, it is important to make sure that in any individual case there is a good match between the willingness of the client and therapist to opt for internet-based psychotherapy. This means that for the near future this kind of therapy should be an option and not become an obligatory standard.

Practical Considerations and Tips

- Since in EDT a central focus of the therapist is the way emotions and feelings are expressed at the body level, ideally the whole body of the client should be visible. So, best would be if the client (and therapist!) sat at some distance from the camera. If that is not possible, second best would be to have a clear picture of the head and shoulders of the client.
- Eye contact: in line with what was said above, direct eye contact is very important. Ideally speaking, the camera should be in the middle of the screen so that both client and therapist can look at each other and see each other. Although nowadays one can purchase mid-screen cameras, most therapists and clients probably will not yet buy those or know how to attach them. Therefore, second best is to find a solution in which the camera is as close to the screen picture of client and therapist is possible. Increasing the distance between the camera and the user can also help (due to the parallax effect).
- According to Murphy's Law 'If anything can go wrong, it will'. It is necessary to have a backup available that one can immediately use when something goes wrong in the connection between client and therapist (i.e., cellular phone, landline). Self-understood but worthwhile re-emphasizing: both sides need to have good quality cameras including good quality

microphones and speakers, a solid computer and good enough connections.

- Given the emphasis in EDT therapy on teaching the client to notice feelings and emotions as they appear here and now in the body, it is desirable to record sessions (with the written permission of the client) and to suggest to the client that he or she watches the session in between the Zoom-therapy sessions. At the beginning of a new session, the therapist should explicitly ask the client about his or her thoughts and feelings watching the recorded material.
- To prevent 'Zoom-fatigue', which has a negative effect on concentration, therapists should schedule somewhat shorter sessions than normally and leave more time in between sessions.
- As far as possible therapists should begin therapy with a face-to-face session in their clinic before moving on to video-conferencing sessions.
- Since the 'real relationship' is a crucial element of EDT and since also the emotions of the therapist as expressed in his body and on his face are a necessary part of the therapy, therapists should make sure that their clients can see them clearly. When recording sessions by Zoom (which is easy to do) they should record in such a way that their picture will appear next to the one of the client.
- Since it is easy to record sessions, there is an excellent opportunity to get a copy of the session and in between sessions review the session and reflect on what was said and how both therapist and client reacted non-verbally. To my surprise, in my practice, very few clients used this opportunity and even if they received a copy on their request, did not 'do' the homework they had said they wanted to do, i.e., they never watched the session.

Last, but not least, it is advisable to see to it that, as a therapist, one has in-person sessions and not only Zoom sessions, even if Zoom-therapy turns out to be as effective as in-person therapy. As therapists we also have to take care of our own mental and physical health and in order to prevent burn out and Zoom fatigue, we would do well to now and then also be in the three dimensional space of two bodies who can see, hear and smell (yes … smell) each other. Zoom can do a lot, but communication of body-odors is a vision for the future.

References

Békés, V., & Aafjes-van Doorn, K. (2020). Psychotherapists' attitudes toward online therapy during the COVID-19 pandemic. *Journal of Psychotherapy Integration, 30*(2), 238. https://psycnet.apa.org/doi/10.1037/int0000214

Berryhill, M. B., Halli-Tierney, A., Culmer, N., Williams, N., Betancourt, A., King, M., & Ruggles, H. (2019). Videoconferencing psychological therapy and anxiety: A systematic review. *Family Practice, 36*(1), 53–63. 10.1089/tmj.2018.0058

Carlbring, P., Andersson, G., Cuijpers, P., Riper, H., & Hedman-Lagerlöf, E. (2018). Internet-based vs. face-to-face cognitive behavior therapy for psychiatric and somatic disorders: An updated systematic review and meta-analysis. *Cognitive Behaviour Therapy, 47*(1), 1–18. 10.1080/16506073.2017.140111

Davanloo, H. (1995). *Unlocking the Unconscious*. Wiley.

Derdikman Eiron, R. (2021). Play therapy for children inspired by experiential dynamic therapy (EDT). *Journal of Infant, Child, and Adolescent Psychotherapy*, 1–16. 10.1080/15289168.2021.1912535

Evans III, F. B. (2006). *Harry Stack Sullivan: Interpersonal Theory and Psychotherapy*. Routledge.

Johansson, R., Frederick, R. J., & Andersson, G. (2013). Using the internet to provide psychodynamic psychotherapy. *Psychodynamic psychiatry, 41*(4), 513–540. 10.7717/peerj.102

Lilliengren, P., Johansson, R., Lindqvist, K., Mechler, J., & Andersson, G. (2016). Efficacy of experiential dynamic therapy for psychiatric conditions: A meta-analysis of randomized controlled trials. *Psychotherapy, 53*(1), 90. 10.1037/pst0000024

Lindegaard, T., Hesslow, T., Nilsson, M., Johansson, R., Carlbring, P., Lilliengren, P., & Andersson, G. (2020). Internet-based psychodynamic therapy vs cognitive behavioural therapy for social anxiety disorder: A preference study. *Internet Interventions, 20*, 100316. 10.1016/j.invent.2020.100316

Malan, D. (1995). *Individual Psychotherapy and the Science of Psychodynamics*. Taylor and Francis.

McCullough, L. (1997). *Changing Character*. Basic Books.

Murphy, K. (2020). Why zoom is terrible. *The New York Times, 23*. https://nyti.ms/35hnfN7

Osimo, F. (2003). *Experiential Short-Term Dynamic Psychotherapy: A Manual*. 1st Book Library.

Osimo, F., & Stein, M. J. (Eds.). (2018). *Theory and Practice of Experiential Dynamic Psychotherapy*. Routledge.

Rousmaniere, T. (2016). *Deliberate Practice for Psychotherapists: A Guide to Improving Clinical Effectiveness*. Taylor & Francis.

12 Online-IPT – Not Necessarily a Second Best

Brunstein Klomek Anat and Anaelle Benistri

Interpersonal Psychotherapy (IPT)

IPT is a structured, time-limited manualized therapy that was originally developed for the treatment of depression (Cuijpers et al., 2016; Klerman & Weissman, 1994). IPT is based on the principle that symptoms such as depression occur within an interpersonal context, therefore the intervention focuses on symptomatic recovery while helping patients improve the quality of their relationships (Weissman et al., 2017). IPT's primary interpersonal thrust and focal strategies are inherently trans-diagnostic, therefore it has been used to treat a wide range of disorders (Cuijpers et al., 2016; Lipsitz & Markowitz, 2013).

The foundation of IPT is based on attachment theory and interpersonal theory making it relevant and useful for people in all cultures around the world (Klerman et al., 1974). The theoretical basis of IPT is rooted in the assumption that humans are inherently relational and develop patterns of connecting to others in varying attachment styles (Bowlby, 1969). These attachment styles influence expectations one has about his or her relationships as well as how these attachment needs are communicated and are likely to be responded to by others. According to the basic premise of IPT, psychological distress is related to problems in relational functioning; challenges in interpersonal relationships may cause direct psychopathology and psychological distress. At the same time, psychopathology and psychological distress interfere with adaptive interpersonal functioning. Therefore, IPT serves to address both interpersonal functioning and psychopathology/emotional distress. Other therapy modalities all deal with interpersonal aspects but IPT has a unique focus on that, combined with associated emotional components.

Generally, IPT includes 12 to 16 acute treatment sessions. It consists of four fundamental treatment phases: initial, middle, termination, and maintenance. Across the four phases, the primary goals of treatment are to reduce psychological symptoms, improve interpersonal functioning, and learn about the association and interaction between one's symptoms and his or her interpersonal functioning. One of the IPT unique aspects is its focus on a problems area (or a few of them). The problem area is formulated at the end of the initial phase and then worked on during the middle phase. The problem areas

DOI: 10.4324/9781003205029-15

will be described below. The middle phase of IPT includes learning and practicing skills within the problem area. The termination phase includes summarizing the process, focusing, on relapse prevention and discussing the need for future therapy. In the adolescent adaptation of IPT (IPT-A; Mufson et al., 2004), work with parents and school staff is incorporated into treatment. IPT has proven efficacy across multiple randomized controlled trials (RCTs) (Cuijpers et al., 2011).

Online IPT

IPT has advanced dramatically, with one of its key developments being the ability to deliver it online (Bennett, 2020). There is growing evidence for its online use (indicated below). Further, current consensus guidelines prescribe IPT as a recommended treatment (e.g., World Health Organization, 2010).

Phases of Online IPT

Initial Phase

The unique elements of online-IPT in each phase of the treatment are described in Table 12.1. In the initial phase of IPT, the clinician works to establish a collaborative, online working alliance with the patient while assessing that patient's psychological symptoms, current social support, relational problems, and communication patterns. This phase aims to achieve three main goals: 1) evaluation of the patient's psychopathology/distress and examination of his or her Interpersonal Inventory – a thorough review of the patient's past and current relationships; 2) conceptualizing and formulating the problem area which guides the focus of treatment, providing the patient with the "sick role" (Parsons, 1951); and 3) receiving the patient's agreement on the treatment plan (Lipsitz & Markowitz, 2013).

The initial phase of online-IPT includes thorough assessment of the patient's psychopathology, including suicide risk assessment when needed (Stanley et al., 2020). The Interpersonal Inventory, which is conducted in the initial phase, is also easy to administer online; one can use a white board to draw closeness circles (explained in the next sentences) and start the Interpersonal Inventory. The closeness circles are a graphic representation of the patients' significant relationships. The circles are drawn by therapist and patient together in a way that the patient's name is in the middle circle and his or her significant others are written according to their level of significance to the patient. The instructions are to place the person on the circle in a way that will represent how significant this person is for the patient, with their influence being either negative or positive. After outlining them on the white board, the patient and therapist can begin discussing each of the significant others the patient indicated as part of the Interpersonal Inventory. Using the closeness circles and the interpersonal inventory helps the therapist identify the patient's

Table 12.1 The unique elements of online-IPT in each stages of the treatment

Fundamental Treatment Phases on IPT	Classical Stages on IPT	The Unique Efforts and Possibilities that the Online Work Demands and Allows in Online-IPT
Initial Sessions	Diagnosis and sick role	The therapist can send the patient's self-report questionnaire via e-mail or do an online semi-structure interview. The assessment of the sick role can be performed via messaging using the chat tool. A family member can join the assessment via video conference.
	Detailed assessment of the interpersonal environment	The closeness circle can be drawn on a shared white board followed by the Interpersonal Inventory. The therapist assesses the significant others that were written on the white board.
	Relate depression to the interpersonal context: focus selection	The therapist can refer to the figure of a dynamic model between interpersonal aspects and depression symptoms via a shared screen. Interpersonal ⟲ Depression
	Formulation and contract setting	The formulation can be provided as a recorded session or as a document that was written on a shared interactive document. The treatment contract should include the online setting such as how to deal with technical challenges and privacy.

(Continued)

Table 12.1 (Continued)

Fundamental Treatment Phases on IPT	Classical Stages on IPT	The Unique Efforts and Possibilities that the Online Work Demands and Allows in Online-IPT
Middle Sessions	Interpersonal Role Transition	In a session discussing the positive and negative aspect of the new role, the therapist can open a table and write the different aspects in a shared document.
	Interpersonal Role Dispute	In an online session of a role dispute, the therapist can suggest an interactive role play session in which he switches roles and practices interpersonal challenges. When conducting communication analyses, the patient can easily access and share social media conversations. Therapist and patient can also summarize the maladaptive communication patterns in a shared document. Therapist can display the written Teen Tips used in IPT via the chat tool so he can practice together with the patient in real time during the session. It is also relatively easy to add a family member and get a joint analysis of the dispute.
	Grief	Using digital emotional cards, the patient can better accept and express negative emotions.
	Interpersonal Deficits	Decision analyses in various social situations can be done using the written stages that the patients can follow via a shared screen. Therapist can also show examples of video vignettes, so the patients realize that in different social situations there are various options to react.
Final Sessions: Termination	Review the course of treatment and progress with the patient	Therapist and patient can summarize in writing the progress and achievement of the therapy in a shared document. The online writing and editing strengthens the collaborative aspect.
	Evaluate the treatment and assess future needs	Writing the summary in the shared document should include points to work on.
	Assess early warning signs and discuss procedures for re-entry into treatment if necessary	A relapse prevention plan can be jointly writing. Family members can easily join the online meeting.

interpersonal patterns and interpersonal/emotional issues that may be causing the depression/psychopathology or worsening his or her symptoms.

At the end of the initial phase, a problem area is collaboratively formulated so that patient and therapist agree on what they should focus on during the middle phase of treatment. The interpersonal problem area formulation identifies factors that cause and maintain the psychopathology and provides a rationale for treatment by emphasizing the role of interpersonal and emotional factors.

There are four problem areas in online-IPT: grief, interpersonal disputes, role transitions, and interpersonal deficits. The work in these four problem areas is equivalent to offline IPT except for the delivery format.

1   Grief – is chosen in IPT when the onset of major depressive disorder coincides with an actual death, or an anniversary event related to the death of a significant other. IPT facilitates grieving and examination of the positive and negative aspects of the relationship with the lost loved one in order to achieve a more realistic view of the person and the patient's relationship with him or her. In the middle phase, patients are encouraged to replace aspects of what was lost in the relationship and begin moving forward in their lives. In online-IPT patients often show pictures or other objects of the deceased from their house.

2   Interpersonal disputes – Interpersonal disputes are the main problem area when there is a serious conflict between the patient and a significant other that is causing the patient's distress. Often these are challenges in the relationships with close family members (e.g., a parent and a teen) that tend to be characterized by poor communication and/or unrealistic expectations. Interpersonal and emotional patterns are often revealed, elucidating how the patient frequently interacts with the significant other in a non-adaptive manner. The therapist and patient examine communication patterns within relationships in order to facilitate more adaptive interpersonal paradigms. In online-IPT, just as in offline, the therapist can offer a significant other to join the sessions and encourages the patient to employ various IPT techniques (see below) to address the patient's miscommunication with this person.

3   Role transitions – refer to the problem area when there is a major life event that leads to interpersonal changes. Examples might include divorce, receiving a medical diagnosis, moving, changing jobs, going to college, retiring etc. The tasks of the therapy in this problem area involve exploring both positive and negative aspects of the old role in addition to examining the difficulties and opportunities of the new role.

4   Interpersonal deficits- this problem area is formulated when the patient lacks interpersonal and social skills. This problem area does not include a specific life event as defined in the above problem areas. The patients' social deficits are associated with the onset, exacerbation, or perpetuation of current symptoms. The aim of this problem area is to help the patient

connect with social supports and improve the quality of his or her relationships. A therapist examines these interpersonal deficits in the online relationship that they establish.

Middle Phase

The middle phase of IPT is easily conducted online since IPT is a skills-based intervention. The patient and therapist discuss the issue the patient is presenting by connecting it to the problem area and using a range of IPT techniques to improve and practice emotional and interpersonal skills to address it. Below we describe the main IPT techniques, which are employed online. Online-IPT also enables significant others to become part of treatment sessions via video conferencing. This is commonly used in online- IPT-A when the therapist offers the parents and adolescent to meet jointly in one or more of the sessions, so they can learn and practice together. Adolescents and parents can sit in front of the same camera or use different cameras, depending on their needs and desires. Each IPT session starts with a brief review of how things have been going since the last session as well as self-monitoring of the symptoms.

Communication analysis is one of the most common techniques of IPT. Communication analysis focuses on helping patients develop awareness of their communication patterns, particularly those which are maladaptive. Patients develop more effective ways of communicating by learning new communication skills and strategies and practicing these in role-play exercises and home experiments. The patient is encouraged to adopt realistic expectations for their relationships. When conducted offline or online, the therapist asks the patient to describe a specific argument or fight and to report the details of the interaction (e.g., verbal and nonverbal communications, feelings generated and responses given). This may be done by writing on a white board, via the chat tool or by watching the argument itself using the "share screen" tool if it occurred on social media. The patient and therapist jointly review the goals of the communication and assess whether these goals were achieved. They discuss what was intended to be communicated as well as what he or she thinks/feels was communicated. During this process, the therapist can also educate the patient about the nature of ineffective communication styles (e.g., using hostile communication, which leads to either hostile or passive responses from those with whom they are interacting) so that he or she is more aware of these in future interactions. In addition, the therapist can teach and practice alternative, more adaptive communication strategies with the patient. The various strategies include communicating feelings, expectations and opinions directly and clearly without blame; clarifying misperceptions made by the other communication partner; seeing the other person's point of view and using empathy appropriately; communicating when calm rather than when angry; and making use of "I" statements to express one's feelings (Mufson et al., 2004).

Decision analysis is another IPT technique which can easily be conducted online. In a decision analysis, the patient learns to make decisions that are associated with the patient's interpersonal problem area. The therapist's role is to help the patient consider a range of alternative actions that can be taken and to assess the possible consequences associated with each of those actions. Decision analysis is composed of multiple steps, which can be presented to the patient in a shared document so that the patient and therapist can review it together. The patient can use this shared document in management of on-going interpersonal situations during the week (i.e., between treatment sessions). The general steps involved in decision analysis are to: identify the decision that needs to be made; determine a goal; generate a list of alternative actions; evaluate the options by thoroughly examining their consequences; select and implement the best available option; and, lastly, to evaluate the outcome and potential need to select a second option (Mufson et al., 2004).

Emotional work in online-IPT includes fostering skills that increase emotional awareness, developing acceptance of negative emotions, cultivating emotion regulation, etc. Encouragement and exploration of affect in IPT refers to a range of techniques used to help the patient express, explore, and understand the nature of their emotions (Mufson et al., 2004). The therapist can facilitate this process by normalizing the experience of negative emotions, helping the patient identify, acknowledge and accept painful affective states, as well as encouraging the patient's development of new, desirable affects that may facilitate change and growth. While some patients' may need minimal training in identifying their emotional states, others may require substantial therapeutic support (Mufson et al., 2004). The emotional work can be done using emotion cards (Mufson et al., 2004). Emotion cards are cards which each have a different type of emotion written on it. These cards can be digital and permit to assist the patient in identifying his or her emotions and learning how to deal with them. Patients may use emotion cards to master how to communicate one's emotions to others and how to regulate them, so they do not act on them impulsively.

Role plays are practiced online by the patient and the therapist in almost every IPT middle-phase session. They are usually performed to rehearse agreed-upon topics discussed during the sessions. Within an online role play, patients can perform a challenging conversation with the therapist in a safe, risk-free environment. During role plays, the therapist attempts to challenge the patient, so he or she will be prepared to successfully manage similar situations in life between sessions. During online sessions, the therapist can provide feedback by writing it in the chat. In addition, the therapist may often record part of the session so that they can analyze it together as well as let the patient watch it and practice between sessions. An important aspect of role play in IPT is expressing one's feelings or needs to the therapist as if he were the significant other that the patient experiences difficulties with.

Home experiments between sessions should be agreed upon in online-IPT. Patients are encouraged to practice techniques learned in treatment during the time between the meetings. Interpersonal experiments should be developed by the clinician and patient based on situations and skills that are practiced in the session. The emphasis should not be on failure or success of these experiments, but rather on venturing and attempting the incorporation of interpersonal skills learned and discovering what happens when the interaction is or is not attempted.

In IPT, the therapeutic relationship functions as a mini laboratory, by providing both an example of the patient's relationships and a place in which skills can be practiced and feedback is provided. The therapist often links what happens in the session to similar patterns that occur in the patient's other relationships and models direct communication between two people about their feelings. For example, the therapist can demonstrate in session that expressing negative feelings within a relationship can improve the quality of the relationship, even when it's not easy. In the online world after the exposure to COVID-19, examining the online interactions with the therapist can assist in understanding the online interactions the patient has with others in his/her world.

Termination Phase

The termination phase of online-IPT includes a review of the therapeutic gains as well as relapse prevention planning. Relapse prevention includes psychoeducation that normative sadness is different from clinical depression as well as an identification of interpersonal challenges that may trigger depression in the future. The therapist models direct communication, which includes discussion of the feelings associated with the ending of therapy and what aspects of treatment did not work as expected. Further, it is crucial to consider the need for further treatment; therapy may be extended, or the patient may be referred to a different form of treatment (e.g., an offline intervention may be recommended).

Lastly, treatment should include a maintenance phase. This phase generally consists of sessions that occur post-acute treatment. Initially, these should occur bimonthly. Later, monthly sessions may suffice for maintenance of care. The aim of this phase is to maintain recovery from the previous symptoms, prevent recurrence of new symptoms, reduce the risk of suicide when relevant, and promote psychosocial functioning.

Studies on Online-IPT

Existing research on the efficacy of online-IPT is limited. Future studies, particularly RCTs of IPT via technology platforms (e.g., mobile- and internet-based programs) are needed. Another alternative to traditional, face-to-face IPT, is IPT delivered by telephone, a format that has been found to be considerably effective in depression (Mohr et al., 2008). Below is a review of available studies evaluating contemporary formats of delivering IPT (i.e., by online or mobile platforms).

Donker and colleagues (2013a) examined the efficacy of a fully self-guided internet-delivered IPT compared to an online version of cognitive behavioral therapy (CBT). The internet based IPT intervention consisted of the four problem areas mentioned above and a personal workbook (containing 13 different exercises and assessments). The internet delivered IPT was performed completely independently, without the guidance and assistance of a therapist. The various modules of the intervention and the practice exercises were displayed on the left side of the screen in an accessible manner so that it was easy for patients to navigate between the various topics. The online intervention included illustrations showing examples of social interactions and of thoughts that participants may experience in each case. The authors demonstrated a significant reduction in depressive symptoms posttreatment and at 6-month follow-up for both CBT and IPT (Donker et al., 2013a). A follow-up study (Donker et al., 2013b) found that younger participants (16–24) who received IPT made greater improvements in depression scores that those who were treated with online-CBT.

Dagöö and colleagues (2014) developed an IPT treatment for social anxiety disorder adapted for mobile phone administration. Unlike face-to-face IPT, participants worked with all four problem areas described earlier. The intervention consisted of nine modules. Participants could not practice with a therapist and were encouraged to role-play problematic situations with a close friend. The authors found this mobile-based version of IPT for social anxiety disorder led statistically significant improvements in social anxiety symptoms (Dagöö et al., 2014).

In addition, project CATCH-IT is an internet-based preventive intervention for depression for adolescents in primary care (Landback et al., 2009). This intervention consisted of 14 modules based on behavioral activation, CBT and IPT. In the IPT component of the intervention, adolescents learned to identify and manage difficult relationships and life transitions as well as strengthen social support in family, school, and peer settings. Each module began with a summary of the previous module as well as specific learning goals for the current module. Each module lesson included "teen stories," skill building exercises, and behavior change assignments. At the completion of each module, patients received an internet-based "reward" (Landback et al., 2009). CATCH-IT was found to be associated with declines in depressed mood (Gladstone et al., 2018; Van Voorhees et al., 2009).

In addition, several telephone-IPT (tele-IPT) studies have also demonstrated promising results. In a large RCT, postpartum women with major depression were randomly assigned to 12 weekly 60-minute nurse-delivered tele-IPT sessions or standard locally available care (Dennis et al., 2020). The tele-IPT intervention included the first three phases of IPT and the content of the sessions was similar to treatment administered face-to-face. Study results indicated that depressive symptoms, attachment avoidance, and comorbid anxiety decreased more so than the control group (Dennis et al., 2020). These findings are in line with Posmontier and colleagues' study (2016).

In addition, a recent RCT tested whether tele-IPT acutely relieved depressive symptoms in a diverse sample of individuals suffering from HIV and depression (Heckman et al., 2017). Patients who participated in the nine sessions of individual tele-IPT reported significantly lower depressive symptoms and interpersonal problems than controls who received standard, usual care (Heckman et al., 2017). Similarly, Neugebauer and colleagues (2007) showed a decline in depressive symptoms in an open trial among miscarrying women after receiving one to six weekly sessions of manualized, telephone-administered interpersonal counseling (IPC), a variant of IPT. Recently, Kobak and Lipsitz (2017) have developed the first empirically validated comprehensive internet therapist training program for IPT. Their findings support the efficacy and feasibility of employing technology in training clinicians in performing IPT.

Practical Tips and Consideration

IPT can be easily conducted online. The online therapist should know the IPT manual and have experience in online therapy. The online therapist should be able to administer all four treatment phases of the original IPT model as well as implementation of all its relevant therapeutic techniques. The therapist needs to ensure that in each technique delivered online there is also online role playing and home experiments. In addition, family members should be involved online, as we would do offline. The major consideration to take is that although research demonstrates promising results for the efficacy of online IPT, the literature on online-IPT is modest.

References

Bennett, C. B., Ruggero, C. J., Sever, A. C., & Yanouri, L. (2020). eHealth to redress psychotherapy access barriers both new and old: A review of reviews and meta-analyses. *Journal of Psychotherapy Integration, 30*(2), 188–207. 10.1037/int0000217

Bowlby, J. (1969). *Attachment and Loss: Vol. 1.* Basic Books.

Cuijpers, P., Donker, T.,Weissman, M. M., Ravitz, P., & Cristea, I. A. (2016). Interpersonal psychotherapy for mental health problems: A comprehensive meta-analysis. *American Journal of Psychiatry, 173*(7), 680–687. 10.1176/appi.ajp.2015.15091141

Cuijpers, P., Geraedts, A. S., van Oppen, P., Andersson, G., Markowitz, J. C., & van Straten, A. (2011). Interpersonal psychotherapy for depression: A meta-analysis. *American Journal of Psychiatry, 168*(6), 581–592. 10.1176/appi.ajp.2010.10101411

Dagöö, J., Asplund, R. P., Bsenko, H. A., Hjerling, S., Holmberg, A., Westh, S., Öberg, L., Ljótsson, B., Carlbring, P., Furmark, T., & Andersson, G. (2014). Cognitive behavior therapy versus interpersonal psychotherapy for social anxiety disorder delivered via smartphone and computer: A randomized controlled trial. *Journal of Anxiety Disorders, 28*(4), 410–417. 10.1016/j.janxdis.2014.02.003

Dennis, C. L., Grigoriadis, S., Zupancic, J., Kiss, A., & Ravitz, P. (2020). Telephone-based nurse-delivered interpersonal psychotherapy for postpartum depression: Nationwide randomised controlled trial. *The British Journal of Psychiatry, 216*(4), 189–196. 10.1192/bjp.2019.275

Donker, T., Bennett, K., Bennett, A., Mackinnon, A., van Straten, A., Cuijpers, P., Christensen, H., & Griffiths, K. M. (2013a). Internet-delivered interpersonal psychotherapy versus internet-delivered cognitive behavioral therapy for adults with depressive symptoms: Randomized controlled noninferiority trial. *Journal of Medical Internet Research, 15*(5), e82. 10.2196/jmir.2307

Donker, T., Batterham, P. J., Warmerdam, L., Bennett, K., Bennett, A., Cuijpers, P., Griffiths, K. M., & Christensen, H. (2013b). Predictors and moderators of response to internet-delivered interpersonal psychotherapy and cognitive behavior therapy for depression. *Journal of Affective Disorders, 151*(1), 343–351. 10.1016/j.jad.2013.06.020

Gladstone, T. R., Terrizzi, D. A., Paulson, A., Nidetz, J., Canel, J., Ching, E., ... & Van Voorhees, B. W. (2018). Effect of internet-based cognitive behavioral humanistic and interpersonal training vs internet-based general health education on adolescent depression in primary care: A randomized clinical trial. *JAMA Network Open, 1*(7), e184278–e184278. 10.1001/jamanetworkopen.2018.4278

Heckman, T. G., Heckman, B. D., Anderson, T., Lovejoy, T. I., Markowitz, J. C., Shen, Y., & Sutton, M. (2017). Tele-interpersonal psychotherapy acutely reduces depressive symptoms in depressed HIV-infected rural persons: A randomized clinical trial. *Behavioral Medicine, 43*(4), 285–295. 10.1080/08964289.2016.1160025

Klerman, G. L., Dimascio, A., Weissman, M., Prusoff, B., & Paykel, E. S. (1974). Treatment of depression by drugs and psychotherapy. *American Journal of Psychiatry, 131*(2), 186–191. 10.1176/ajp.131.2.186

Klerman, G. L., & Weissman, M. M. (1994). *Interpersonal Psychotherapy of Depression: A brief, focused, specific strategy.* Jason Aronson, Incorporated.

Kobak, K. A., Lipsitz, J. D., Markowitz, J. C., & Bleiberg, K. L. (2017). Web-based therapist training in interpersonal psychotherapy for depression: Pilot Study. *Journal of Medical Internet Research, 19*(7), e257. 10.2196/jmir.7966

Landback, J., Prochaska, M., Ellis, J., Dmochowska, K., Kuwabara, S. A., Gladstone, T., Larson, J., Stuart S., Gollan, J., Bell, C., Bradford, N., Reinecke, M., Fogel, J., & Van Voorhees, B. W. (2009). From prototype to product: Development of a primary care/internet-based depression prevention intervention for adolescents (CATCH-IT). *Community Mental Health Journal, 45*(5), 349–354. 10.1007/s10597-009-9226-3

Lipsitz, J. D., & Markowitz, J. C. (2013). Mechanisms of change in interpersonal therapy (IPT). *Clinical Psychology Review, 33*(8), 1134–1147. 10.1016/j.cpr.2013.09.002

Mohr, D. C., Vella, L., Hart, S., Heckman, T., & Simon, G. (2008). The effect of telephone-administered psychotherapy on symptoms of depression and attrition: A meta-analysis. *Clinical Psychology: Science and Practice, 15*(3), 243–253. 10.1111/j.1468-2850.2008.00134.x

Mufson, L. H., Dorta, K. P., Moreau, D., & Weissman, M. M. (2004). *Interpersonal Psychotherapy for Depressed Adolescents (2nd ed.).* Guilford Press.

Neugebauer, R., Kline, J., Bleiberg, K., Baxi, L., Markowitz, J. C., Rosing, M., Levin, B., & Keith, J. (2007). Preliminary open trial of interpersonal counseling for subsyndromal depression following miscarriage. *Depression and Anxiety, 24*(3), 219–222. 10.1002/da.20150

Parsons, T. (1951). *The Social System.* Routledge & Kegan Paul.

Posmontier, B., Neugebauer, R., Stuart, S., Chittams, J., & Shaughnessy, R. (2016). Telephone-administered interpersonal psychotherapy by Nurse-Midwives for postpartum depression. *Journal of Midwifery & Women's Health, 61*(4), 456–466. 10.1111/jmwh.12411

Stanley, B., Brodsky, B., Labouliere, C. Telehealth tips: Managing suicidal clients during the COVID-19 pandemic. *Center for Practice Innovations at Columbia Psychiatry and the New York State Psychiatric Institute.* Retrieved March 25, 2020, from https://practiceinnovations.org/I-want-to-learn-about/Suicide-Prevention

Van Voorhees, B. W., Fogel, J., Reinecke, M. A., Gladstone, T., Stuart, S., Gollan, J., ... & Bell, C. (2009). Randomized clinical trial of an Internet-based depression prevention program for adolescents (Project CATCH-IT) in primary care: Twelve-week outcomes. *Journal of Developmental and Behavioral Pediatrics: JDBP, 30*(1), 23. 10.1097/DBP.0b013e3181966c2a

Weissman, M. M., Markowitz, J. C., & Klerman, G. L. (2017). *The Guide to Interpersonal Psychotherapy: Updated and Expanded Edition.* Oxford University Press.

World Health Organization (2010). *mhGAP Intervention Guide for Mental, Neurological and Substance Use Disorders in Non-Specialized Health Settings: Mental Health Gap Action Programme (mhGAP).* World Health Organization.

13 Online EMDR Therapy in the COVID-19 Era and Beyond

Udi Oren and Isabelle Meignant

The COVID-19 pandemic has proven to be not only a life threatening global event, but also one that has had a major psychological impact on millions of people around the world. The fact that many individuals experienced anxiety, depression, loneliness, and post-traumatic symptoms, led to a greater need for psychological services. Demand for therapeutic support increased, yet at the same time, the feasibility of meeting clients in-person dropped drastically. For this reason, many therapists began offering psychotherapy online. One group facing this challenge was that of therapists practicing Eye Movement Desensitization and Reprocessing (EMDR) Therapy. This chapter will introduce the reader to EMDR Therapy and to the Adaptive Information Processing (AIP) Model. It will review the literature regarding the current provision of online EMDR Therapy and make clinical recommendations for its use.

The Adaptive Information Processing (AIP) Model

The AIP model is the theoretical framework that guides EMDR's clinical practice (Shapiro, 2001). It is a model that focuses on the development of both human health and human pathology, as well as explaining how change occurs (or fails to occur) within life in general and in the context of psychotherapy. Shapiro (2002) sees AIP as "an inherent system in all of us that is physiologically geared to process information to a state of mental health". While AIP is a psychological model, it is also clearly rooted within the body, suggesting that sensory, cognitive, emotional, and somatic information is processed in the brain and integrated into the memory system. The system is seen as adaptive, since in normal functioning it is able to learn from the information to support human growth and development. The relevant sensory, cognitive, emotional, and somatic information is stored in memory networks that will be used to adaptively guide the person's reactions to experiences in the future.

Some events seem to overwhelm the AIP system and thus prevent their adaptive assimilation. Unprocessed memories contain the disturbing emotions, physical sensations, and perspectives experienced at the time of the event. These events are at times significant traumas, but more often are daily negative events that people may experience, such as humiliations, rejections, failures, etc. When

DOI: 10.4324/9781003205029-16

these memories are formed, the information regarding the negative event is maladaptively encoded and is unable to connect with the adaptive memory networks. Present-day situations may then trigger the earlier memory, causing the person to experience some or all of its sensory, cognitive, emotional, and somatic aspects. This results in maladaptive or symptomatic behavior. The AIP model views negative beliefs, behaviors, and personality characteristics as resulting from maladaptively processed memories (Shapiro, 2001). From this perspective, a negative self-belief (e.g., "I am stupid"), a negative emotional reaction (e.g., fear in the presence of an authority figure), and a negative somatic reaction (e.g., stomach pain before an exam), are symptoms rather than causes of current problems. Instead, the causes are seen as the memories of unprocessed life events that are activated in the present. This view of psychological pathology is the theoretical core of EMDR Therapy and guides the clinician in understanding the client, forming a treatment plan, and building therapeutic interventions. It is possible to integrate the AIP model with the concept of pathogenic memories (Centonze et al., 2005) which can be seen as the basis for understanding mental and psychosomatic disorders (Hase et al., 2017). EMDR Therapy provides tools to target these memories and reprocess them, leading to long-lasting change.

One of EMDR Therapy's reprocessing tools is bi-lateral stimulation (BLS). This includes visual BLS (helping the client move their eyes from side to side), auditory BLS (making sounds in alternate sides of their head), and tactile BLS (tapping alternate hands/knees/shoulders).

Eye Movement Desensitization and Reprocessing (EMDR) Therapy

EMDR Therapy is a trans-diagnostic, comprehensive, integrative, and flexible psychotherapy approach which is guided by the AIP Model. While being an evidence-based psychotherapy for PTSD (World Health Organization, 2013), it also has scientific support as a treatment for affective disorders, anxiety disorders, chronic pain, and addictions(Valiente-Gómez et al., 2017). Recently EMDR Therapy has been found to be the most cost-effective treatment for PTSD in adults (Mavranezouli et al., 2020).

The eight phase "Standard EMDR Protocol" (Shapiro, 2001) addresses and processes (1) memories of past events that are seen as the foundation of current patterns of difficulties and dysfunction; (2) current stimuli that trigger these patterns and lead to their activation; (3) imagined templates of appropriate future responses to triggers. The eight phases of the protocol will be described later in the chapter, with specific recommendations for use in an online format.

Online EMDR Therapy

EMDR Therapy, as other forms of therapy, has been used for years in online settings. There are many reasons for delivering therapy in an online capacity rather than in-person. These include: geographical distance between client and therapist, the opportunity to continue therapy when a client or therapist relocates, clients' wish to be in therapy with a therapist who speaks their mother tongue, personal circumstances that limit the client's ability to travel, and access to a therapist with the desired specialty. The COVID-19 pandemic compelled people to isolate, preventing social contact for long stretches of time. This gave a great boost to the delivery of online therapy and EMDR online therapy specifically. Both therapists and clients who would never have previously considered online work, found themselves open to it. The use of online EMDR Therapy grew exponentially, with many training workshops offered to clinicians to support the change. This period also saw the development of specific online platforms for the use of EMDR Therapy (e.g., remotEMDR, activeEMDR). These platforms enabled therapists and clients to have online interactions (visual and auditory), while also providing options for visual and auditory bilateral stimulation. In addition, multiple EMDR Therapy apps and computer programs were developed.

Two of the major issues that arose during this rapid growth of online EMDR Therapy, were the safety and effectiveness of this format (Fisher, 2021). These questions were raised despite the fact that multiple meta–analyses indicated that face-to-face and online therapies had similar clinical outcomes and user satisfaction (Simpson & Reid, 2014; Varker et al., 2019). TF-CBT (Trauma-Focused Cognitive Behavioral Therapy) and EMDR Therapy have been found to have similar outcomes in multiple studies (de Jongh et al., 2019) and since online TF-CBT has been found to be effective (Acierno et al., 2017), one could surmise that online EMDR Therapy would be effective too.

Several studies have looked at the questions of safety and effectiveness of online EMDR. One should keep in mind that all these studies were published during the 2020–2021 COVID-19 period and that each study has significant limitations.

Of the studies carried out to date, none have evaluated a full online EMDR Therapy process. All the studies have used populations suffering from Acute Stress Disorder (ASD) or Post Traumatic Stress Disorder (PTSD). They have used AIP/EMDR based protocols that were developed specifically for acute interventions (Black et al., 2021, Perri et al., 2021; Perez et al., 2020; Smyth-Dent et al., 2021; Tarquinio et al., 2020). Many of the studies used group EMDR protocols for acute situations (Perez et al., 2020; Smyth-Dent et al., 2021), and all the studies used short interventions, with many of them having only one therapy session (Yael et al., 2021; Smyth-Dent et al., 2021). None of the studies investigated the use of online EMDR Therapy with children and adolescents.

Despite these limitations, the outcomes of these studies point in only one direction: online EMDR Therapy is safe and effective. The results of the different interventions showed a significant reduction in the level of disturbance associated with the target memories that were processed and reduction in symptoms of PTSD, anxiety, and depression. The results were maintained at follow-up (up to 90 days post treatment), in both individual and group online EMDR Therapy interventions.

Several studies looked specifically at computerized EMDR Therapy interventions (Moench & Billsten, 2021; Nakano, 2013, 2015), while others applied self-help procedures based on the AIP model and EMDR Therapy (Karadag et al., 2021; Maxfield, 2021; Spence et al., 2013). All of them reported positive results.

Recommendations for the Use of Online EMDR Therapy During the COVID-19 Pandemic

During 2020, guidelines for the implementation of online EMDR Therapy during the COVID-19 epidemic (and beyond) were released. These were published by both the EMDR Europe Association (EMDR Europe) which acts as an umbrella organization for over 30 national EMDR associations (EMDR Europe, 2020), as well as by the EMDR International Association (EMDRIA), the EMDR association in the U.S. (Rollins et al., 2020).

EMDR Europe took a position based on existing research, stating that it is not possible to conclude whether or not there are any differences between in-person and online EMDR therapy. In accordance with anecdotal evidence, their guidelines recommended the use of online EMDR therapy following the standard EMDR therapy protocol with all clients (children, adults, ongoing clients, or new clients) who are appropriately assessed. In addition, they suggested that the association's members consider using EMDR Therapy protocols that are specific to crisis situations and those that focus on enhancing internal resources. Therapists were also asked to apply caution when working with complex clients. They were urged to follow the EMDR Europe Code of Ethics, as well as national regulations.

The guidelines made a clear recommendation not to alter the standard EMDR Therapy protocol when practicing in an online setting. It also concluded that there is no higher risk present in online EMDR Therapy in comparison to its use face-to-face. Clinicians were asked to continue working only with clients who are within their present level of competence and to learn the technical and practical skills needed to provide effective online EMDR Therapy.

One of the major concerns held by members of the EMDR Europe Standards Committee, as well as by many other members of the EMDR Therapy community, was the issue of how to establish and maintain the therapeutic relationship in an online therapy setting. In their review of therapeutic alliance in online therapy, Simpson and Reid (2014) concluded that despite findings that online psychotherapy is associated with high levels of client satisfaction and acceptability, there is a negative bias among psychologists against online therapy. They pointed to the fact that client-rated therapeutic alliance is high across diagnostic groups and interventions, while therapist-rated therapeutic alliance is only moderate to high in online psychotherapy. Based on their own personal clinical experience and that of their supervisees, the authors of this chapter concur with these findings. In most cases, clients report a positive experience while the therapists are, at times, concerned about the possible negative impact of the online setting on the therapeutic relationship.

The EMDR Therapy Protocol and Recommendations for Its Online Use

The EMDR Therapy protocol (Shapiro, 2001) is composed of eight phases. While the first two phases are performed usually once, the other phases are used for each of the target memories that are processed.

Phase 1 – History taking. The clinician obtains general psychological background focusing on current strengths and difficulties, past events that are related to the current problems, situations in the present in which the problems are triggered, and positive future goals.

History taking and the formation of the treatment plan that follows can be done easily in an online format. The EMDR therapist needs to also find out where the client is planning to have the sessions, who is going to be around, whether he will be able to have privacy during the session, as well as who are the people that can be helpful if he needs support.

Phase 2 – Preparation. The clinician prepares the client for the processing of memories by establishing a therapeutic relationship. Preparation involves psycho-education regarding both the EMDR process and the role of the client. In addition, the "safe place" exercise (Shapiro, 2001) is offered as a means of introducing EMDR Therapy, testing the client's resources and forming a grounding experience. The therapist also teaches the client the different bilateral stimulation (BLS) options.

While for most clients this phase is short, when conducted in an online format it is recommended that the therapist spends more time in getting to know the client, his surroundings, and to have a conversation on what can be done if the internet connection fails, and if the client experiences a strong emotional/somatic reaction. It is also recommended for the therapist to take more time to make sure the client fully understands the technical aspects of the BLS. Some clients will need a longer preparation phase that will include using one or more resourcing/grounding techniques, before moving on to trauma processing. The use of these techniques in an online format has been found to be possible and effective (Fisher, 2021).

Phase 3 – Assessment. The clinician helps the client to identify details of the memory chosen to be processed ("Target Memory"). This includes identifying the central image, the currently held negative cognition, the desired positive cognition, the currently felt emotion and physical sensation, as well as several baseline measurements.

This is a relatively short phase that is not challenging for the online format.

Phase 4 – Desensitization. The clinician follows and guides the client's processing of the target memory. During this phase, bilateral stimulation is used while the client is also asked to notice his internal experience. This dual attention seems to activate the client's AIP system. The processing usually leads to changes in sensory, cognitive, emotional, and somatic information. The goal of this phase is to bring the disturbance associated with the memory to the lowest possible level. It aims to connect clients with their resources and to help them develop a more adaptive view of the event and of themselves.

The desensitization phase, where most of the memory processing takes place, is the center of the EMDR Therapy protocol. Putting aside the general and technical issues that must be addressed by the online EMDR therapist (e.g., room setting, internet connection, distance from the camera, direction of lighting etc.), the therapist must also consider how best to perform bilateral stimulation. The simplest way this can be carried out, is for the therapist to move their hand in front of the computer camera, while asking the client to follow this movement with his eyes. The therapist can also ask the client to do self-tapping, instead of, or in addition to the eye movements. Several online platforms have also been found to be helpful, providing visual and auditory stimulations. As with all other elements of online EMDR Therapy, most therapists have been able to adjust to the online options for bilateral stimulation, in a relatively short period of time.

While the EMDR therapist is not supposed to interfere with the way the client is processing the memory, he is asked to be focused on the client and to support him. That is even truer in an online setting. The therapist is asked to be even more supportive, especially when the client experiences strong emotional/somatic associations. Statements like "this is part of the process", "these are just things from the past", "you are here now" and others tend to ground the client, support the needed dual attention, and enable him to continue processing the memory.

If the internet connection fails, the therapist will use another form of communication (usually a cell phone) to continue the session. While computers are preferred, it is possible to conduct EMDR Therapy sessions by using smart phones.

Phase 5 – Installation. The clinician helps the client to identify the current desired positive self-belief in relation to the memory and then to strengthen it. In this way, the memory is integrated into the adaptive memory network.

This short processing phase brings with it less challenges since most clients will not experience difficult emotions or body sensations while focusing on a positive statement.

Phase 6 – Body scan. The clinician facilitates the client's identification and processing of any residual somatic sensations associated with the target memory, aiming for a complete somatic resolution.

The last processing phase is usually brief. In an online format, since the therapist does not see the client's entire body, it is important to ask the client to give a longer description of his somatic experience.

Phase 7 – Closure. The clinician gives the client feedback about the session and what to expect after its completion. If needed, the clinician will use relaxation techniques to help the client stabilize before he leaves the session.

This phase is conducted in a similar way in both in-person and online formats. In online formats the phase becomes even more important and at times longer (than in-person), because many times the client moves to other activities immediately after the end of the session. Usually the client is asked to be the one leaving the online platform.

Phase 8 – Reevaluation. The clinician assesses the client at the beginning of the following session, focusing on changes that took place in between the sessions. The phase also includes re-accessing the previously processed target memory to evaluate maintenance of treatment effects. The information is used by the clinician to determine the next step(s) in the course of the treatment (Oren & Solomon, 2012).

Conclusions

Online psychotherapy and specifically online EMDR Therapy have been used by therapists for a number of years. The COVID-19 pandemic has required many therapists to begin using the online setting as their main, and at times only, form of therapy delivery. Both current research and clinical experience suggest that online EMDR Therapy is as effective as in-person EMDR Therapy. While most clients seem to feel comfortable receiving EMDR therapy online and report being able to develop a positive therapeutic alliance, it is in fact the therapists who report some concerns relating to therapy delivery in the online setting.

In their presentation at the EMDR Europe Trainers' meeting, de Jongh and Oren (2020) concluded that online EMDR Therapy is indeed possible and effective. It also contributes to both clients and therapists and is un-doubtedly part of EMDR Therapy's future.

The authors believe that online EMDR Therapy will remain in demand, beyond the COVID-19 era. Therapists are encouraged to learn the ins and outs of online platforms and to develop their comfort in employing them for online work with their clients. Developing such experience will expand the therapists' ability to provide EMDR Therapy comfortably with a wide variety of clients, diverse needs and in a range of locations.

References

Acierno, R., Knapp, R., Tuerk, P., Gilmore, A. K., Lejuez, C., Ruggiero, K., … & Foa, E. B. (2017). A non-inferiority trial of prolonged exposure for posttraumatic stress disorder: In person versus home-based telehealth. *Behaviour Research and Therapy, 89*, 57–65.

Black, R., Sinclair, M., Reid, B., Mc Cullough, J., Miller, P. W., Tesler Stein, M., & Farrell, D. (2021). *Effectiveness of online psychotherapy interventions for perinatal mental health: A systematic review.* Poster session presented at Faculty of Nursing and Midwifery 40th annual international nursing & midwifery research and education virtual conference, Dublin.

Centonze, D., Siracusano, A., Calabresi, P., & Bernardi, G. (2005). Removing pathogenic memories. *Molecular Neurobiology, 32*(2), 123–132.

de Jongh, A., Amann, B. L., Hofmann, A., Farrell, D., & Lee, C. W. (2019). The status of EMDR therapy in the treatment of posttraumatic stress disorder 30 years after its introduction. *Journal of EMDR Practice and Research, 13*(4), 261–269.

de Jongh, A., & Oren, U., (2020). *Online EMDR therapy in corona times, and not only*, a presentation in the online EMDR Europe's Trainers' meeting.

EMDR Europe Association (2020). Recommendations for the use of online EMDR therapy during the COVID-19 pandemic. Unpublished document.

Fisher, N. (2021). Using EMDR therapy to treat clients remotely. *JEMDR, 15*(1), 73–84.

Hase, M., Balmaceda, U. M., Ostacoli, L., Liebermann, P., & Hofmann, A. (2017). The AIP model of EMDR therapy and pathogenic memories. *Frontiers in Psychology, 8*(1578), 1–5.

Karadag, M., Topal, Z., Ezer, R. N., & Gokcen, C. (2021). Use of EMDR-derived self-help intervention in children in the period of COVID-19: A randomized-controlled study. *Journal of EMDR Practice and Research, 15*(2), 114–126.

Mavranezouli, I., Megnin-Viggars, O., Grey, N., Bhutani, G., Leach, J., Daly, C., ... & Pilling, S. (2020). Cost-effectiveness of psychological treatments for post-traumatic stress disorder in adults. *PloS One, 15*(4), 1–22.

Maxfield, L. (2021). Low-intensity interventions and EMDR therapy. *Journal of EMDR Practice and Research, 15*(2), 86–98.

Moench, J., & Billsten, O. (2021). Randomized controlled trial: Self-care traumatic episode protocol (STEP), computerized EMDR treatment of COVID-19 related stress. *Journal of EMDR Practice and Research, 15*(2), 99–113.

Nakano, K. (2013). Evaluation of the eye movement desensitization procedure through the Internet for resolving distressing memories. *International Journal of Psychology and Counselling, 5*(4), 72–79.

Nakano, K. (2015). Efficacy of eye movement desensitization treatment through the internet. *European Journal of Psychological Research, 2*(1) 63–72.

Oren, E., & Solomon, R. (2012). EMDR therapy: An overview of its development and mechanisms of action. *European Review of Applied Psychology, 62*(4), 197–203.

Perez, M. C., Estevez, M. E., Becker, Y., Osorio, A., Jarero, I. et al. (2020). Multisite randomized control trial on the provision of the EMDR integrative group treatment protocol during the COVID-19 pandemic. *International Journal of Psychology and Behavioral Science, 15*(4), 1–12.

Perri, R. L., Castelli, P., La Rosa, C., Zucchi, T., & Onofri, A. (2021). COVID-19, isolation, quarantine: On the efficacy of internet-based eye movement desensitization and reprocessing (EMDR) and cognitive-behavioral therapy (CBT) for ongoing trauma. *Brain Sciences, 11*(5), 579, 1–8.

Rollins, S., Hughes, T., Cordes, G., Cohen-Peck, M., & Watson-Wong, J. (2020, January). Guidelines for virtual EMDR therapy. *A report of the virtual training and therapy task group.*

Shapiro, F. (2001). *Eye Movement Desensitization and Reprocessing – Basic Principles, Protocols, and Procedures.* 3rd Edition. New York, NY: Guilford.

Shapiro, F. E. (2001). *EMDR as an Integrative Psychotherapy Approach: Experts of Diverse Orientations Explore the Paradigm Prism* (pp. vii-444). American Psychological Association.

Simpson, S. G., & Reid, C. L. (2014). Therapeutic alliance in videoconferencing psychotherapy: A review. *Australian Journal of Rural Health, 22*(6), 280–299.

Smyth-Dent, K., Becker, Y., Burns, E., & Givaudan, M. (2021). The acute stress syndrome stabilization remote individual (ASSYST-RI) for telemental health counseling after adverse experiences. *International Journal of Psychology and Behavioral Science, 16*(2), 1–7.

Spence, J., Titov, N., Johnston, L., Dear, B. F., Wootton, B., Terides, M., & Zou, J. (2013). Internet-delivered eye movement desensitization and reprocessing (iEMDR): An open trial. *F1000Research, 2,* 1–11.

Tarquinio, C., Brennstuhl, M. J., Rydberg, J. A., Bassan, F., Peter, L., Tarquinio, C. L., … & Tarquinio, P. (2020). EMDR in telemental health counseling for healthcare workers caring for COVID-19 patients: A pilot study. *Issues in Mental Health Nursing,* 1–12.

Valiente-Gómez, A., Moreno-Alcázar, A., Treen, D., Cedrón, C., Colom, F., Perez, V., & Amann, B. L. (2017). EMDR beyond PTSD: A systematic literature review. *Frontiers in Psychology, 8*(1668), 1–10.

Varker, T., Brand, R. M., Ward, J., Terhaag, S., & Phelps, A. (2019). Efficacy of synchronous telepsychology interventions for people with anxiety, depression, posttraumatic stress disorder, and adjustment disorder: A rapid evidence assessment. *Psychological Services, 16*(4), 621–635.

World Health Organization. (2013). *Guidelines for the Management of Conditions that are Specifically Related to Stress.* World Health Organization.

Yael, B., Elena, E. M., Cristina, P. M., Amalia, O., Ignacio, J., & Martha, G. (2021). Longitudinal multisite randomized controlled trial on the provision of the acute stress syndrome stabilization remote for groups to general population in lockdown during the COVID-19 pandemic, *16*(2), 555931.

14 Getting a Little Closer in Every Session: The Unique Contribution of Remote Biofeedback to Psychotherapy

Yossi Ehrenreich, Arnon Rolnick, and Adam Leighton

Introduction

Therapy from a distance imposes considerable limitations on basic treatment premises. The elementary settings of therapy: space and time have changed. In part, this kind of change challenges the therapist and client's ability to sense each other's presence. Moreover, that might hinder the creation of intimacy. Biofeedback therapy stands out in its reliance on aiding imaging technology, opening a window to one's internal behavior.

One of biofeedback's tasks is the joint query of the relevance of information gathered from the client's body to the client's issues and the therapeutic goal. This chapter will focus on the art of sharing as a building block of online intimacy creation particularly in the context of remote therapy. We explicitly illuminate the unique contribution of psychophysiological monitoring to establishing therapist-client intimacy. We will illustrate how psychophysiology enriches and augments the therapeutic interaction, emphasizing its relevance to intimacy creation. We will also highlight a few elements in our biofeedback procedure that are somewhat neglected: Creating a mutually shared experience and creating intimacy in psychophysiological therapy.

The advantages of remote Biofeedback have been known for many years. Nearly two decades ago, Folen et al. (2001) described how Biofeedback via telehealth could provide accessibility to patients in rural and remote areas. However, we will present at first Biofeedback therapy's unique features.

Biofeedback: Psychophysiologically Driven, and Technology-Aided Psychotherapy

Biofeedback therapy is a well-established form of psychophysiological psychotherapy. Biofeedback therapy evolved from self-regulation training into a psychotherapeutic approach that stands for its own merits (Frank et al., 2010; Moss, 2008). At first, Biofeedback therapy relied on behavioral theory and methodologies. Neal Miller, Joe Kamiya, John Basmajian, and others were inspired by possibilities revealed by the first clinical experiments demonstrating

DOI: 10.4324/9781003205029-17

volitional regulation of visceral processes developed through operant learning enabled by feedback given. Thus, giving hope to developing new ways for healing medical and psychological ailments (Moss, 1998). Their accomplishments expanded the known boundaries of operant learning at their times (Peper & Shaffer, 2018).

On the other hand, Biofeedback therapy is easily integrated with other therapeutic approaches such as CBT, Hypnosis, Dyadic psychotherapy, Mentalization-based treatment, and Compassion-Focused Therapy (Hamiel & Rolnick, 2017; Moss, 2020, 2019; Ehrenreich, 2018, 2021; Ehrenreich & Rolnick, 2019). The common denominator of all treatments is Biofeedback therapy's technological advantage: imaging and feedback.

The uniqueness of Biofeedback therapy is its reliance on monitoring client physiological occurrence by applying non-invasive sensors on the client's body. Usually, outside conscious awareness, the physiological occurrence is displayed on a screen visible to both client and therapist. This imaging quality was termed a "psychophysiological mirror" (Peper et al., 2009). Using that mirror, the client gains insight into his physiological patterns, a bodily reaction to external and internal events.

The stream of data from the screen to the client opens a door for new learnings to occur. The client can 'experiment' with different cognitive, affective, and behavioral patterns and receive feedback. The client simultaneously receives feedback from his body, otherwise termed as embodied knowledge (Tanaka, 2011), and display (usually computer or mobile phone screen). Thus, making the implicit explicit and enabling a learning process otherwise not possible.

Let us consider the following exchange. A therapist is commenting that the client seems tense. The client responds with a deep sigh, stating rejecting the therapist's observation. This exchange might be considered a mismatch. First, the therapist's comment related to an occurrence outside the client's awareness; was then rejected. Now, consider a similar exchange, which Biofeedback therapists are familiar with. A client sits hooked to a surface electromyography (SEMG) sensor attached to his trapezius muscles. The therapist asks the client to note that the reading on the screen is relatively high. The client becomes curious and inquires about the possible meanings of elevated muscle activity. He is becoming aware that the graphs on the screen are displaying his tensed shoulders—he then notices altogether that his muscles are tensed indeed.

We will discuss these two short exchanges further on. Meanwhile, it will suffice to say that they portray a clear picture of the feedback nature given to the client. He receives visual feedback on-screen and bodily feedback – noticing the tensed shoulders. That, in turn, enables client learning. Further experimenting with new emotional, cognitive, and behavioral patterns and noticing the connection between the graphic description of the internal occurrence and bodily sensation that results from these new patterns strengthens an embodied yet explicit learning.

The client learns how the mind and body relate to each other. He also learns that physiological patterns are lent to conscious influence. Given that imaging possibilities are various, his psychophysiological 'image' portrayed on screen is mind intriguing, offering new ways of minding the body. Skin response (SR), surface electromyography (sEMG), electroencephalography (EEG), blood pressure (BP), heart rate (HR) and heart rate variability (HRV), blood volume pulse (BVP), respiration (RESP), skin temperature of body extremities (TEMP), end-tidal CO_2, are only limited and partial list of modalities by which the client can know oneself. New modalities are discovered continuously, opening doors for the client's body.

Wearables and Domestic Biofeedback Devices a Path for Quantified Self

Consumer tracking devices are now available and can continuously measure physiological activity. These devices are used alongside clinical level Biofeedback devices. For a full review of devices available, refer to Rolnick, Ehrenreich, and Leighton (2021). We shall introduce the most common ones.

Heart rate variability (HRV) is currently the foremost popular Biofeedback measurement. HRV relates to interbeat interval variation of heartbeats measured moment by moment (Moss & Shaffer, 2016). It is considered an index of resilience and positive health (Geisler et al., 2013; Singer, 2010) and possible disease risk (McCraty & Shaffer, 2015).

Skin response is a variable aspect of electrodermal activity measured by applying electrodes placed on hand palms or finger digits and measuring the electrical velocity of low-level electrical current applied using these electrodes. Skin response reflects sympathetic activation (Shaffer et al., 2019). It is still the most common in use. Many affordable, accurate devices are available, most using finger or ear sensors (or both). The low price, ease of use, and affordability allow patients to purchase and use these devices easily. The critical disadvantage is that the sensors require the patient to be relatively stationary and are less suited for continual daily monitoring.

The term "Quantified Self" was coined in 2007 to describe data acquisition of oneself, mainly physiological or behavioral. Using smartphone apps, one can track, monitor, and change health-related habits. Using these apps, mountains of data are gathered and stored in personal cellphones and virtual clouds. Sophisticated algorithms were developed to utilize the acquired data using data mining and artificial intelligence. Analyzing that data unveils aspects of self, such as eating, sleeping, exercising, and physiological activity previously unknown to the self. The continuous data stream affords feedback on behavior change that leads to behavior optimization. Whether it is health behavior or athletic performance, tracking and shaping such behaviors creates feedback loops. By receiving ongoing feedback on behavior, behavior is changing.

In the following parts of this chapter, we will explore the clinical impact of the "Quantified Self". We will present the theme of sharing and its relevance to remote therapy and remote Biofeedback therapy. We will conclude by addressing the question of privacy through the lens of sharing.

Sharing: Time and Space

Time and space are the fundamental features of clinical settings. Within these agreeable constraints, therapy occurs. The therapist shares his designated space in favor of client healing. The time spent together is also for the client's benefit under certain constraints. Online therapy changed these features, as therapy can happen everywhere. Yet, each of them can choose how much of their current surrounding is disclosed. While in, so called, normal conventional treatment setting, client's sense of control is lessened. Both client and the therapist gained the ability to manipulate time and space in remote therapy. We shall discuss some of them in detail.

Space

Online therapy enables both parties – therapist and client – to manipulate their visibility. By adjusting the camera's angle, each can decide which part of him the other will see. In addition, communication apps allow users to change the background of their images. Thus, affording the users to pretend they are somewhere else – in a real or imagined place. Altogether, these features promote the freedom of each part of the therapeutic act – therapist and client – to customize his presence in the therapy "room". The camera brings the client and therapist closer together and mirrors them to oneself. Rolnick and Ehrenreich (2020) proposed that purposeful camera use remedies online therapy violations of space constraints. We shall elaborate on two viable options for expanding camera use.

First, extracting data from the camera, such as facial skin color changes and respiration detected by the rise and fall of the client's chest, is another use of the camera for imaging and feedback. Such applications are already researched (e.g., Tezuka & Nakamura, 2018). Products such as Philips VitalSigns Camera algorithms use skin color change and chest movement to measure HRV and respiration rate. This data at hand allows the therapist to either share it with the client or use it to tune his interventions. By sharing such data, the human feedback (on behalf of the therapist) is meaningful and facilitates another opportunity for expanding the client's awareness and behavior change. At the time these lines are written, the above option is yet to be common.

Second, purposeful camera manipulation turns the camera into a feedback device from a mere mirroring appliance. Inviting the client to play with camera zoom and to focus her/his attention on his/her own face and not the therapist's face, and identify the emotion reflected from his/her face (mirror feedback) yields countless options for intervention. It can be used to promote emotional awareness and trigger emotional reactions to the client's current emotions. Another intervention might be promoting the client's compassion towards his emotional reaction. Evoking and promoting compassionate states and reactions is evident in current Biofeedback therapy through physiological facilitation (HRV training) (Ehrenreich, 2021). Using the camera adds another dimension of feedback to that practice by allowing the client to watch how his facial expression softens.

Time

Examination of the therapeutic setting time dimension emphasizes its synchronous aspect. Synchronicity is a two-end term. At the one extreme as synchronous – a constant real-time flow of information usually during a limited time frame (e.g., a session) and at the other; asynchronous – fragmented, intermittent ongoing communication. A reflection of the synchronicity aspect appears in communication mode and content. Meeting applications concede synchronous treatment – while at a distance, bringing therapist and client closer in time. The importance and impact of synchronicity are accentuated when a poor internet connection disrupts therapy flow. It hinders our ability to be tuned to client mood changes.

Asynchronous communication using various applications can strengthen the therapeutic bond. We make ourselves available for clients by letting them make contact at will. Furthermore, we have the opportunity to plan and fine-tune our response, not bound to a time restriction.

Different types of information collected about the client are considered part of the treatment regarding communication content. For example, a client who practices relaxation techniques aided by a home unit or a wearable device may share data collected in training with his therapist. it corresponds with familiar types of information commonly gathered in cognitive-behavioral therapy – journals tracking mood, stress, thoughts.

Nevertheless, data collected through journals differ from psychophysiological data accumulated by a wearable device, both quantitatively and qualitatively. Vast amounts of psychophysiological information accumulate in a wearable device compared to thoughts or mood record keeping. While personal data describing mental activity is considered subjective information, psychophysiological data, on the other hand, is deemed to be objective. In other words, wearable devices grant the therapist exposure to personal and intimate information about internal occurrences in the client's life. From the client's perspective, along with other selves, he brings to therapy his "Quantified Self".

Using wearable device data is becoming a prevalent practice in Biofeedback Therapy. Some manufacturers of Biofeedback devices offer real-time information sharing. Thus, the therapist can access the client's private occurrence – Quantified Self – despite the distance. Here, the two sides of the synchronicity aspect of time settings come into play. The therapist can analyze data accumulated and identify the unforeseen pattern of behavior. Indeed, he is acquainting the client asynchronously. Thus, therapist access to client's data redefines therapy time settings, broadening their time spent together. The physiological data can be presented in real-time during a synchronous session using home-based biofeedback devices, as described. These graphs or animations can be shared with the patient via video conference programs (Zoom, Skype, Meet, etc.), using the share screen ability.

Sharing and Intimacy: The Building Block of Therapy

At the beginning of this chapter, we introduced two clinical exchanges between therapist and client related to the client's tense position. The so-called traditional exchange is liable for a mismatch by commenting on a client's private occurrence outside the client's awareness, in which the client cannot 'find' himself. On the other hand, a similar exchange within the Biofeedback session facilitated client awareness – "finding" himself on screen. Now we shall reflect on the function of sharing – the therapist's decision to share a piece of information known only to the therapist.

Cordova and Scott (2001) define intimacy as a sequence of events in which another person's response reinforces behavior vulnerable to interpersonal punishment – suggesting intimacy as a function of sharing. Determining the degree of exposure is bound to the extent of possible vulnerability by information shared. Kanter et al. (2020) further expanded this definition to a complete model of intimate relations. Their model, which relates to verbal and non-verbal aspects, describes three distinct relations within an intimate relationship: non-verbal emotional expression and safety, verbal self-disclosure and validation, and asking and giving. In a nutshell, the model describes a cascade of interpersonal exchanges, both verbal and non-verbal. These are reciprocal exchanges, where one part self-discloses and receives a safety-providing and validating response. Upon getting the response, he is further encouraged to ask what he needs and receives (once again) an "empathically accurate and tailored response" (Kanter et al., 2020).

Kanter's model describes the circumstances within which therapy occurs. The therapist is committed to providing safety and validation and meeting the client's emotional needs. At the same time, the client is sharing his personal needs.

Implementing Kanter's model to online therapy stresses the unique features of remote treatment. As described earlier, the client's total control of his camera, thus enabling manipulation of the amount of information flowing through the camera. That ranges from no disclosure – blurring the entire surroundings, hiding any detail of his current private place – to full disclosure – exposing the client's messy room. The therapist sees merely what the client discloses about his surroundings and appearance. That diminishes the probability of receiving punishment for non-verbal self-disclosure. At the same time, lowering this risk reduces the likelihood of validation and, therefore, safety – this kind of exchange compromises the opportunity for an intimate relationship. Behaviorally speaking, online biofeedback therapy potentially challenges building a solid therapeutic bond, which is essential for therapy success. Biofeedback therapy involves sharing, as well, and adding a third type of self-disclosure (besides verbal and non-verbal emotional expression) to Kanter's model – psychophysiological data.

The "share screen" option of the various video conferencing programs is very useful in remote therapy. This type of sharing emphasizes the "therapeutic triangle" in each biofeedback session (patient, therapist, and physiological data presentation). The therapeutic triangle's impact can be understood using the "joint attention" concepts in developmental psychology literature. Joint attention or shared attention exists when two individuals look at the same object (Corkum, 1995). This ability to attend to an aspect of one's environment is fundamental to developing relationships by sharing experience and knowledge. Thus, the client's internal occurrence is at the center of the therapist and client's joint attention. Indeed, Biofeedback done from a distance highly emphasizes shared physiological data presentation. The shared physiological data narrows the distance between therapist and client, bringing them closer together.

We place great importance on this sharing process of the subjective elements and the verbal interaction accompanying biofeedback therapy. Rolnick and Rickles (2010), adopting an intersubjective point of view of Biofeedback in-session interaction, suggest that the therapist and client's interaction should be the center of attention. The therapist interacts with clients regarding their self-regulating efforts, bringing awareness of the mind-body connection and verbalizing it. Else, making the subjective visible by attending psychophysiology of regulation process. Therefore, a replication of early interaction between a parental figure and a helpless child occurs within a biofeedback session where the parental figure attends its offspring's self-regulation trials and verbalizes them.

Biofeedback case studies usually describe the progression between sessions (i.e., what we achieved in the first session, in the second, and the last). Somewhat less attention is given to the description of the therapy within the session. Specifically, there is rarely a script of the step-by-step interaction between the therapist and the patient during a one-hour session. Hamiel and Rolnick (2017) suggested a model of integrating psychotherapy and Biofeedback. In this model, they identified macro stages of treatment. They also divided each therapeutic session into alternating specific phases of practicing with the biofeedback equipment followed by sharing phases.

The designation of sharing phase facilitates interaction between the client and the practitioner. Its purpose is to gain some insight into the client's internal processes. The client is asked to tell the Biofeedback therapist whether he felt he could relax and what was going on in his mind during the previous exercise.

At a superficial level, this is the client's way of telling the therapist what helped him regulate his physiology and what hampered the process. A highly valuable therapeutic procedure commences at a more profound level during this stage. The dialogue between the mother and her baby facilitates our self-control processes from birth. The baby is overwhelmed by physical and emotional discomfort and by the experience of incompetence. The mother "listens to her baby's complaints" and comforts him by responding to his pain. Sharing between client and practitioner resembles this very primary process between child and caregiver.

To facilitate sharing the subjective process, after the training period, the client should share with the Biofeedback Therapist what else went on in his mind during practice and how he felt. Several points may arise during this phase. He/she may also speak of being frustrated about not fulfilling the relaxing assignment. On the other hand, the client may reveal, for the first time, how eager he was for a chance to "let go" and how much he missed having a warm and tender significant other.

Intimate interactions bridge intimate experiences and intimate relationships (Prager, 1997). Interactions primarily consist of behaviors and experiences, which can be emotional, cognitive, social, and physical. The act of sharing in the context of Biofeedback entails all the elements of a shared intimate experience.

In order to achieve the level of sharing in which the patient is willing to volunteer information that can be potentially 'punishable,' the therapist needs to gradually build a level of trust that will allow open sharing.

As suggested by Hamiel and Rolnick (2017), we suggest that following the therapy stages becomes increasingly important as the ownership of the physiological data shifts from therapist to patient. In this light, we can see that the Biofeedback therapist's role will increasingly emphasize intimacy building.

Conclusion

We asserted the importance of sharing in remote Biofeedback. We demonstrated that the Biofeedback therapist has two sets of information shared with the client: asynchronous and synchronous. These sets of information and the client's self-disclosure are the content of sharing. The client is willing to disclose his thoughts, feelings, overt behavior (manipulating the camera), and visceral behavior. On the other hand, the therapist shares his thoughts (interpretation), feelings, and overt behavior (by manipulating the camera). The client is affording the therapist insight into his unseen occurrence between sessions. In return, the therapist shares his insight – observation of unforeseen patterns. This mutual sharing and reinforcement sharing process (by counter sharing) creates intimacy between client and therapist in Biofeedback Therapy.

Remote Biofeedback Therapy is practiced in either one or both ways: asynchronous and synchronous. The asynchronous way utilizes data (visceral and subjective) aggregated between sessions, mirroring its analysis and feedback. This process ties together the client's life and the therapist's mind. The synchronous way uses various data (visceral, visual, auditory, subjective) flow to create a place designated by time, space, and data sharing that encapsulate client and therapist closer together.

References

Cordova, J. V., & Scott, R. L. (2001). Intimacy: A behavioral interpretation. *The Behavior Analyst, 24*(1), 75–86.

Corkum, V., & Moore, C. (1995). Development of joint visual attention in infants. In C. Moore & P. J. Dunham (Eds.), *Joint Attention: Its Origins and Role in Development* (pp. 61–83). Lawrence Erlbaum.

Ehrenreich, Y. (2021). A happy heart comes first: Heart based compassion training. *Biofeedback, 48*(4), 73–80.

Ehrenreich, Y. (2018). Attachment-informed biofeedback – The next generation of biofeedback therapy. *Biofeedback, 46*(3), 52–59.

Ehrenreich, Y., & Rolnick, A. (2019). Mentalization-based psychophysiological therapy. *Biofeedback, 47*(4), 81–84.

Folen, R. A., James, L. C., Earles, J. E., & Andrasik, F. (2001). Biofeedback via telehealth: A new frontier for applied psychophysiology. *Applied Psychophysiology and Biofeedback, 26*(3), 195–204.

Frank, D. L., Khorshid, L., Kiffer, J. F., Moravec, C. S., & McKee, M. G. (2010). Biofeedback in medicine: Who, when, why and how?. *Mental Health in Family Medicine, 7*(2), 85–91.

Geisler, F. C., Kubiak, T., Siewert, K., & Weber, H. (2013). Cardiac vagal tone is associated with social engagement and self-regulation. *Biological Psychology, 93*(2), 279–286. 10.1016/j.biopsycho.2013.02.013

Hamiel, D., & Rolnick, A., (2017). *Biofeedback and Cognitive Behavioral Interventions: Reciprocal Contributions, in Schwartz MS, Andrasik F. Biofeedback, A Practioner's Guide*, 4nd Edition. New York: Guilford Press.

Kanter, J. K., Kuczysnki, A. M., Manbeck, K. E., Corey, M. D., & Wallace, E. C. (2020). An integrative contextual behavioral model of intimate relations. *Journal of Contextual Behavioral Science, 18*, 75–91.

McCraty, R., & Shaffer, F. (2015). Heart rate variability: New perspectives on physiological mechanisms, assessment of self-regulatory capacity, and health risk. *Global Advances in Health and Medicine, 4*(1), 46–61. 10.7453/gahmj.2014.073

Moss, D. (1998). Biofeedback, mind-body medicine, and the higher limits of human nature. In: D. Moss (Ed.), *Humanistic and Transpersonal Psychology: A Historical and Biographical Sourcebook*. Westport, CT: Greenwood Publishing.

Moss, D. (2008). 15 Grundsätze für die Anwendung von Biofeedback in einer psychosomatische Psychotherapie [15 principles for the application of biofeedback in a psychosomatic psychotherapy]. In I. Pirker-Binder (Ed.), *Biofeedback in der praxis, Band II. Erwachsene [Biofeedback in practice: Vol. 2. Adults]* (pp. 108–114). Springer Medizin.

Moss, D. (2019). The most beautiful man: An integration of hypnosis and Biofeedback for depression and dissociation. *American Journal of Clinical Hypnosis, 62*(4), 322–334. 10.1080/00029157.2018.1517082

Moss, D. (2020). Physiological monitoring to enhance clinical hypnosis and psychotherapy. *International Journal of Clinical and Experimental Hypnosis*. 10.1080/002 07144.2020.1790992

Moss, D., & Shaffer, F. (Eds.). (2016). Foundations of heart rate variability: A book of readings. *Association for Applied Psychophysiology and Biofeedback*.

Peper, E., Harvey, R., Takabayashi, N., & Hughes, P. (2009). How to do clinical Biofeedback in psychosomatic medicine: An illustrative brief therapy example for self-regulation. *Japanese Journal of Biofeedback Research, 36*(2), 1–16.

Peper, E. & Shaffer, F. (2018). Biofeedback History: An Alternative View. *Biofeedback*, 46(4), 80–85. 10.5298/1081-5937.46.4.80

Petrocchi, N., Ottaviani, C., & Couyoumdjian, A. (2016). Compassion at the mirror: Exposure to a mirror increases the efficacy of a self-compassion manipulation in enhancing soothing positive affect and heart rate variability. *The Journal of Positive Psychology*, 1–12.

Prager, K. J. (1997). *The Psychology of Intimacy*. Guilford Press.

Rolnick, A. & Rickles W. (2010). Integrating biofeedback with psychodynamic, relational and intersubjective approach. *Biofeedback*, *38*(4), 131– 13.

Rolnick, A., Ehrenreich, Y., Leighton, A. (2021). Psychophysiological Therapy from a Distance: The Art of Sharing. *Biofeedback*, 49(1), 18–24.

Rolnick, A., & Ehrenreich, Y. (2020). The Role of the Body, Its Absence, and Its Measurement in Online Video Psychotherapy. *Biofeedback*, 48(1), 20–23.

Shaffer, F., Combatalade, D., Peper, E., & Meehan, Z. (2019). A guide to cleaner electrodermal activity measurements. In D. Moss & F. Shaffer (Eds.), *Physiological Recording Technology and Applications in Biofeedback and Neurofeedback* (pp. 233–246). Association for Applied Psychophysiology and Biofeedback.

Singer, D. H. (2010). High heart rate variability, marker of healthy longevity. *American Journal of Cardiology*, *106*(6), 910. 10.1016/j.amjcard.2010.06.038

Tanaka, S. (2011). The notion of embodied knowledge. In P. Stenner, et al. (Eds.), *Theoretical Psychology: Global Transformations and Challenges* (pp. 149–157). Concord: Captus University Publications.

Tezuka, T., & Nakamura, T. (2018). Contactless vital sensing technology using video imaging and its applications. *Japanese Journal of Biofeedback Research*, *45*(1), 3–9.

15 Interactive Hypnosis and Hypnotic Psychotherapy Online

Joseph Meyerson

Video conferencing and internet technology have advanced therapists' ability to make psychotherapy more accessible to distanced and specific populations and during emergencies. Online psychotherapy was found to be especially relevant for treating relocated patients, patients with accessibility issues, and professionals with busy schedules, as well as during personal and collective health or security crises. Although online conferencing procedures somewhat challenged the familiar psychotherapeutic props of empathic and therapeutic presence and interventions, online psychotherapy is manifested in everyday therapeutic practice and in the scientific literature (Weinberg & Rolnick, 2019). Yet, the majority of professionals who applied hypnosis during psychotherapy in face-to-face interactions in their clinical practice hesitated to use the online platform for performing hypnotic interventions and therapy. As the online therapeutic arena became divided into three geographically and conceptually distant locations (the therapist location, the patient location, and the digital interconnecting space) (Meyerson, 2020), technological, geographical, and psychological obstacles challenged well-known principles of hypnotic art. The present chapter deals with the task of converting hypnotic psychotherapy (H-psychotherapy) into a safe psychotherapeutic endeavor with distant patients online. The first section relates to some objective factors of online hypnotic interactions. They include the setting of an online therapeutic arena as design and utilization of the therapists' and patients' physical locations and operation of peripheral equipment (for broadening see Meyerson, 2020). The second part of the chapter discusses the set of interactive online H-psychotherapy, addressing therapists' and patients' personal preferences, as well as specific hypnotic strategies and techniques for handling hypnotized patients online. Finally, the chapter addresses the therapist's ability to hold patients (Baker, 2000) when they are silent and to contain their abreactive expressions, remotely.

Online, Interactive Hypnosis

Tele-hypnosis (hypnosis with patients by phone) was introduced about 50 years ago and was described as a feasible practice (Weitzenhoffer, 1972). Two decades have passed since the first trials using video conferencing

DOI: 10.4324/9781003205029-18

hypnosis (video-hypnosis) were introduced (Simpson et al., 2002); since then, literature on the subject has been scarce (Hasan et al., 2019; Meyerson, 2020).

Video conferencing has been recognized and used in many therapeutic arenas, including individual, couple, and group psychotherapy, as well as in psychoanalysis (Weinberg & Rolnick, 2019). Therapeutic video conferencing is helpful for patients located at a distance from their therapists, for patients who are physically and/or psychologically challenged as well as in emergencies and for busy professionals (Simpson et al., 2002; Weinberg & Rolnick, 2019). Lately, during COVID-19-pandemic distancing policies it was useful to close the gap between therapists and their patients (Crowe et al., 2020). It can also liberate psychotherapy participants from geographical or material stagnation (regarding fixed living and working places). In light of this, the scarce of clinical and scientific literature on online H-psychotherapy is even more conspicuous. Hypnotists are usually innovators who aspire to improve their professional performance and are not easily intimidated by the unexpected and the unknown (Meyerson et al., 2013; Strauss, 1997). So, their avoidance of online hypnosis interventions cannot not be explained exclusively by technology anxiety or by tendency to cling to traditional ways of conducting hypnotherapy. The neglect of online H-psychotherapy practice can be attributed to the genuinely challenging nature of H-psychotherapy for both therapist and patient. I discuss the challenges mentioned above in the following sections, and present some solutions.

It is noteworthy that on-demand, pre-recorded, online hypnotherapy is in use by internet frequenters (Kittle & Spiegel, 2021) and can be used experimentally, prophylactically, and can even promote self-hypnosis practices (Farrell-Carnahan et al., 2010; Flynn, 2019), but it is no different from pre-recorded video/audio sessions used by therapists for decades (Hoslin et al., 2019; Weitzenhoffer, 1972). This chapter does not focus on this type of hypnotherapy, but on online **interactive** hypnosis and H-psychotherapy. Interactive hypnosis, as emphasized further on, includes in-person bidirectional communication between the hypnotist and the hypnotized patient, not only in pre- and post-hypnotic parts of therapy, but also during the hypnotic trance phase. This style of hypnosis implementation in therapy requires the therapist to help the hypnotized patient to develop automatic, dissociative speech, and is characteristic of patient-centered hypnotic psychotherapy (Erickson & Rossi, 1979; Rossi, 1997).

The Development of the Setting During Online H-Psychotherapy

Face-to-face H-psychotherapy has specific characteristics, agreed-upon rules, and roles that can be referred to as a setting (Mayer, 2006). The therapist is usually responsible for defining and safeguarding the setting and by doing so, assist the patient to feel safe and protected. This experience of safety enables the patient to enter into hypnotic state more easily and swiftly, allowing effective psychotherapy to be performed (Erickson & Rossi, 1979; Yapko & Sheehan, 2012).

During the online therapeutic session, the hypnotist has to develop a safe therapeutic space in which to work hypnotically with patients by interconnecting three geographically and conceptually distant spaces: the therapist's location, the patient's location, and the digital interconnecting medium. It is helpful for the therapist to remember that every psychotherapeutic setting, including H-psychotherapy, has concrete and subjective elements (Lunn, 2002). During hypnotic psychotherapy, the concrete aspects of the setting are dominant at the beginning and at the end of a hypnotic phase (patient with eyes open), and subjective elements are seminal during that phase of the session (patient with eyes closed, concentrating on internal realities). For the sake of clarity, I address concrete and subjective elements of H-psychotherapy separately.

The Concrete Elements of Online H-Psychotherapy (Setting)

Preparing a therapeutic setting for online H-psychotherapy requires consideration of two physical locations – of the therapist and of the patient. The therapist's clinic must be arranged in such a way that what is visible on the screen projects the atmosphere that the therapist wishes to create. This includes adequate lighting and the option of varying the therapist's distance from the online camera, e.g., using a wheeled chair in a spacious room. The camera's position is also important. An eye-level position creates an atmosphere of person-to-person communication as opposed to the atmosphere created by one-down or one-up positions – either above or below eye level. During therapy sessions, unplanned disturbances by people or domestic animals should be minimized.

The patient arranges the patient's side of the setting. In order to shape an atmosphere conducive to the therapeutic process, the therapist needs to be flexible and creative while using the patient's contribution. In addition, some basic ground rules should be observed that require discussion and agreement with patients: starting the sessions on time, guiding the patient to find a safe, private place without interference from household members, and with good lighting that must be switched on before evening darkness falls.

Additionally, the patient must prepare a comfortable place, with some pillows, and either sit or lie down in front of the camera, leaving a considerable part of the body visible. During a hypnotic trance, due to muscular relaxation, a patient's face is sometimes less expressive than peripheral body parts, where movement may be detected. Since patients sometimes remain in the same posture throughout the hypnotic trance, it is helpful to ask them to place a dynamic, moving object (such as a large clock) in the background and visible to the therapist. This can help the therapist to differentiate between the patient's static posture and the frozen state of the image on the screen resulting from internet problems.

Good quality headphones and microphone are essential when preparing an online hypnosis session setting, allowing therapists and patients to be more attuned to verbalizations and less distracted by external noises. In addition, with good quality headphones and a sensitive microphone, patients can be more receptive to the paraverbal quality of therapeutic interaction – essential information for hypnotized patients whose eyes are closed. All these seemingly technical remarks are vital to the development of a safe, appropriate therapy setting.

The Safety Protocol for Online Interactive Hypnosis

To ensure safe online H-psychotherapy, it is essential to set a protocol for unexpected internet disturbances, and to include it when preparing the patient for hypnosis. In addition to regular preparatory procedures (Meyerson, 2017b), patients may be guided in the following manner: "Sometimes, the online communication can get cut off. So, if you [the patient] are uncertain whether I [the therapist] am with you, you can call me [the therapist] by name. If, after calling **twice**, you receive no answer, proceed with de-hypnotizing procedures: count from five down to one, open your eyes, and reconnect with me." This concrete, agreed-upon safety measure helps patients feel more comfortable during their sessions in a digital world and grants legitimacy to their uncertainties (transferential or realistic) concerning development of a safe, appropriate therapeutic environment. The last comment links us naturally with the next part of the chapter that deals with the subjective elements of online H-psychotherapy.

The Subjective Elements of Online H-Psychotherapy (Set)

The belief that eliciting hypnotic trance necessitates proximity and contact between the hypnotist and the hypnotized patient is firmly rooted in patients' cultural expectations and the professional approach of some hypnotists (Levitan & Johnson, 1986). The assumption that the hypnotic process and hypnotists-patient influence have tangible and substantial presence in addition to interpersonal interaction and communication (Green, 2003; Meyerson, 2017b), are fueled by the history of hypnosis, onstage hypnosis performances, TV shows, and YouTube demonstrations of hypnosis (Pintar & Lynn, 2008). In my view, they contribute significantly to the withdrawal from online interactive hypnosis. For effective online H-psychotherapy, these therapists' and patients' misconceptions need to be exposed and changed.

The additional belief cultivated not only by hypnosis bystanders but also by some hypnotists is that to reach patients' unconscious, the patients have to be in a receptive, quiet state, or at least not verbally communicating their experiences during hypnotic trance. This belief is fueled by the conviction that verbal communication during hypnotic trance impairs its quality and effectiveness by involving more cognitive and conscious mental processes. Verbal communication as an obstacle to effective hypnotic therapy is a misconception. It disregards a hundred years of psychodynamic psychotherapy experience and the understanding that the unconscious expresses itself in every human behavior, especially in verbalizations, and that psychotherapy is an interactive, bilateral process (Alter, 2020). Verbal interactions with patients during hypnotic psychotherapy, when searching for patients' unconscious language cues, are widely accepted in the Ericksonian approach. This approach encourages active and vocal patient participation not only during hypnotic intervention but also in developing and monitoring hypnotic trance (Meyerson, 2017a).

After the aforementioned misconceptions have been detected and corrected, it should be noted that hypnotists who use an online platform for therapy are genuinely challenged by the difficulties it poses. These difficulties, inter alia, include two-dimensional on-screen vision; sometimes-unreliable online communication that distorts images, words, para-verbal intricacies, and body language, including minimal cues that are so useful for hypnosis facilitation and handling. Consequently, the H-psychotherapist has to develop and reinforce special techniques and strategies to bypass and overcome these complications.

Specifics of Online H-Psychotherapy: Techniques and Strategies

The challenge of online interactive hypnosis and H-therapy is the need to rely heavily on verbal interactive communication with the hypnotized patient. This can be achieved by teaching patients dissociative automatic speech (Zeig, 1985) and offering suggestions in the form of questions (Battino, 2005; Yapko & Sheehan, 2012). These strategies for handling the online hypnotic process can help patients verbally communicate with a therapist without interrupting the hypnotic trance state essential for effective therapeutic interventions. To achieve this goal, the following techniques are recommended.

Dissociative Automatic Speech

At the beginning of the hypnotic session, after the induction, you may offer this suggestion to the patient:

> "… you can speak freely during the trance … and with every word, you will go further and deeper into hypnosis … Your speech will remain intact, and at the same time, your body and your mind will continue to go deeper and deeper into a hypnotic trance … "

Suggestions in the Form of Questions

During the hypnotic session, suggestions will be offered to the patients in the form of questions.

"How do you feel right now? Can you now talk about …? Is it possible for you to concentrate on …? Can you imagine yourself in …? Can you release yourself from …? What can be done about this problem …? etc."

These techniques channel patients' attention toward the therapist and to participate more actively in developing and utilizing a hypnotically created therapeutic space.

To complete their adaptation to online hypnosis, therapists must hone their abilities and skills to develop and use a self-induced, externally oriented hypnotic state, usually referred to as the therapist trance. Adopting the externally directed, patient-oriented therapist trance both focuses and refines hypnotists' attentive capabilities, thus helping to prevent them from missing information completely when audio and video is fuzzy. After the patient's trance has developed sufficiently and the therapist has used the external patient-oriented hypnotist trance, the next step in H-psychotherapy is patient–therapist synchronization by entering a mutual co-trance, sometimes called attunement (Baker, 2000).

The Intersubjective Elements of Online H-Psychotherapy

H-psychotherapy is an interactive, intersubjective process, and this understanding has slowly but steadily penetrated professional discourse (Alter, 2020; Diamond, 2000). Synchronized co-trance between the hypnotist and the hypnotized patient has not only been theoretically discussed (Varga et al., 2006), but has also been empirically researched (Varga & Kekecs, 2014). During a face-to-face interaction, the patient's trance meets and synchronizes with the hypnotist's trance, allegedly through neurocognitive mechanisms of mirror neurons (Wickramasekera, 2015; Rossi & Rossi, 2006). These are mediated by vocal prosody, interpersonal synchrony, and nonverbal communication between the hypnotist and the hypnotized. The video conference setting and online disturbances weaken visual and auditory cues, which are so important during face-to-face communication and serve as the basis of the therapist–patient attunement during online H-psychotherapy. To synchronize the patient's and therapist's hypnotic trances, we must rely on trance elements that are not usually located in the spotlight of clinical attention. The patient's externally oriented trance (p-EOT) and the therapist's internally oriented trance (t-IOT) can become leading instruments of attunement (Baker, 2000) throughout H-psychotherapy with a distant patient. During hypnosis implementation, specifically after the induction, the therapist usually directs the patient's attention to the internal body–mind processes (p-IOT), while simultaneously attentively self-orienting toward the patient's verbal and physical behavior (t-EOT). Parallel to this process, the patient's externally focused attention (p-EOT) directed toward the hypnotist's communication and the therapist's sensitivity to therapist internal processes (t-IOT) are almost automatically developed. These processes require more attention during induction and development of the hypnotic trance as they are essential elements of online H-psychotherapy. An externally oriented trance can help the patient to be more attuned to the therapist. The therapist's internally oriented trance can facilitate the therapist's use of reminiscences of past hypnotic face-to-face interactions, to complete the missing or Web-distorted elements of the current hypnotic interaction. An internally oriented hypnotist trance can also enhance the hypnotist's clinical intuition by effectively using reverie experiences (Ogden, 1997).

The patient's silence or intense emotional expression (abreaction) during online H-psychotherapy can be very challenging for both the patient and the psychotherapist. A hypnotic trance can intensify the patient's and the therapist's emotional expressions. Physical distance from the therapist can cause the patient to feel abandoned by the therapist, and the therapist can sense a lack of control. Appropriate coping with those hypnotherapeutic interactions can enable the creation of a safe hypnotic and therapeutic space beyond the technological, physical, and psychological barriers. In face-to-face hypnotic interaction, silence is usually a unidirectional process: the patient remains silent and the therapist talks, or vice versa. The therapist's ability to be quiet during the patient's silence develops the patient's ability to be alone in the presence of others (Winnicott, 1958), thus increasing the patient's confidence and ability to work online. During hypnotic psychotherapy, patients, generally, spontaneously take some time to be silent and to process some critical issues that have arisen during the hypnotic session (Rossi et al., 2013). The therapist is responsible for recognizing and allowing this meaningful silence without premature interruption. Imagine a case in which the patient uses hollow verbalizations, masking anxiety about remaining silent. In such cases, it is useful to initiate quietness and invite patients to be quiet for a moment or two, allowing themselves to internalize issues addressed during the session. Additionally, the therapist's ability to be calm and empathic during online H-psychotherapy, while a patient forcefully expresses emotions, signals to the patient that, although the therapist is distant, he or she can handle and contain the patient's emotional expressions.

Reservations

Online H-psychotherapy is a fruitful but somewhat complicated therapeutic modality, and, as with every type of therapy, some safety measures are vital. First, all online newcomers will require some guidance, and supervision is essential for a therapist who feels incompetent in or uncertain about implementing hypnosis remotely. It is preferable to work with a patient who has prior experience with face-to-face H-psychotherapy. Patients with PTSD, personality disorders, or suicidal tendencies should be treated only by specialists in these very sensitive mental health areas. Appropriate precautions are needed, such as ensuring that trusted family members, friends, or neighbors are available to be contacted during the session, if necessary. Ethical guidelines concerning telemedicine, provided by the American Society of Clinical Hypnosis (ASCH) and local professional hypnosis communities, can be very useful for orienting and securing online hypnotherapy.

Conclusions

After erupting into most therapists' consciousness during the COVID-19 pandemic, online H-psychotherapy is here to stay. The opportunities that it reveals will gradually spread among clinicians and their patients. Our ability, as professionals, to be flexible in applying the modes of therapy that we promote and deliver to our patients will define our future relevance as specialists in the mental health arena.

Practical Considerations and Tips

- Use only high-quality web cameras and headphones, and ensure high bandwidth connectivity.
- Be sure to set a safety protocol for online connection problems prior to starting the hypnosis session.
- Offer suggestions in the form of questions and help patients develop dissociative automatic speech for interactive communication during the hypnosis session.
- Be prepared to handle the patient's silence or intensive emotional abreactive expressions.
- Implement online interactive H-hypnotherapy with caution, using appropriate ethical guidelines.

References

Alter, D. S. (2020). In the intersubjective space: Hypnosis through a neuropsychological lens. *American Journal of Clinical Hypnosis*, *62*(1–2), 74–94. 10.1080/00029157. 2019.1581049

Baker, E. L. (2000). Reflections on the hypnotic relationship: Projective identification, containment, and attunement. *The International Journal of Clinical and Experimental Hypnosis*, *48*(1), 56–69. doi: 10.1080/00207140008410361

Battino, T. L. S. R. (2005). *Ericksonian approaches: A comprehensive manual* (2nd ed.). Crown House.

Crowe, M., Inder, M., Farmar, R., & Carlyle, D. (2020). Delivering psychotherapy by video conference in the time of COVID-19: Some considerations. *Journal of Psychiatric and Mental Health Nursing*. 10.1111/jpm.12659

Diamond, M. J. (2000). The long and winding road from concept to practice: The intersubjective shaping of psychoanalytically informed technique in contemporary hypnosis--a commentary upon and extension of Baker's "reflections on the hypnotic relationship." *The International Journal of Clinical and Experimental Hypnosis, 48*(1), 70–85. 10.1080/00207140008410362

Erickson, M. H., & Rossi, E. L. (1979). *Hypnotherapy: An exploratory casebook* (Har/Cas ed). Ardent Media.

Farrell-Carnahan, L., Ritterband, L. M., Bailey, E. T., Thorndike, F. P., Lord, H. R., & Baum, L. D. (2010). Feasibility and preliminary efficacy of a self-hypnosis intervention available on the web for cancer survivors with insomnia. *E-Journal of Applied Psychology, 6*(2), 10–23. https://psycnet.apa.org/record/2011-01464-003

Flynn, N. (2019). Effect of an online hypnosis intervention in reducing migraine symptoms: A randomized controlled trial. *International Journal of Clinical and Experimental Hypnosis, 67*(3), 313–335. doi: 10.1080/00207144.2019.1612674

Gallese, V., Eagle, M. N., & Migone, P. (2007). Intentional attunement: Mirror neurons and the neural underpinnings of interpersonal relations. *Journal of the American Psychoanalytic Association, 55*(1), 131–175. 10.1177/00030651070550010601

Green, J. P. (2003). Beliefs about hypnosis: Popular beliefs, misconceptions, and the importance of experience. *International Journal of Clinical and Experimental Hypnosis, 51*(4), 369–381. 10.1076/iceh.51.4.369.16408

Hasan, S. S., Pearson, J. S., Morris, J., & Whorwell, P. J. (2019). Skype hypnotherapy for irritable bowled syndrome: Effectiveness and comparison with face-to-face treatment. *International Journal of Clinical and Experimental Hypnosis, 67*(1), 69–80. doi: 10.1080/00207144.2019.1553766

Hoslin, L., Motamed, C., Maurice-Szamburski, A., Legoupil, C., Pons, S., & Bordenave, L. (2019). Impact of hypnosis on patient experience after venous access port implantation. *Anaesthesia Critical Care & Pain Medicine, 38*(6), 609–613. 10.1016/j.accpm.2019.02.013

Kittle, J., & Spiegel, D. (2021). Hypnosis: The most effective treatment you have yet to prescribe. *The American Journal of Medicine, 134*(3), 304–305. doi: 10.1016/j.amjmed.2020.10.010

Levitan, A. A., & Johnson, J. M. (1986). The role of touch in healing and hypnotherapy. *American Journal of Clinical Hypnosis, 28*(4), 218–223. 10.1080/00029157.1986.10402657

Lunn, S. (2002). The psychoanalytic room. *Scandanavian Psychoanalytic Review*, 135–142. doi: 10.1080/01062301.2002.10592738

Mayer, A. (2006). Lost objects: From the laboratories of hypnosis to the psychoanalytic setting. *Science in Context, 19*(1), 37–64. doi: 10.1017/s026988970500075x

Meyerson, J. (2017a). Self-talk monitoring and utilization for enhancing hypnotic induction. *American Journal of Clinical Hypnosis, 60*(2), 149–158. doi: 10.1080/00029157.2017.1289465

Meyerson, J. (2017b). Presenting hypnosis to patients. In G. R. Elkins (Ed.), *Handbook of medical and psychological hypnosis* (pp. 29–34). Springer. doi: 10.1891/9780826124876

Meyerson, J. (2020). Online hypnotic psychotherapy with distant patients. *International Journal of Complementary & Alternative Medicine, 13*(6), 238–242. doi: 10.15406/ijcam.2020.13.00522

Meyerson, J., Gelkopf, M., Golan, G., & Shahamorov, E. (2013). What motivates professionals to learn and use hypnosis in clinical practice? *The International Journal of Clinical and Experimental Hypnosis, 61*(1), 71–80. 10.1080/00207144.2013.729437

Ogden T. H. (1997). Reverie and interpretation. *The Psychoanalytic Quarterly*, *66*(4), 567–595. https://psycnet.apa.org/record/1997-43805-001

Pintar, J., & Lynn, S. J. (2008). *Hypnosis: A brief history*. Wiley-Blackwell.

Rossi, E., Mortimer, J., & Rossi, K. (2013). Therapeutic hypnosis, psychotherapy, and the digital humanities: The narratives and culturomics of hypnosis, 1800–2008. *American Journal of Clinical Hypnosis*, *55*(4), 343–359. 10.1080/00029157.2012.696078

Rossi, E. L., & Rossi, K. L. (2006). The neuroscience of observing consciousness and mirror neurons in therapeutic hypnosis. *American Journal of Clinical Hypnosis*, *48*(4), 263–278. 10.1080/00029157.2006.10401533

Rossi, E. L. (1997). The symptom path to enlightenment: The psychobiology of Jung's constructive method. *Psychological Perspectives*, *36*(1), 68–84. 10.1080/00332929708403330

Simpson, S., Morrow, E., Jones, M., Ferguson, J., & Brebner, E. (2002). Video-Hypnosis—The Provision of Specialized Therapy via Videoconferencing. *Journal of Telemedicine and Telecare*, *8*(2_suppl), 78–79. doi: 10.1258/135763302320302136

Strauss, B. S. (1997). Operator variables in hypnotherapy. In J. W. Rhue, S. J. Lynn, & I. Kirsch (Eds.), *Handbook of clinical hypnosis* (3rd ed., pp. 55–72). American Psychological Association.

Varga, K., Józsa, E., Bányai, É. I., & Gősi-Greguss, A. C. (2006). A new way of characterizing hypnotic interactions: Dyadic Interactional Harmony (DIH) questionnaire. *Contemporary Hypnosis*, *23*(4), 151–166. 10.1002/ch.320

Varga, K., & Kekecs, Z. (2014). Oxytocin and cortisol in the Hypnotic Interaction1. *International Journal of Clinical and Experimental Hypnosis*, *62*(1), 111–128. https://doiorg/10.1080/00207144.2013.841494

Weinberg, H., & Rolnick, A. (2019). *Theory and practice of online therapy: Internet-delivered interventions for individuals, groups, families, and organizations* (1st ed.). Routledge.

Weitzenhoffer, A. M. (1972). Open-ended distance hypnotherapy. *American Journal of Clinical Hypnosis*, *14*(4), 236–248. doi: 10.1080/00029157.1972.10402191

Wickramasekera, I. E. (2015). Mysteries of Hypnosis and the Self Are Revealed by the Psychology and Neuroscience of Empathy. *American Journal of Clinical Hypnosis*, 57, 330–348 10.1080/00029157.2014.978495.

Winnicott, D. W. (1958). The Capacity to be Alone. *International Journal of Psychoanalysis*, *39*, 416–420. https://www.pep-web.org/document.php?id=ijp.039.0416a

Yapko, M. D., & Sheehan, P. (2012). *Trancework: An introduction to the practice of clinical hypnosis* (4th ed.). Routledge.

Zeig, J. K. (1985). *Teaching seminar with Milton H. Erickson* (1st ed.). Routledge.

Section III

Couples & Families

16 An Introduction to Online Couple and Family Therapy

Arnon Rolnick, Adam Leighton, and Haim Weinberg

A recent study by Morgan et al. (2021) found that marital and family therapy (MFT) cases were significantly less likely to transition to teletherapy than individual cases, although couples and families suffered significant stress during the COVID-19 pandemic (see below). Not enough has been written about online MFT. An important exception is Teletherapy & Telesupervision Guidelines II, published recently by the Association of Marital and Family Therapy Regulatory Boards.

The Effects of National or Universal Crisis on Couples and Families: COVID-19 as a Case Study

The extensive isolation, separation, and loss caused by the COVID-19 pandemic increased the risk to the quality and stability of couples' relationships. According to Lebow (2020), the reasons for this include loss of loved ones due to the pandemic, unemployment and financial stress, caregiving responsibilities, children's remote learning, and exacerbation of distressing relational dynamics, resulting in an increased need for therapy. In addition, pandemic stressors were found to exacerbate domestic conflict (Arenas-Arroyo et al., 2021).

The Uniqueness of Online Couple and Family Therapy

The fundamental difference between individual and couples/family therapy is clear. Unlike individual therapy, which involves one client and one therapist**, online couple therapy involves at least one therapist and a multi-participant system, i.e., the family or the couple.** This requires the development of fundamentally more complicated methods for meeting with a couple or family online.

Online therapy can involve different types of distance settings:

1   The therapist is in one place, and the couple is in a different place.
2   Each participant is in a different place. This may occur when the couple is in a long-distance relationship or prefers not to meet in the same place due to a painful breakup.

DOI: 10.4324/9781003205029-20

3   In family therapy, the couple meets a therapist remotely, while the couple is in one place and other family members are in a third location.
4   Theoretically, the therapist can be in the same room as one of the partners, while the other partner is in a different location (we usually do not recommend this asymmetrical setup).

In couples/family therapy, there is **always a conflict in the background**. Some types of misunderstandings or even disputes or quarrels are common-place in family therapy meetings. The therapist's role is very often to guide the conversation or to serve as a "traffic cop" and stop the partners' angry re-actions. This means the family therapist takes a leadership role in minimizing angry hostility.

Conflicts of this kind between couples are usually correlated with phy-siological arousal that might not be noticed online, as these bodily reac-tions might not be detected. When working with couples in general, and online in particular, each partner must feel understood and acknowledged as an individual. The therapist must therefore find ways to produce in-timacy not only between the partners, but also with each of them in-dividually.

The therapist's role in online couple therapy is more complicated, due to the need to intervene and ensure that each family member has the oppor-tunity to speak separately. This means that the therapist assumes the role of a conductor in the orchestra who signals to the different instruments and invites them to play their musical role or to listen silently to the other instruments in the orchestra (the same situation occurs in group therapy). This can become quite complicated in online multi-participant therapy settings. While in the same physical space, the therapist can use cues like moving physically closer to one partner with his/her chair or slightly touching the other, this cannot be done in video-based therapy.

The fact that the whole body is not seen in online therapy constitutes a major disadvantage in individual and family/couple therapy. It prevents the therapist from viewing interactions between family members and notingnon-verbal bodily interaction, which is very important in couple relationships.

In an in-person setting, where everyone is in the same room, it is evident to whom the therapist is referring, as the therapist's head and body face one participant or another. When using video, the therapist should be aware that the couple cannot identify who is being addressed, so the therapist must find alternative ways of indicating this. Moreover, eye contact is lost in online couple and family meetings, making it difficult for the participants to know which of them is the focus of the therapist's intervention. The authors of the chapters that deal with MFT review this shortcoming of online therapy and suggest some solutions.

Despite the many challenges, we believe there are certain advantages to online couple and family therapy.

Advantages of Working with Couples and Families Online

Expanding the Concept of Home Visits

The concept of home visits is quite common in the field of social work, and is used with families contending with complex, multiple problems (Hogue et al., 2020).

We can adapt this well-documented approach for online MFT to enhance therapeutic interventions. This method can give therapists more information about the human and physical environment in which the couple/family live. We can ask the couple/family to use the computer camera to allow us to "visit their home" and to see their space and the other members of the family.

Another advantage is that online MFT allows the couple/family members to receive psychotherapy sessions without the stigma of going to a mental health clinic.

The Internet Allows Us to Incorporate Wider Family Circles into the Therapy Program

Many leading family therapists incorporate the entire "clan" of the family of origin, suggesting that they can serve as "consultants" for therapy. Framo (1976) proposed that marital and family difficulties are extensions of relationship problems the spouses experienced in their original families. According to this view, couples who seek therapy would need to deal directly with past and present issues related to their families of origin to allow reconstructive changes in their present family relationships.

Whitaker (1976) argued that every family member is vital to the process and that if families "elect" to attend therapy without a particular family member, it is a significant decision that might reveal important information and some secrets about the family.

Due to geographic distance and other technical constraints, classical recommendations to involve extended family members are not often implemented in regular face-to-face family therapy. In most cases, the therapist works with the couple or the immediate family members who live in the same household and overlooks the value of other family members who live further away.

A related issue is the possibility of using co-therapy. Since family and couple therapy involves more interactions and conflicts than individual therapy, using two therapists might be an advantage. However, this may be quite difficult to organize for face-to-face sessions due to practical issues of time and space. This issue can easily be resolved in online family/couple therapy, which allows more opportunities for co-therapy. Some of the advantages of this format are that it expands creativity, range of interventions, and techniques; enhances transference and improves control of counter-transference; and provides a model for interpersonal cooperation (Hoffman et al., 1994).

Online Meetings can be Easily Recorded

Recording sessions are highly recommended in MFT, but can be somewhat cumbersome. The therapist would have to bring multiple cameras to shoot various angles, and place microphones near himself/herself and the couple/family. This procedure is distracting, and draws much attention from the participants. As a result, many therapists prefer not to record their sessions. In online therapy, however, recording is seamless.

Viewing session recordings allows participants to identify habitual patterns and catch subtle signs that can predict escalation. Video recording can be an intervention in and of itself. Replaying specific moments of the couple's interaction might give the partners a new perspective on their maladaptive responses. Observing video recordings is valuable for therapists as well, as it allows them to monitor their interventions and learn from their mistakes.

Recordings are the Best Tool for Supervision

Video recordings allow supervisors to monitor trainees' therapy sessions and follow their progress and abilities in steering couple therapy. Supervision of a recorded session makes it possible to monitor the verbal and nonverbal behaviors of the couple and the therapist, which may be more precise and objective than the classical methods of reading psychotherapy notes.

Real-Time Supervision Using Breakout Rooms

Live, real-time supervision via a one-way mirror is common practice in couple and family therapy (Cade & Cornwell, 1983). However, this requires a special place and special arrangements for at least four people: the therapist, the couple, and the supervisor. As was explained earlier regarding co-therapy, the internet overcomes barriers of time and space, and enables practical live supervision without a one-way mirror. Moreover, the breakout room option in the video applications can be used for quiet consultations between the supervisor and the trainee, which is more elegant than calling the trainee by phone or entering the therapy room.

Using the Share Screen Feature to Enhance Couple and Family Therapy

Most videoconference meeting applications allow participants to share their screens with the other participants. This function creates new possibilities that are difficult to apply in face-to-face settings. For example, many couple therapy interventions suggest that the couple begin by focusing on the early days of their relationship. Revisiting those days can be a reminder of what is good about their relationship and why they are together. The therapist may ask the couple to use the share screen feature to share pictures or video clips of the days they felt satisfied in their relationship. Sharing such moments can be very moving. Similarly, the therapist might ask the couple to upload and share pictures of their children. Our experience is that the virtual presence of the children can help the couple focus on the shared values in their lives and reduce fights and quarrels.

Sharing Psychoeducation Materials Related to the Couple's Problems

A major step in couple therapy is identifying the processes that result in misunderstanding, pain, and fights. This identification is usually based on a specific model (e.g., the four horses of the eclipse and its countermeasures in the Gottman approach; schemas in schema-focused therapy for couples; and Sue Johnson's EFT cycles diagram). Keeping this model visible to the couple can help them try a new means of interaction.

Using the Whiteboard for Couple Drawing

Many couple therapists who use art therapy techniques ask the couple to draw together to help them analyze and demonstrate their interaction patterns. The whiteboard, a tool that is available in most video apps, enables participants to draw together. It can be used in couple therapy for creating a couple drawing.

Homework

Most couple therapy methods suggest some type of homework that the couple should do.

In our first book, we differentiated between two ways in which the internet has affected psychotherapy: One involves the option of video-based conversations with a therapist, and the second involves the use of stand-alone applications that do not involve a therapist. Although the latter is not the focus of our book, we would like to mention some hybrid programs that are based on work done with therapists that is complemented by an application.

Several of the methods described in this book have been used to develop internet-based applications that complete the work that is done with the therapist. Gottman developed the Couple Builder, Sue Johnson created the Hold Me Tight website that uses EFT methods, and Imago Relation Therapy developed a program named Couplehood – A New Way to Love. Apart from these applications, there are thousands of applications claiming to help enhance relationships, but they are beyond the scope of this book.

One type of hybrid intervention presented as an example is an internet-based process-management system named The Resonator (Rolnick & Gronich, 2019), which follows the couple during their daily routine, allowing them to incubate the therapeutic content in their consciousness so that it can be processed more extensively and evolve between therapy sessions. Resonators include images, audio and video, and supporting text, as well as tools for collecting important information on the couple's status. "Resonate" means that partners and the therapist synchronize their focus to understand the issues on which they are working, define a common language for describing these issues, and determine what may help the patients overcome their issues. This is an intriguing example for a hybrid intervention that works between meetings to continuously recalibrate the couple's focus of attention with the spirit of the therapeutic process. It also means that therapeutic content remains effective between meetings.

Summary

In this introduction, we discussed the uniqueness of online couple and family therapy and pointed out some of the obstacles in MFT from a distance. However, we also presented the possible advantages of meeting with families via the internet. As you read Chapters 17, 18, 19, 20, and 21, you will likely draw conclusions similar to ours – there are obstacles to online MFT, but following Galileo, "E pur si muove!", namely online couple and family therapy is possible and does work!

References

Arenas-Arroyo, E., Fernandez-Kranz, D., & Nollenberger, N. (2021). Intimate partner violence under forced cohabitation and economic stress: Evidence from the COVID-19 pandemic. *Journal of Public Economics, 194*, 104350.

Cade, B. W., & Cornwell, M. (1983). The evolution of the one-way screen. *The Australian Journal of Family Therapy, 4*, 73–80.

Clinical Child and Family Psychology Review (2021) 24: 244–266 10.1007/s10567-02 0-00340-2

Framo, J. L. (1976). Family of origin as a therapeutic resourcefor adults in marital and family therapy: You can and should go home again. *Family Process, 15*, 193–210.

Hoffman, S., Gafni, S., & Laub, B. (1994). *Cryotherapy with individuals, families and groups.* Northvale, N. J.: Jason Aronson.

Hogue, A., Becker, S. J., Fishman, M., Henderson, C. E., & Levy, S. (2020). Youth OUD treatment during and after COVID: Increasing family involvement across the services continuum. *Journal of Substance Abuse Treatment, 120*, 108159. 10.1016/j.jsat.2020.108159

Mclean etal. (2021). Exploring the efficacy of telehealth for family therapy through systematic, meta-analytic, and qualitative evidence.*Clinical Child and Family Psychology Review, 24*, 244–266. 10.1007/s10567-020-00340-2

Morgan, A., et al. (Apr. 2021). The transition to teletherapy in marriage and family therapy training settings during COVID-19: What do the data tell us?. *Journal of Marital and Family Therapy, 47*(2), Blackwell Publishing Ltd., 320.

Pietromonaco and Overall (2022). Implications of social isolation, separation, and loss during the COVID-19 pandemic for couples' relationships. *Current Opinion in Psychology, 43*, 189–194.

Rolnick, A., & Gronich, D. (2019). Schrödinger's cat turns to therapy: A tool for enhancing therapy. Proceedings of the Technology, Mind, and Society, Washington, DC, USA.

Whitaker, C. (1976). A family is a four-dimensional relationship. In P. J. Guerin (Ed.), *Family therapy: Theory and practice* (pp. 182–192). New York: G Gardner press.

17 Emotionally Focused Couple Therapy Online: Handholding from a Distance

Lorrie Brubacher and Ting Liu

Emotionally Focused Therapy (EFT), has reshaped the field of psychotherapy to be focused on the healing power of emotional connection. Initially designed as a model of couple therapy, EFT is now broadly used across three modalities of individual (EFIT), family (EFFT) and couple therapy (EFCT) (Johnson, 2019). Emotional connection is the primary mechanism of change in EFT. Creating and maintaining empathic responsiveness and emotional connection between therapist and clients, towards the goal of shaping emotional connections within clients' relationships, are tasks that are fostered in EFT whether in-person or online.

In this chapter, we illustrate how EFT, by its very nature, is adaptive to online therapy. We focus on the modality of EFCT and briefly comment on the modality of EFIT (Brubacher, 2017b; Johnson, 2009; 2019; Johnson & Campbell, 2022), which is similarly amendable to an online format. We discuss how the attachment-orientation of the model and the experiential and systemic interventions aptly meet the challenges of online therapy. The three core ingredients shown to be associated with success in EFT therapy – therapeutic alliance, deepening of emotional experiencing, and shaping affiliative encounters (Brubacher & Wiebe, 2019; Greenman & Johnson, 2013) can all be created online. To operationalize these ingredients online or in-person, an EFT therapist needs to be solidly grounded in the model, consciously and deliberately aware of their presence in the therapeutic collaboration, and empathically attuned to the clients. We argue that there is little different or additional that an EFT therapist needs to do when working online that they would not already be doing in-person.

Emotional Proximity: Handholding from a Distance

Bowlby (1988) first put forth the view that the need for a secure base with reliable others from which to venture forth into the world endures throughout a lifetime. *From the cradle to the grave*, humans need emotional connection to survive. Infants require the physical presence of their primary attachment figure, and the older a child gets, the less need there is for continual physical presence to feel the security of the bond. The need for secure attachment

DOI: 10.4324/9781003205029-21

extends into adulthood and has been well-documented in adult attachment literature, which illustrates that adults can experience the security of an attachment bond in a representational manner at times when the attachment figure is not physically present (Cassidy & Shaver, 2016).

Adult attachment bonds differ from parent-child attachment in that adult attachment bonds are *representational*, meaning that adults can experience the soothing effects of the bond in spite of physical distance. Coan et al. (2006) demonstrated in a series of handholding studies with subjects in an fMRI machine, that proximity to a human touch regulates negative affect by buffering the perception of threat. In the globalizing world, however, physical distance has become a fact and a stressor in many couples' lives. To adapt to this reality, loved ones, as well as clinicians, need to develop both technical and emotional strategies to maintain emotional proximity without physical togetherness. How can the attachment foundation and the need for emotional proximity and co-regulation be realized in online therapy? EFT therapists create *representational* hand-holding with EFT interventions online.

Accessibility, responsiveness, and engagement (A.R.E.) as in "Are you there for me?" are the central attachment behaviors that determine security or distress in close relationships. Research specific to couples and attachment suggests that these supportive behaviors predict both secure attachment and relationship satisfaction (Feeney, 2002; Rholes et al., 2001). Therapists operationalize A.R.E. behaviors by their attunement, validation, empathic responsiveness, and collaboration, thereby serving as a secure base for clients.

The EFT macro-intervention, the EFT Tango is an almost formulaic guide, albeit used with flexibility and artistry once the moves are familiar to the therapist, for shaping this secure base. The five moves of the EFT Tango are: mirroring and reflecting present process; assembling elements of emotion and deepening; shaping engaged encounters; processing the impact of the encounters; integrating and validating. Each macro move is made up of various micro-skills: empathic attuning and responding, validation, evocative questioning, heightening, empathic conjecturing, therapist transparency or self-disclosure, reflecting and tracking patterns, reframing, refocusing, shaping encounters. Specially designed reframes and conjectures to heighten the impact of the in-session encounters are known as *slicing thinner, catching bullets*, and *seeding attachment*. (For more detail on the interventions see Allan et al., 2021; Brubacher, 2018; Furrow et al., 2022; Johnson, 2019, 2020.) These interventions are used across modalities, with the only difference being that in EFIT, the engaged encounters are shaped between client and therapist, between client and an imagined other (such as an attachment figure or an abusive other) or between two parts of self (such as between a vulnerable part and a more nurturing part.)

EFT is Naturally Adaptive to Online Therapy

We argue that working online compels therapists to do their very best EFT. Working online requires paying exquisite attention to nonverbal cues and to the state of the therapeutic alliance. Attuning to nonverbal elements of communication is a vital part of all three tasks of EFT: building and maintaining alliance especially task alliance; deepening emotional experiencing; shaping encounters (Brubacher & Wiebe, 2019; Greenman & Johnson, 2013). EFT therapists attune carefully to the nonverbal cues they can see online, typically only from the waist up – and intentionally follow and explicitly comment on verbal and nonverbal expressions. They can also invite clients to tell them what may be happening, for example, with a couple, "I can't see – but did you just reach over and take her hand?" They engage clients to help them in attending to nonverbal, somatic experiencing, thereby slowing the pace and heightening explicit awareness of the links between verbal and bodily communication, totally important for an experiential therapy like EFT (Kailanko et al., 2021). The need to be very focused when working online can help a therapist to remember to use a deliberately slow pace to keep partners or individuals emotionally engaged in the present moment.

Working online compels therapists to prioritize building and maintaining trust in the therapeutic alliance – a staple of EFT. It is inherent in EFT, that therapists focus on building and maintaining an alliance both in terms of creating a trusting bond and confidence in the tasks of therapy, both very important elements for creating emotional proximity online. Emotional proximity is built in the personal, nonpathologizing way that EFT therapists seek to create and maintain the therapeutic alliance: To collaborate, to communicate empathic understanding, and make conjectures on the attachment leading edge of what clients have articulated, always with tentativeness, inviting clients to check whether the therapist's words accurately match their experience, and to make corrections wherever necessary. The safety created in a trusting therapeutic alliance helps with engaging clients more and more explicitly in their present-moment process. The task element of the alliance – whether clients are finding the tasks of therapy to be relevant to their goals is particularly important for the success of EFT (Brubacher & Wiebe, 2019; Johnson & Talitman, 1997). Online therapy may be unfamiliar to clients, thus working online, EFT therapists' are compelled to check on client's comfort with the process – another vital element of good EFT.

Attuning to the fine nuances of client's expressions, both verbal and nonverbal, to the state of the therapeutic alliance, and to clients' comfort with the key tasks of deepening emotional experience and participating in therapist directed encounters – are the basic components of EFT. They are the processes that can create safety and emotional proximity in the physical distance of working online. In other words, what makes for effective online therapy is simply doing good EFT.

Online EFT therapy actually has some benefits over in-person therapy. Change in EFT begins with identifying, accepting, and validating precisely where people are, and online therapy is inherently oriented towards meeting people where they are and is responsive to people's needs during the added stressors of the pandemic. Online therapy reduces travel costs for clients and office costs for therapists, thus making it more available to serve clients who may be financially strained and otherwise unable to attend therapy. Aside from pandemic restraints for meeting in person, working online is helpful for couples who are not in close physical proximity to a therapist's office. In situations where cost is not an issue, being able to do sessions from home is beneficial for many clients because it reduces travel time. It is also a resource for spouses who, due to work requirements are not in the same location but can join in online from different locations. If partners are in different locations, online therapy combats the deleterious health effects of loneliness (Greenman & Johnson, 2022). Meeting online makes it more viable to do couple sessions with an infant or variations of older children who may be in the house but engaged independently in an activity. Given EFT's effectiveness is changing relationship satisfaction and individual depression (Wittenborn et al., 2019) online EFT has the added benefit of being accessible for couples where one partner may be too depressed to go to a therapy session.

Resources that can complement couple therapy, whether in-person or online are the online *Hold Me Tight* <https://holdmetightonline.com> program as well as the print or audio book *Hold Me Tight* (Johnson, 2008). Couples can follow the exercises, called *conversations for a lifetime of love* to create more contact between therapy sessions or use it as self-help program to improve the emotional connection in their relationship.

EFT's Response to Therapist Questions and Anxiety of doing EFT online

The EFT therapeutic stance and interventions seamlessly address therapists' questions and fears of doing EFT online. Many of these questions could arise with couple (EFCT) or individual (EFIT) online therapy, however several are specific to couple therapy.

How can I Work Deeply Online if I am Uncomfortable with Emotions or Intimacy?

For therapists who are not comfortable working with emotions, starting with online EFT may provide a natural shield that protect the therapists from feeling overwhelmed and flooded by intense emotions. This can help a therapist to pay attention to their own emotional balance, and slowly and patiently, take increasing risks of emotional engagement within themselves and with their clients. Good therapists will not hide behind the computer screen, rather they will continuously explore what may be blocking them from engaging in the present-moment emotional experience of their clients. They will also read and practice the micro-skills needed for assembling and deepening emotional processes and explore self-of-the-therapist issues to increase their level of comfort about and competency for working with emotions.

How do I Manage Distractions in Clients' Home?

Distractions can be helpfully integrated into the therapy process. They are an opportunity for therapists to demonstrate the EFT accepting, empathic stance towards clients in their current distress. For example, in couple therapy, a therapist tracking the cycle in Stage 1 says, "I noticed when the baby started crying, you looked at Mark and he immediately jumped up to tend to the baby (reflecting and tracking interpersonal process). How is it to have him so quickly respond to your look?" Or "How is it for you Mark when Karla glances at you? What do you see on her face?" A therapist could also explore the baby's crying as part of their cycle, "What usually happens when the baby starts crying in the middle of your fight?" Or "What do you typically do when your fight is interrupted by the baby's crying?"

We can make distractions part of the process during engaged encounters as well. A dog who suddenly shows up during an emotionally heightened moment – of warm intimacy or conflict – can be part of heightening the present moment emotional experiencing in Tango Move 2 assembly.

> How is it for you, that right now, your dog nuzzled his way between you, as you were taking in each other's soft gazes in response to Isaiah sharing with you that his turning away and sleeping for two days was the way he coped with the arrow through his heart at your threat to leave?

Jessica with a warm smile: I just thought Isaiah didn't care … but our dog always senses the warm moments of truth! Similarly a family pet interrupting a moment of escalation, can be a moment the therapist uses to help the couple stand back and observe what is happening in the room – "What must the dog notice is happening here" can be a way to step back and explicitly evoke the threatening triggers and the reactive responses of both partners.

What if the Internet Connection Freezes?

EFT therapists are adept at *going back* to moments rife with attachment emotion. After reestablishing an internet connection, after it freezes or breaks, an EFT therapist is nonplussed, doing what is frequently done in EFT. They check their notes for a significant *emotional handle* (phrase or image) and replay the present process. "Let's go back to the moment when … ." Whatever stage of change clients are in, an EFT therapist knows it is an important key ingredient of change to deepen present moment experiencing (Klein et al., 1986). Replaying a moment, particularly a moment of interpersonal contact or a moment of a client accessing a new element of emotion will be helpful.

What if My Voice is Too Loud and Harsh?

Many therapists have a tendency to project their voice louder than necessary on video calls. EFT therapists working online can slow their pace and monitor their volume, which will help with softening one's voice. Regularly listening to one's recorded sessions is a good way for therapists to monitor their tone and voice on video calls.

How can I Build Trust when Working Online with Couples I have Never Met Before?

Individual sessions, usually held after the first one or two couple sessions and the deliberately slow pacing, soft, soothing voice (unless matching strong assertive affect) helps with building trust. Being transparent and inviting clients to discuss any challenges they feel about the therapy, are built into EFT and help to make online work safer and more alive.

How do I Contain Escalation Between Partners?

First, EFT therapists interrupt and intervene as soon as they see signs of escalating conflict, especially when couples are clearly stuck in their persistently vicious cycle. Second, EFT therapists contain escalation by reflecting present process as part of their cycle, soothing and validating reactive emotions and *catching bullets* (reframing aggression). Third, after validating reactivity, to contain and communicate empathic understanding, EFT therapists reflect with RISSSSC to zoom in on clients' vulnerable emotions underneath the conflict to provide soothing and comfort. Containing escalation is particularly important for online EFT sessions, to prevent clients from leaving the meeting or shutting down the computer to cope with intense negative emotions.

How do I Build and Hold Emotional Intensity?

There are two responses to this question. First, similar to in-person EFT, to deepen and maintain engagement with some newly accessed emotional experiencing in Stage 1 or to deepen vulnerable engagement with a core attachment fear or need in Stage 2, EFT therapists will heighten with the micro-skills of RISSSSC (repetition, images, simple, soft, slow voice, with specifics, and using client's words). This helps a client *risk* deepening emotional experience. Therapists will not, however, heighten beyond a client's *window of tolerance*.

An EFT therapist seeking to deepen the sadness a partner expresses, validates, "It makes a lot of sense that you are feeling sad, when you experience Andrea to be cold and distant and you feel it as rejection and when you start to believe that she has fallen out of love with you." The client keeps her head down, remains silent, and the therapist is unclear what she is experiencing. Using an evocative question the therapist asks, "Paula, as I was talking about your deep sadness, you became very quiet. Can you help me understand what is happening?" Paula buries her head deeper, remaining silent. The therapist waits a short moment to give her space, then validates and conjectures to repair the alliance, "This may be too much for you right now? Perhaps we are moving too fast? It is ok if you don't want to go there." Paula whispers, "Not now – too much – too fast." The therapist responds, "I am glad that you can let me know when I move too fast. We can return to this sadness and fear when you are ready.

Secondly, to hold emotional intensity, and create corrective emotional experiences, an EFT therapists will *shape* dialogues between partners, called *engaged encounters*. Direct sharing between partners heightens emotional intensity. SHAPE provides a simple acronym for the delicate choreography.

S to Simplify and sharpen the core message to share. "When you see your partner engaged on his computer game, you walk away quietly, fuming and stewing all alone, cooking up a stew of rage, never telling him how afraid you are that he is tired of being with you."

H to Heighten. Using repetition of elements of emotion already distilled, "Do you feel that ache in your heart – that feels like it will break? So afraid to share your fear, that you just slink away quietly, cooking up a stew of rage for later. Yes? – you feel that ache in your heart?"

A to Anticipate. "Imagine turning to your partner and sharing this new awareness – that under all your fuming inside that feels so lonely and tumultuous, in your fear that your partner is happier without you! Just notice in your body how it feels to anticipate sharing this with them."

P to directing client to Present message "Turn and tell him about your aching heart filled with fear that he is happier without you – your fear that never gets shared but gets all mixed up in a stew of rage for later."

E to Engage. If she gets distracted or exits – bring her back to the heightened emotion. "Can you look at me again – you got distracted there, yes? Can you feel your aching heart again? Can you look at your partner and feel that fear that your partner has not heard – the fear and heartbreak you hide when you walk away fuming – your fear that just maybe he is happier without you? And can you tell him, 'I do walk away from you when I get so afraid you'd rather be anywhere but with me. I slink away and don't show you my heart ache – I come back later with a stew of rage.' Can you let him know, please?"

How do I Handle Difficulty Hearing with the Awkwardness of Online Seating Arrangements?

Facilitating open, responsive dialogues between partners is a hallmark of EFT. Online, partners are typically sitting beside each other, facing the camera, rather than sitting in two separate chairs facing each other, as is typical in an EFT therapist's office. For engaged encounters a therapist will ask them to turn and face one another. "If I cannot hear you well because you are turned away from the camera, that is ok." While processing the impact of the encounter – the therapist can elicit their help. "I couldn't quite hear you, so can you repeat what you said to her?" Or to the one receiving the disclosure, "Even though I couldn't hear all of what he said to you – can you let me know how his words and the look on his face landed inside of you?" This repetition and slower pace of processing encounters has the added benefit of engaging partners more in the impact of the encounter, deepens emotional experiencing, and mines the moments of each disclosure. If partners are joining the online call from two locations – the difficulty of partners looking directly at the other as they speak is alleviated. Therapists can temporarily turn off their camera to "leave the partners alone with each other in cyber space" during the encounter if they wish.

How do I let Partners Know whom I am Addressing?

At times it is helpful to use clients' names when switching from one to the other to reflect on their experience. Without addressing partners by name, it can be confusing for couples to differentiate which partner the therapist is addressing. This also helps to keep the process personal, present-moment focused, and engaging.

The effectiveness of EFT has been established as an empirically validated model that goes beyond creating relationship satisfaction to strengthening the attachment bond and changing the brain (Burgess-Moser et al., 2015; Doss et al., 2022; Johnson et al., 2013; Rathgeber et al., 2019; Wiebe and Johnson, 2016). Online EFT, specifically, has not yet been researched – but our position in this chapter as well as our personal experiences as therapists are that we are doing the same therapy online as in person. The experience of working online can give EFT therapists an opportunity to be even more mindful of how they are impacting their clients and to check that the therapeutic alliance is solid. In particular, EFT therapists need to confirm that the two key ingredients of successful EFT – deepening emotional experiencing and shaping open and responsive dialogues – are a regular part of each therapy session and that these tasks feels helpful to the clients. If clients do not find the process relevant to their goals, therapists listen intently, validate clients' experience, and engage openly to repair the alliance. We do this in-person and online.

Distinguishing the Individual Modality of EFT (EFIT) from Other Emotion-Focused Approaches

Since this chapter highlights EFCT and also includes EFIT it is important to distinguish EFIT from other emotion-focused approaches and in particular from the emotion-focused model developed by Greenberg and colleagues (Elliott et al., 2004; Goldman & Greenberg, 2015; Goldman et al., 2021). While both models are experiential humanistic models that focus on empathic responding and creating change through working with engaged emotion in session, there are significant differences between the two approaches.

Given that the two individual approaches have different views of the problem, the route towards change is different. In EFIT the problem is seen as rigid, ineffective patterns of emotion regulation, whereas in Greenberg's model the problem is rooted in maladaptive emotion. The patterns of emotion regulation are normative attachment strategies of hyperactivation or suppression that have become rigidly self-reinforcing

EFIT, in accordance with attachment theory neither distinguishes between adaptive and maladaptive primary emotions, nor differentiates emotions as dysfunctional or functional emotion as in Greenberg's model. In EFIT, all primary emotional responses are framed as normal survival reactions in the face of what Bowlby called "separation distress" (Bowlby, 1980, 1988; Cassidy & Shaver, 2016).

EFIT is *interpersonal* first and foremost – consonant with neuroscience and attachment theory where co-regulation precedes self-regulation and effective dependency is the basis for change. Change is created in-session in relationship first by discovering and stabilizing the patterns of emotion regulation, in depression and anxiety for example, and secondly by restructuring co-regulation through engaged encounters with therapist, with imagined or between two parts of self, such as a vulnerable part and a compassionate part (Brubacher, 2017a; 2017b; 2018; Johnson, 2019). By contrast, Greenberg's model retains a focus on individual identity and self-soothing before co-regulation and prioritizes self-soothing, intrapsychic growth and differentiation from others (Goldman & Greenberg, 2015). In Greenberg's model, change in self is the starting point to prepare clients to form better relationships.

EFIT therapist interventions are captured in the parsimonious macro-intervention of five basic EFT Tango moves, described above. The simplicity of this approach potentiates deep emotional engagement on part of the therapist while they help clients to restructure rigid strategies of hyperactivating or deactivating to regulate emotion into effective strategies of co-regulation. In this process clients reshape models of self and other and move into the accessibility/openness, responsiveness and full engagement that characterizes secure attachment with others. Greenberg's model, on the other hand is more complex, having different categories emotion, needs, emotional processing difficulties, types of empathy, eleven different markers for four types of therapy tasks, and an emotion schematic system that is seen to be the base of dysfunction and ultimately the road to cure (Goldman & Greenberg, 2015). EFIT focuses not on dysfuction but upon growth and strengths, validating that, "Clinical conditions are best understood as disordered versions of what is otherwise a healthy response" (Bowlby, 1980, p. 245). For more on the comparison of the two models, see Brubacher (2017a) and Johnson, (2019). Training video examples of EFIT and EFCT online sessions can be found at www.steppingintoeft.com and at www.iceeft.com.

Practical Considerations and Tips for Doing EFT Online

While most tips below are relevant to couple and individual therapy, a few are directed to couples.

1   Have a comfortable workspace where you are at ease. Be confident with the security of your online platform and your room if working from home. Have a warm, non-distracting backdrop in your office and no disturbances.

2   Monitor your own arousal during sessions. Calm with your own breathing by recalling a supportive colleague or consultant who believes in you.

3   Discuss with clients how to create best arrangements possible, such as lighting on their faces so you can see them, sitting up as opposed to lying on their bed, and phones turned off. As in all EFT – the alliance is key. Be patient – knowing all circumstances may not be ideal.

4   Have a clear plan for how to reconnect if the internet goes down. Have an alternate way of connecting. Sessions can be done via speaker phone if the connection goes down. Remember, you are there to serve the clients.

5   Pace, pace – very important to keep a slow pace. Monitoring pacing is very important for experiential therapy and since it is automatic to project one's voice online, slowing one's pace can also help to moderate tone and maintain a calming prosody.

6   Basic empathic responsiveness (Agosta, 2020) and validation of differences between partners in couple therapy are the EFT therapist's greatest tools for creating safety, containing escalation, and deepening emotional experiencing. You don't need to be clever or perfect. You just need to be fully present. A.R.E. you fully present for each client (accessible, responsive, emotionally engaged)?

7   Be prepared, in couple therapy, for the awkwardness of partners facing forward rather than in two facing chairs – the way EFCT is best done.

8   Recognize that if you talk at the same time – you cannot be heard. Perhaps negotiate a hand sign for interruption if needed with escalated couples.

References

Agosta, L. (2020). Empathy in cyberspace: The genie is out of the bottle. In H. Weinberg & A. Rolnick, (Eds.), *Theory and practice of online therapy: Internet-delivered interventions for individuals, groups, families, and organizations* (pp. 34–46). Routledge.

Allan, R., Wiebe, S. A., Johnson, S. M., Piaseckyj, O., & Campbell, T. L. (2021). Practicing emotionally focused therapy online: Calling all relationships. *Journal of Marital & Family Therapy, 47*(2), 424–439.

Bowlby, J. (1980). *Attachment and loss: Vol. 3. Loss, sadness and depression.* Basic Books.

Bowlby, J. (1988). *A secure base.* Basic Books.

Brubacher, L. L. (2017a). Distinguishing emotionally focused therapy from emotion-focused therapy. Unpublished manuscript. Retrieved from https://www.lbrubacher.com/wp/wp-content/uploads/Distinguishing-Emotionally-Focused-from-Emotion-focused-1.pdf

Brubacher, L. (2017b). Emotionally focused individual therapy: An attachment-based experiential/systemic perspective. *Person-Centered and Experiential Psychotherapies, 16*(1), 50–67.

Brubacher, L. L. (2018). *Stepping into emotionally focused couple therapy: Key ingredients of change.* Routledge.

Brubacher, L. L., & Wiebe, S. A. (2019). Process-research to practice in Emotionally Focused Couple Therapy: A map for reflective practice. *Journal of Family Psychotherapy, 30*(4), 292–313.

Burgess-Moser, M., Johnson, S. M., Dalgleish, T., Lafontaine, M., Wiebe, S., & Tasca, G. (2015). Changes in relationship-specific attachment in emotionally focused couple therapy. *Journal of Marital and Family Therapy, 42*(2), 231–245.

Cassidy, J., & Shaver, P. R. (Eds.) (2016). *Handbook of attachment: Theory, research, and clinical applications* (3rd ed.). Guilford.

Coan, J. A., Schaefer, H. S., & Davidson, R. J. (2006). Lending a hand: Social regulation of the neural response to threat. *Psychological Science, 17*(12), 1032–1039.

Doss, B. D., Roddy, M. K., Wiebe, S. A., & Johnson, S. M. (2022). A review of the research during 2010–2019 on evidence-based treatments for couple relationship distress. *Journal of Marital and Family Therapy, 48*, 283– 306.

Elliott, R., Watson, J. C., Goldman, R. N., & Greenberg, L. S. (2004). *Learning emotion-focused therapy: The process experiential approach to change.* American Psychological Association.

Feeney, J. A. (2002). Attachment, marital interaction, and relationship satisfaction: A diary study. *Personal Relationships, 9*(1), 39–55.

Furrow, J., Johnson, S. M., Bradley, B., Brubacher, L., Campbell, T. L., Kallos-Lilly, V., Palmer, G., Rheem, K., Woolley, S. (2022). *Becoming an emotionally focused therapist: The workbook* (2nd ed.). Routledge.

Goldman, R. N., & Greenberg, L. S. (2015). *Case formulation in emotion-focused therapy: Co-creating clinical maps for change.* American Psychological Association.

Goldman, R. N., Vaz, A., Rousmaniere, T. (2021). *Deliberate practice in emotion-focused therapy.* American Psychological Association.

Greenman, P., & Johnson, S. (2013). Process research on EFT for couples: Linking theory to practice. *Family Process, Special Issue: Couple Therapy, 52*(1), 46–61.

Greenman, P., & Johnson, S. M. (2022). Emotionally focused therapy (EFT): Attachment, connection, and health. *Current Opinion in Psychology, 43*, 146–150.

Johnson, S. M. (2008). *Hold me tight: Seven conversations for a lifetime of love.* Little Brown.

Johnson. (2009). Attachment theory and emotionally focused therapy for individuals and couples. In J. H. Obegi & E. Berant (Eds.), *Attachment theory and research in clinical work with adults* (pp. 410–433). Guilford Press.

Johnson, S. M. (2019). *Attachment theory in practice: Emotionally focused therapy with individuals, couples and families.* Guilford.

Johnson, S. M. (2020). *The practice of emotionally focused therapy: Creating connection* (3rd ed.). Routledge.

Johnson S. M., & Campbell, T. L. (2022). *A primer for emotionally focused individual therapy (EFIT): Cultivating fitness and growth in every client.* Routledge.

Johnson, S. M., & Talitman, E. (1997). Predictors of success in emotionally focused marital therapy. *Journal of Marital and Family Therapy, 23*(2), 135–152.

Johnson, S. M., Burgess Moser, M., Beckes, L., Smith, A., Dalgleish, T., Halchuk, R., Hasselmo, K., Greenman, P. S., Merali, Z., & Coan, J. A. (2013). Soothing the threatened brain: Leveraging contact comfort with emotionally focused therapy. *PLOS ONE, 8*(11), e79314.

Kailanko, S., Wiebe, S. A., Tasca, G. A., & Laitila, A. A. (2021). Impact of repeating somatic cues on the depth of experiencing for withdrawers and pursuers in emotionally focused couple therapy. *Journal of Marital and Family Therapy, 00*, 1–16.

Klein, M. H., Mathieu-Coughlan, P., & Kiesler, D. J. (1986). The experiencing scales. In L. S. Greenberg & W. M. Pinsof (Eds.), *The psychotherapeutic process: A research handbook* (pp. 21–71). Guilford.

Rathgeber, M., Bürkner, P., Schiller, E., & Holling, H. (2019). The efficacy of emotionally focused couples therapy and behavioral couples therapy: A meta-analysis. *Journal of Marital and Family, 45*(3), 447–463. 10.nn/jmft.12336

Rholes, W. S., Simpson, J. A., Campbell, L., & Grich, J. (2001). Adult attachment and the transition to parenthood. *Journal of Personality and Social Psychology, 81*(3), 421.

Wiebe, S. A., & Johnson, S. M. (2016). A review of the research in emotionally focused therapy for couples. *Family Process, 55*(3), 390–407.

Wittenborn, A. K., Liu, T., Ridenour, T. A., Lachmar, E. M., Rouleau, E., & Seedall, R. B. (2019). Randomized controlled trial of emotionally focused couple therapy compared to treatment as usual for depression: Outcomes and mechanisms of change. *Journal of Marital and Family Therapy, 45*, 395–409.

18 Adapting Emotion Focused Therapies for Online Delivery

Mirisse Foroughe and Prakash Thambipillai

Before the COVID-19 pandemic, mental health clinicians and therapists conducted therapy online for clients unable to access in-person care (Norman, 2006; Richardson et al., 2009; Simpson, 2009). However, stay-at-home public health measures required therapists to adapt their practices to an entirely virtual format. As social distancing guidelines ease and in-person sessions resume, many clients are opting to continue online video-conferencing therapy due to its accessibility (Geller, 2020). Guidance is needed for adapting different therapeutic approaches to online formats.

For therapists practicing process-experiential based approaches such as Emotion Focused Therapy (EFT) and Emotion Focused Family Therapy (EFFT), adapting to an online therapy environment is particularly challenging[1]. This is because the therapeutic process and interventions used in these modalities require moment-to-moment parallel emotional processing with the client to facilitate therapeutic change (Greenberg, 2004; McGuinty et al., 2016). Considering the importance of in-session processes in EFT, it is crucial that therapeutic techniques are properly adapted for online delivery to approximate the core macro and micro processes that are hallmarks of emotion focused therapies. This chapter will describe specific online adaptations and considerations for the practice of emotion focused modalities online.

Emotion Focused Therapy

EFT is rooted in person-centered and gestalt principles (Greenberg, 2010, 2015). The approach to the therapeutic relationship is person-centered in that it involves ongoing empathic attunement and validation (McGuinty et al., 2016). This relational style is then complemented with a process-directive gestalt approach using experiential exercises to bring about therapeutic change (Greenberg, 2010). Client markers, or specific problematic emotional-processing states, are identifiable by in-session behaviors and common narratives. These markers indicate specific emotion processing difficulties which each have corresponding interventions (Greenberg, 2004, 2010; Greenberg et al., 1996). For example, when a person expresses that they have an emotion or feeling that they cannot describe, a task referred to as *focusing* can be used.

DOI: 10.4324/9781003205029-22

In this exercise the client is asked to reflect on how they experience the emotion or feeling in their body and to approach it with curiosity to verbalize what they are feeling. There are several experiential exercises used within emotion focused approaches and they have been described in previous works (Elliott et al., 2004; Foroughe, 2018; Greenberg et al, 1996; Greenberg & Watson, 2006). The main exercises are summarized and practical adaptations for online delivery are also outlined.

Emotion Focused Family Therapy

EFFT is a transdiagnostic family therapy model that actively engages caregivers of individuals with mental health difficulties to be the primary drivers of change in their loved one's recovery (Foroughe et al., 2019; Lafrance et al., 2020). EFFT is based on the same principles of awareness, emotional expression, emotion regulation, reflection, and transformation that inform EFT (Dolhanty & Lafrance, 2019; Lafrance Robinson et al., 2015).

Due to the caregiver stress that often accompanies supporting a child with mental health difficulties, caregiver emotions such as fear, shame, or helplessness can lead to emotionally avoidant responses including caregiver denial, accommodation, enabling, unproductive criticism, and anger (Cordeiro et al., 2018; Strahan et al., 2017). These *emotion blocks* hinder the successful implementation of necessary behavioral strategies, diminish caregiver self-efficacy, and block the experience of more adaptive emotions that would help caregivers effectively support the treatment process (Foroughe & Goldstein, 2018; Foroughe et al., 2019; Strahan et al., 2017). Therefore, EFFT aims to process caregivers' maladaptive *emotion blocks* so that they may access emotions that support their child's emotional processing (Cordeiro et al., 2018; Foroughe & Goldstein, 2018). This may allow the child to become aware of their own emotions and process them adaptively, resulting in improved behavior and emotional regulation (Foroughe & Goldstein, 2018; Robinson et al., 2015).

Adapting EFT and EFFT for Online Delivery

Adapting EFT Exercises

While the core tasks and steps of emotion focused experiential exercises remain the same, there are some important adaptations in the way they are implemented. In Table 18.1 below, some of the main emotion focused exercises are summarized and their corresponding online-delivery adaptations are outlined.

Adapting EFFT Exercises

In online video-conferencing, the psychoeducation components of EFFT are relayed through direct dialogue, anecdotes, metaphors, and visual images

Table 18.1 Experiential exercises used in EFT and adaptations to consider for online delivery

EFT Experiential Exercise	Brief Description	Adaptations for Online Delivery
Focusing	When a client mentions an *unclear felt sense*, therapist guides client to pay attention to the way this unclear emotion feels in their body. The client is encouraged to approach these embodied aspects of their experience with curiosity and to verbalize their bodily felt sense.	1 Use softer, reverent tone and direct client's attention to their body. Provide time and clear a space for client to access bodily felt-senses. 2 Ensure cameras of both therapist and client are focused such that the faces and upper bodies of both parties are visible as much as possible; helpful to see hands; if second camera, set up whole body view to see lower body
Systematic evocative unfolding	The detailed recall of a problematic reaction or memory in the present moment. Client is guided in reexperiencing situation and associated emotions in session to explore and acknowledge the associations between the situation, cognitions, & emotions experienced. Implicit meaning of the situation is uncovered.	1 Ensure optimal timing for client – no major tasks immediately after so that client does not return to home/work environment emotionally charged, without enough time to process task. 2 Secure back up audio in case of lost connection – cell or home phone line to keep dialogue if needed. 3 Have client prepare regulation-focused supports (water, tissues, fidget items) 4 Use verbal guidance, imagery, repetition, and references to specific details of events to anchor in client's memory.
Affirming empathic validation	Client marker is expressions of vulnerability or insecurity. Requires empathic attunement on the part of the therapist to acknowledge and normalize the client's experience. Noting what the client is feeling and mirroring the embodied aspects of the client's experience, matching their tone and body language to communicate genuine understanding.	1 Consider audio delay, using visual cues to mitigate: a. moving closer to the screen to approximate "leaning in," b. affirmative nod, c. mirror client's tone as usual, as well as their visible upper body – check your face + body as you go. 2 Move small window with client's video directly under your camera to simulate natural eye contact for both therapist and client. 3 Pay more attention than usual to mirroring client's own words, volume, and intonation in your speech.

(Continued)

Table 18.1 (Continued)

EFT Experiential Exercise	Brief Description	Adaptations for Online Delivery
Clearing a space	This intervention is utilized when a client is overwhelmed by multiple worries or painful experiences. Therapist helps the client mentally set aside various issues or problems so that client can experience the sense of a clear and safe internal space that they may feel and express their emotions in.	1 Invite client to look away from the screen to allow for greater internal focus – looking down or closing their eyes may be helpful. 2 Check in about your volume level and adjust if too low/high for client. Consider switching from headphones to built-in or externals speakers. 3 May need to repeat emotion focused prompts more prominently.
Empty-chair intervention	For clients that express *unfinished business* with a significant other. The client is guided to engage in a dialogue with an empty chair in which they imagine the significant other from their perspective.	1 Consider and implement tips and steps provided for other experiential exercises. 2 Ask client to use any chair, bench, stool, or other seating near them. 3 Have client turn camera or move chairs to allow you to see them in both places. 4 Check how well you hear client and they hear you from both chairs.
Two-chair work (Self-critical/Self-interruptive splits)	If a self-critical or self-interruptive split is expressed, the client is guided in enacting two aspects of the self that conflict with one another. Client takes turns switching between chairs, embodying, expressing, and exploring the thoughts, feelings, and needs of these different parts. Resolution is marked by integration of two conflicting parts, or by the expression of blocked emotions.	1 Consider and implement all tips and steps provided for empty-chair intervention 2 Ensure that client can physically move into the other chair and check that the proximity between the two chairs is acceptable to them after the first switch – some clients prefer more space between chairs in order to lessen the degree of emotional intensity. 3 Before the session, ensure privacy and that sound from the room cannot easily travel out.

with screen sharing. In contrast, the process-experiential aspects of EFFT require nuanced adaptations for delivery in an online video-conferencing format, as these are the transformational aspects of the approach. Table 18.2 outlines online adaptions for EFFT experiential exercises (Foroughe & Goldstein, 2018, 2018), of which are based upon clinical experience providing and supervising EFFT online.

The practical adaptations to the experiential exercises discussed above are helpful when guiding a client through specific interventions. There are additional therapist and client considerations that have recently been identified in the practice of emotion focused modalities online. Emotion focused approaches emphasize the importance of an empathic and validating therapeutic relationship that creates a space for clients to engage in therapeutic tasks safely at their optimal level of emotional engagement and activation. Several key considerations can help accomplish these goals when using virtual therapy.

Therapist & Client Preparation

Prior to the first virtual session, the therapist can start collaborating with the client to prepare a safe and private space for them to engage in emotionally intensive therapeutic work (Geller, 2020; Pugh et al., 2020; Simpson et al., 2021). In addition, when reaching out to the client before the session, therapists should make sure that clients are comfortable and competent with the chosen online platform of delivery (Pugh et al., 2020; Simpson et al., 2021). This helps address the client's anxiety about technical issues and ensures they feel comfortable enough with the platform without the technology becoming a distraction. Offering a 5-minute test call with the client can help in building the foundation for a strong online therapeutic relationship. It is also important to establish a clear and stable online connection, as audio or visual delays can hinder the flow of therapeutic processes that require moment-to-moment emotional processing.

Another key aspect of the therapeutic relationship is the embodiment of therapeutic presence in online sessions (Geller, 2020). Therapeutic presence involves engaging their whole selves, physically, emotionally, cognitively, and relationally in the encounter with the client so that they may feel "seen," understood, and safe to engage in therapeutic tasks (Geller, 2017; Geller, 2019). Therefore, to facilitate the expression of therapeutic presence online, optimal camera placement, lighting, and the reduction of ambient sounds should be arranged prior to the session (Geller, 2020). Embodying therapeutic presence in remotely delivered emotion focused interventions is understandably linked to the emotional state of the therapist. Taking some time before each session to deliberately practice and activate one's therapeutic presence can go a long a way. Research has found that engaging in brief mindfulness centering exercises before sessions helped therapists feel more present in sessions and clients feel that their session was more effective (Dunn et al., 2013).

Table 18.2 Brief description of the EFFT experiential activities and the adaptions that can be made for online delivery

EFFT Experiential Exercise	Brief Description	Adaptations for Online Delivery
Shaping	Coaching caregivers through role play to practice setting limits or providing emotional support to their child; providing feedback re: content of speech, tone of voice, body language, and emotional expression.	Having caregivers move their chair so that face and whole body are visible on the camera; zooming in or out to focus on particular area; using visual cue to interject during role play b/c software may suppress therapist's audio when parent is talking. Consider using video feedback to provide concrete feedback and to support the up/down regulation of affect.
Shutdown exercise	Caregiver/therapist each role-play "shutting down" for two minutes and focus on an emotionally upsetting issue while the other tries to provide emotional support. The therapist remains "shut down" for an extended period to illustrate the lack of two-way communication.	When "shutting down," the therapist can turn the chair away from the screen/camera to emphasize the emotional unavailability. Therapist may have to signal emotional unavailability with body language maybe by crossing arms. Shift eye gaze dramatically away from the client, screen, and camera.
Processing caregiver blocks	As caregivers engage in tasks of shaping, providing emotional support & setting limits, emotion blocks may arise (anger, fear, etc.). Working through these emotion blocks is a complex therapeutic process led by a licensed mental health professional.	Therapists may support a caregiver one-on-one or during a role-play exercise. Blocks can be processed through psychoeducation, presentation of an anecdote, analogy, or visual image, direct dialogue, or an experiential exercise (described in Table 18.1).
Therapeutic Apology	Caregivers are coached through a role play delivery of their apology to their child (played by the therapist). The focus is on verbal and nonverbal shaping. Step-by-step instructions are outlined for the caregiver beforehand.	Prepare environment to support emotional distress, ensure privacy, and plan ahead so client has time to debrief with you and does not have a taxing event scheduled immediately after session. In the workshop modality, break-out rooms allow for small groups and more intimate practice.

As emotion focused approaches rely heavily on in-session transformational change requiring authentic client emotional engagement, it is important to help clients prepare themselves and their environment to engage in this therapeutic work. If planning to engage in chair work, it is helpful to ensure that clients have an extra chair to participate in the exercise properly. As these exercises are also very emotionally arousing, a friendly reminder to the client to have tissues close by shows that you care for the client's emotional state and experience and helps the client create a safe space for themselves. In this vein, it is also important to discuss how the client can use different strategies to deal with post-session emotional activation when the therapist is not available to support the client remotely.

In order to stay emotionally attuned to the client, it is important for therapists to track, notice, and clarify the client's micro-expressions (Ekman, 2007; Geller, 2019, 2020). However, as the therapist's focus is on maintaining therapeutic presence, it can be easy to miss these micro-expressions or process markers in the moment. Therefore, to facilitate the noticing and studying of these micro-expressions after a session, it is vital to have a discussion with the client to obtain their consent to record sessions to facilitate the therapeutic process.

Within-Session Considerations

With in-person therapy, the act of travelling to the therapist's office and entering a space specifically meant for therapeutic work allows the client to prepare themselves emotionally for what they are about to do. In remote therapy, clients are often joining sessions from their homes or workplaces, and they may be only a couple rooms away from the very people they are discussing. Acknowledging this and building in some time and space before sessions for clients to debrief is important.

Communication is a vital aspect of the therapeutic relationship and there are many ways that nonverbal communication provides information to both therapist and client that helps foster an empathically attuned relationship (Ogden & Goldstein, 2019). Although interpretation of body language is largely hindered, there are a variety of strategies that therapists can use to overcome these limitations. In terms of interpreting the body language of the client, therapists may find that checking in with the client more regularly improves emotional attunement. It can also be helpful to inquire more often to clarify the meaning of perceived facial expressions or body movements (Simpson et al., 2021). When this is done with a curious and compassionate approach, these can be opportunities to deepen the therapeutic relationship and bring to light what is concealed by the screen.

The divide of the screen may also cloud the client's interpretation of the therapist's behavioral and bodily cues. Virtual therapy necessitates an increased reliance on vocal tone, facial expressions, and complementary gestures (Abbott et al., 2008; Simpson et al., 2021). The therapist's facial expressions may also have to become exaggerated due to poor video quality.

Adjusting the camera so clients can clearly see their facial expressions and body can improve one's therapeutic presence.

General Adaptations for Deepening Emotional Engagement & Experiential Exercises

Within emotion focused modalities, process-experiential tasks support therapeutic change. The depth of in-session emotional experience has been found to correlate with therapeutic change (Johnson & Greenberg, 1988; Pascual-Leone & Yeryomenko, 2017). In addition to the practical advice outlined in the tables, therapists may implement specific adaptations to deepen emotional engagement and optimize the potential benefit for clients using online video-conferencing formats.

Although video quality in most online video-conferencing platforms is acceptable, the use of the body and gestures to communicate emotional attunement and empathy is an area needing close attention and training, particularly for the vast majority of therapists for whom video communication was not a part of professional activities until the COVID-19 pandemic. Without the aid of in-person therapeutic conditions, we lose some of the benefits of in-person attendance that have long been taken for granted including the well-thought-out physical space, social and emotional engagement through nonverbal communication, and the safety of being together in a contained room. Online, the therapist can only optimize what is within their realm of control. Attention to and skill building in these areas can improve the client's experience by enriching therapeutic presence in the areas that are possible to amplify in this mode of interaction.

Voice

The therapist's voice becomes one of the primary means of signalling emotional understanding and empathy. In addition to modulating the tone, pitch, and cadence of one's voice to communicate emotion and accurate empathy, targeted verbalization and direct, supportive statements are also helpful when facilitating experiential exercises. The therapist will likely have to use their voice more often in online formats to provide prompting, indicate togetherness, repeat critical information, or to gently direct the client back on task. This sometimes involves frequent interruptions, which will be easier to experience if the client is told ahead of time to expect this. Indeed, when a therapist provides a reason for interrupting and does so with emotional attunement and unconditional positive regard, clients are often grateful for the coaching and redirection, which are associated with positive outcomes due to an increased level of engagement. For example, during experiential exercises such as focusing, systematic evocative unfolding, and either empty chair or two-chair work, it is crucial to instruct the client to slow down and pay attention to the sensory and interoceptive aspects of their experience;

doing so allows a deeper understanding and familiarity with the physical sensations associated with emotions clients are experiencing (Thompson-de Benoit & Kramer, 2020).

Preparation of Space

As discussed in a previous section and in Table 18.1, preparation can occur to ensure the client is ready and able to engage fully in such an emotionally taxing exercise with as much comfort and support as possible. This preparation involves making sure the client has the appropriate space and chairs needed for the session, advising them of the emotionally demanding nature of the exercises, and leaving more time than usual at the end of the session for debriefing (at least 20 minutes). Within the session, chairs should be placed in the client's room so that they are facing each other, and the side of the client's face and body should be turned slightly towards the screen so that facial expressions are visible through the camera. As engaging in chair work for the first time can be even more confusing online than it is in person, the therapist can mirror the placement of chairs in their room to model the process of the exercise for the client. Persistent redirection of focus to the other chair and its associated role may be necessary because the client may look towards the screen for direction or feedback. Of course, the tendency to look at the therapist and engage directly with them – instead of staying on task by directing attention to the other chair – is not unique to the online environment. Indeed, this happens frequently in person as well. However, it can be more challenging to redirect clients virtually and this makes the preparation conversation with the client all the more valuable and instructive.

Use of Chair Work

When engaged in online-delivered psychotherapy from home or at a workplace, clients may not have a second chair or enough space to move around and arrange optimal conditions. Therefore, in the spirit of reducing barriers to accessing therapy during the pandemic, many therapists have not required clients to have chairs set up. Instead, the emphasis is placed mainly on movement of the whole body to signal both a psychological and physical shift in the client as they move between roles in an enactment (Pugh et al., 2020). Sometimes even just asking the client to shift from one side of their couch to the other facing in opposite directions is enough to create that separation in roles for the client. To deepen the emotional engagement in these cases, the therapist may choose to encourage the use of more specific imagery (e.g., "picture your father the day he moved out – the look on his face when he came to say goodbye to you"). When evoking a detailed visualization of impactful attachment-based memories, therapists will want to be even more careful and attuned in order to ensure that the client experiences a helpful debrief and that they are not left in an emotionally vulnerable situation alone in their space or going to be interrupted by family members immediately after session. Ensuring that the level of emotional activation remains.

Regardless of the constraints of therapy delivered through online video-conferencing, there are surprising benefits that have become apparent through our use of this modality. These benefits include increased access to therapy, increased convenience, and the greater generalizability that may result from practicing skills or emotional experiences within the client's own home. Beyond these, emotion focused approaches offer unique advantages due to the emphasis on therapeutic presence, attunement to emotional process, therapist skill with live emotion processing, and within-session experiential activities. The therapeutic arts have much to learn with respect to ensuring clients' online experience is as close to what clients experience in-person; however, we can offset what is lost in a two-dimensional connection with what can be gained through the online format as well as through the unique elements of emotion focused therapies.

Ending the Session

With remotely delivered therapy, therapists must always be wary of the environment the client is returning to. As the experiential exercises used in emotion focused approaches are emotionally demanding, clients may not have the time to fully process and digest the session before returning back to home or work. Considering this, therapists should allow for enough time for clients to de-role from any enactments and to debrief on the session (Pugh et al., 2020). It is also helpful to inform the client that the levels of emotional arousal may persist even after the online session ends. Discussing tools to self soothe and seek further support can help the client make the transition from the therapeutic environment.

Between-Session Support

Navigating between-session support is a nuanced matter in an online world and just like in-person modalities, upholding boundaries is an active and ongoing process (Hermansson, 1997). This could be done by providing clients with a written document that outlines helpful tools for regulating emotions and self-soothing, while also listing potential avenues of support in their community. If it is early in the therapeutic process, it may be appropriate to discuss a phone call or other exchange to maintain the therapeutic relationship.

All of these considerations in preparation for, during, and at the end of sessions are crucial aspects of creating a space for clients to engage in emotion focused modalities. The adjustments delineated throughout this chapter will help provide guidelines for therapists practicing EFT and EFFT. However, this is a process that will have to continuously be refined and revisited to perfect so that therapists can make the most of the accessibility and convenience that online therapy offers.

Note

1 This chapter provides adaptations for EFFT and for Greenberg's model of in-dividual EFT and does not refer to Couples EFT or to emotionally focused therapy (Johnson, 2015).

References

Abbott, J.-A. M., Klein, B., & Ciechomski, L. (2008). Best practices in online therapy. *Journal of Technology in Human Services, 26*(2–4), 360–375. 10.1080/15228830802 097257

Cordeiro, K., Rependa, S. L., Muller, R. T., & Foroughe, M. (2018). EFFT and trauma: Engaging the dismissing parent. In M. Foroughe (Ed.), *Emotion focused family therapy with children and caregivers: A trauma-informed approach* (pp. 99–119). New York, NY: Routledge/Taylor & Francis.

Dolhanty, J., & Lafrance, A. (2019). Emotion focused family therapy for eating disorders. In L. S. Greenberg (Ed.), *Clinical handbook of emotion focused therapy* (pp. 403–423, Chapter xiv, 534 Pages). American Psychological Association. 10.1037/0000112-018

Dunn, R., Callahan, J. L., Swift, J. K., & Ivanovic, M. (2013). Effects of pre-session centering for therapists on session presence and effectiveness. *Psychotherapy Research: Journal of the Society for Psychotherapy Research, 23*(1), 78–85. 10.1080/10503307.2012.731713

Ekman, P. (2007). *Emotions revealed: Recognizing faces and feelings to improve communication* (2nd edition). Holt Paperbacks.

Elliott, R., Watson, J. C., Goldman, R. N., Greenberg, L. S. (2004). Learning emotion-focused therapy: The process-experiential approach to change (pp. xiii, 366) American Psychological Association.

Elliott, R., Watson, J. C., Goldman, R. N., & Greenberg, L. S. (2018). *Learning emotion focused therapy: The process-experiential approach to change.* American Psychological Association.

Foroughe, M. (Ed.). (2018). *Emotion focused family therapy for children and caregivers: A trauma-informed approach.* NY: Routledge.

Foroughe, M., & Goldstein, A. (2018). *Emotion focused family therapy with children and caregivers: A trauma-informed approach.* Routledge.

Foroughe, M., Stillar, A., Goldstein, L., Dolhanty, J., Goodcase, E. T., & Lafrance, A. (2019). Brief emotion focused family therapy: An intervention for parents of children and adolescents with mental health issues. *Journal of Marital and Family Therapy; Hoboken, 45*(3), 410–430. 10.1111/jmft.12351

Geller, S. (2017). *A practical guide to cultivating therapeutic presence* (1st edition). American Psychological Association.

Geller, S. M. (2019). Therapeutic presence: The foundation for effective emotion focused therapy. In L. S. Greenberg (Ed.), *Clinical handbook of emotion focused therapy* (pp. 129–145, Chapter xiv, 534 Pages). American Psychological Association. 10.1037/0000112-006

Geller, S. (2020). Cultivating online therapeutic presence: Strengthening therapeutic relationships in teletherapy sessions. *Counselling Psychology Quarterly*, 1–17. 10.1080/09515070.2020.1787348

Greenberg, L. S. (2004). Emotion–focused therapy. *Clinical Psychology & Psychotherapy, 11*(1), 3–16. 10.1002/cpp.388

Greenberg, L. S. (2010). Emotion focused therapy: A clinical synthesis. *FOCUS, 8*(1), 32–42. 10.1176/foc.8.1.foc32

Greenberg, L. S., Rice, L. N., & Elliott, R. (1996). *Facilitating emotional change: The moment-by-moment process* (1st edition). The Guilford Press.

Greenberg, L. S., & Warwar, S. H. (2006). Homework in an emotion focused approach to experiential therapy. *Journal of Psychotherapy Integration, 16*(2), 178–200. 10.1037/1053-0479.16.2.178

Greenberg, L. S., & Watson, J. C. (2006). Emotion-focused therapy for depression (pp. viii, 353). American Psychological Association.

Greenberg, L. S. (2015). Emotion-Focused Therapy: Coaching Clients to Work Through Their Feelings(2nd ed.) American Psychological Association.

Hermansson, G. (1997). Boundaries and boundary management in counselling: The never-ending story. *British Journal of Guidance & Counselling, 25*(2), 133–146. 10.1080/03069889708253797

Johnson, S. M. (2015). Emotionally focused couple therapy. In A. S. Gurman, J. L. Lebow, & D. K. Snyder (Eds.), *Clinical handbook of couple therapy* (pp. 97–128). The Guilford Press.

Johnson, S. M., & Greenberg, L. S. (1988). Relating Process to Outcome in Marital Therapy. *Journal of Marital and Family Therapy, 14*(2), 175–183. 10.1111/j.1752-0606.1988.tb00733.x

Lafrance, A., Henderson, K. A., & Mayman, S. (2020). Emotion focused family therapy: A transdiagnostic model for caregiver-focused interventions. In *Emotion focused family therapy: A transdiagnostic model for caregiver-focused interventions* (p. Chapter viii, 212 Pages). American Psychological Association. 10.1037/0000166-000

Lafrance Robinson, A., Dolhanty, J., & Greenberg, L. (2015). Emotion focused family therapy for eating disorders in children and adolescents. *Clinical Psychology & Psychotherapy, 22*(1), 75–82. 10.1002/cpp.1861

McGuinty, E., Nelson, J., Carlson, A., Crowther, E., Bednar, D., & Foroughe, M. (2016). Redefining outcome measurement: A model for brief psychotherapy: Redefining outcome measurement. *Clinical Psychology & Psychotherapy, 23*(3), 260–271. 10.1002/cpp.1953

Norman, S. (2006). The use of telemedicine in psychiatry. *Journal of Psychiatric and Mental Health Nursing, 13*(6), 771–777. 10.1111/j.1365-2850.2006.01033.x

Ogden, P., & Goldstein, B. (2019). Sensorimotor psychotherapy from a distance: Engaging the body, creating presence, and building relationship in videoconferencing. In H. Weinberg & A. Rolnick (Eds.), *Theory and Practice of Online Therapy*. Routledge.

Pascual-Leone, A., & Yeryomenko, N. (2017). The client "experiencing" scale as a predictor of treatment outcomes: A meta-analysis on psychotherapy process. *Psychotherapy Research, 27*, 653–66510.1080/10503307.2016.1152409.

Pugh, M., Bell, T., & Dixon, A. (2020). Delivering tele-chairwork: A qualitative survey of expert therapists. *Psychotherapy Research, 1*–16. 10.1080/10503307.2020.1854486

Richardson, L. K., Frueh, B. C., Grubaugh, A. L., Egede, L., & Elhai, J. D. (2009). Current directions in videoconferencing tele-mental health research. *Clinical Psychology: Science and Practice, 16*(3), 323–338. 10.1111/j.1468-2850.2009.01170.x

Simpson, S. (2009). Psychotherapy via videoconferencing: A review. *British Journal of Guidance & Counselling, 37*(3), 271–286. 10.1080/03069880902957007

Simpson, S., Richardson, L., Pietrabissa, G., Castelnuovo, G., & Reid, C. (2021). Videotherapy and therapeutic alliance in the age of COVID-19. *Clinical Psychology & Psychotherapy*, *28*(2), 409–421. 10.1002/cpp.2521

Strahan, E. J., Stillar, A., Files, N., Nash, P., Scarborough, J., Connors, L., Gusella, J., Henderson, K., Mayman, S., Marchand, P., Orr, E. S., Dolhanty, J., & Lafrance, A. (2017). Increasing parental self-efficacy with emotion focused family therapy for eating disorders: A process model. *Person-Centered & Experiential Psychotherapies*, *16*(3), 256–269. 10.1080/14779757.2017.1330703

Thompson-de Benoit, A., & Kramer, U. (2020). Work with emotions in remote psychotherapy in the time of Covid-19: a clinical experience. *Counselling Psychology Quarterly*, 34, 368–37610.1080/09515070.2020.1770696.

19 Gottman Method: Assessment and Treatment in the Age of Online Therapy

Shoshana Hellman, Don Cole, and Arnon Rolnick

Introduction

Videoconferencing or telehealth therapy became very prevalent during the COVID-19 pandemic, even though it existed years before. Many different therapeutic aspects have been compared between videoconferencing and face to face sessions, for example, the therapeutic alliance, client satisfaction, efficacy of clinical measures, and more (Kaiser et al., 2020). Most of the research studies refer to individual therapy online and not to couple therapy. There has been less research carried out regarding the adaptability of specific approaches to online couple therapy. Since not a lot has been written about online couple therapy, this chapter intends to introduce Gottman's approach to online couple therapy.

Couple therapy online differs from individual online therapy as the therapist must build and maintain a therapeutic alliance with both members of the couple. This presents a need for further research to focus on experiences of the couple in terms of therapeutic alliance building.

Although there is a growing body of empirical evidence demonstrating that the therapeutic alliance is the best predictor of psychotherapy outcome in individual psychotherapy, it was not shown in couple therapy. It is possible that certain approaches such as Gottman theory put the focus on the dyadic nature of the therapy and therefore the therapeutic alliance is less important.

Couple Therapy Online – Literature Review

Couple therapy became especially crucial amid the pandemic, in which many couples experienced "Cabin fever" particularly during the lockdowns (Crawford, 2021).

Couples worked from home and spent most of their time at home together. For many this was a big change which led to tension and challenges in their relationship. In addition, financial worries and job losses increased the increased the uncertainty and therefore increased conflicts. Since many couples experienced an increase in stress and decrease in relationship satisfaction, there was more of a likelihood for affairs (Coop Gordon and Mitchell, 2020).

DOI: 10.4324/9781003205029-23

Ultimately, there was an increase in referrals to couple therapists and mental health providers. On the other hand, the slowed pace that many couples were experiencing during the pandemic, and the fact that many worked from home and stayed together, was an ideal time to work on the relationship, in particular to increase safety and protection and avoid negative cycles (Perle, 2020).

Telehealth therapy is particularly useful for couples as it overcomes some of the barriers that may be more prominent for them, such as the stigma of couple therapy, and physical issues such as childcare and scheduling. Couples in a long-distance relationship and "Living Apart Together" couples (couples who are still married but live apart) can benefit from online therapy, as face-to-face therapy would be more complicated for them.

Hetlelin and Earl (2020) report that according to new research, video-conferencing offers a better opportunity for a couple to express intimacy and reflection in therapy, possibly because the therapist is not physically near the couple, and they feel more free to express their feelings. This is a recurring finding also found by other researchers, such as Kysely et al. (2020). They also found that the connection with the therapist developed faster online, and the dynamics of an online connection created a less threatening space. Some clients have reported an increased sense of empowerment and control resulting from the sharing of a common space that belongs to neither the client, nor the therapist (Lewis et al., 2004). Feeling ownership of a space can empower a client to feel more in charge of the situation and can therefore allow the client to open up more as a result of feeling safe. (Kysely et al., 2020).

Confidentiality is still an issue for couples and individuals in telehealth therapy, but for the most part couples reflecting on their own experience of videoconferencing in the current study by Kysely et al. (2020) did not feel that confidentiality had been a significant issue.

On the other hand, online therapy and the easy use of smartphones can lead to possible over-accessibility when boundaries become harder to maintain (e.g., the possibility to message the therapist at any time). This might deter therapists from using online therapy with couples (Hetlelin & Earl, 2020).

To our best knowledge, no empirical research compared the efficacy of live versus telehealth treatment applying various approaches to couple therapy.

Assessment in Online Therapy

One of the unique features of the Gottman method for couple therapy is the evaluation of the relationship of the couple that is done at the beginning of therapy. This evaluation is part of the therapy. When the concept of evaluation was introduced to Gottman therapists, it was based on a printed questionnaire of over 500 questions which was given to the couples. Later, the Gottman Institute created a secure site for these questionnaires – The Gottman Relationship Check up. Couples are directed to answer online questionnaires in order to assess their relationship. In addition, the Gottman

Love Lab App was developed to enhance the Relationship Checkup site which was used to assess couples. This app also provides analysis of two video conversations (conflict and events of the week) which can be rated for emotional content by the couple themselves.

In this assessment process, the therapist provides information gathered from interviews (both individual interviews of each partner and of the couple together), results of the questionnaires and ratings of the two video clips that the couple provided. A report is generated for the couple and a more detailed report is given to the therapist. The relationship assessment is based on the Sound Relationship Theory, which rose from the years of research conducted by John and Julie Gottman (2018). The theory outlines nine specific areas of functioning that are predictive of relationship strength or weakness. The evaluation allows the therapist to define clearly for couples the areas of dysfunction with which they may be struggling.

The report prepared for the couples includes a copy of the Sound Relationship House Theory as shown in Figure 19.1. Also provided is an indication of the couple's functioning within each area. In online sessions the report can be easily shared with the couple using screen sharing.

In a feedback session, the therapist presents the findings of the evaluation, focusing on the strengths and weaknesses of each of the areas represented by this model. It is best to offer the feedback using the following sequence, as not to overwhelm the couple with too much data. The sequence has four steps for each section of the house model.

a   Define the concept briefly.
b   Discuss the findings as to strength or area of concern for the couple.
c   Check with the couple for questions or comments and see if they accept the finding.
d   Briefly discuss ways therapy will help to improve the area under discussion.

In summary, the process of the assessment nowadays is integrated in the video therapy sessions including a secure site where the couple can videotape and also meet securely with the therapist.

The Use of Video Clips in Online Treatment

The two videos that were taken by the couple for the assessment – the conflict video where they discuss a topic that they have some disagreement on, and the events of the week video in which they describe neutral experiences, can be used later in the sessions as part of the treatment. The counselor can share it on the screen with the couple while in a video session and discuss with them their communication style. A couple can also bring another video clip of a discussion that they videotaped in order to get some feedback from the therapist. This is in addition to the use of these tapes in the assessment and treatment planning.

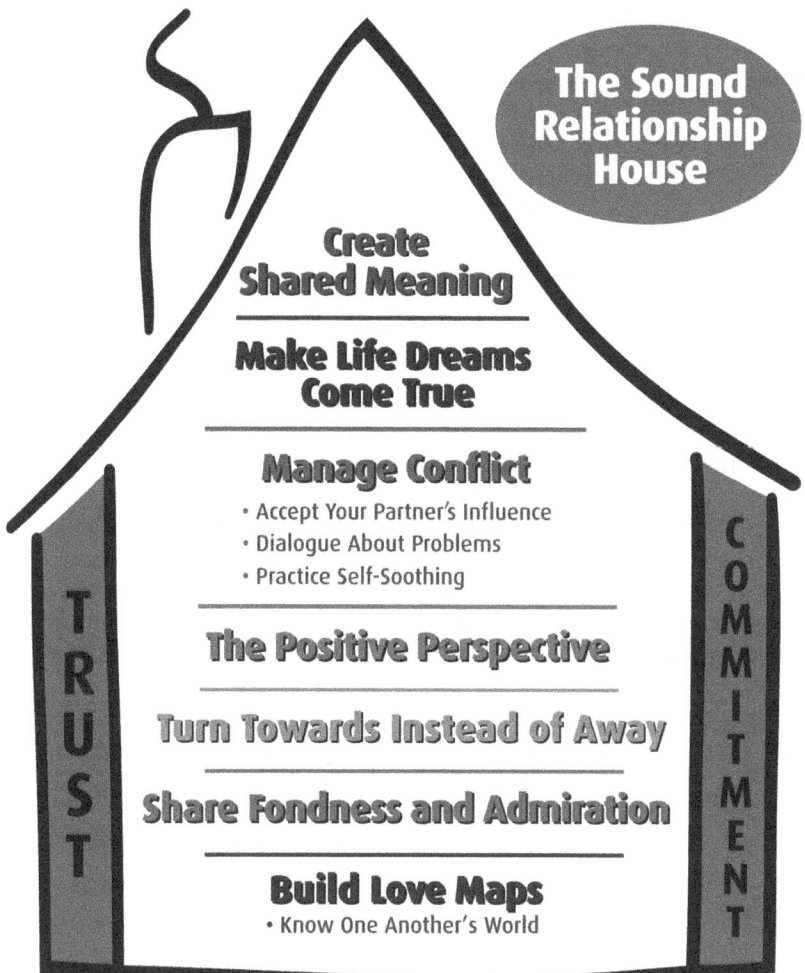

Figure 19.1 The Sound Relationship House.

An important online video resource is the Gottman Relationship Builder, available for therapists to use with couples to enhance their experience of therapy and to reduce relapse after the therapy ends. The Relationship Builder will be discussed in more detail later in this chapter.

Physiology as Part of Gottman's Theory

From the outset, Gottman's research emphasized the importance of physiology and physiological escalation in the functioning of relationships.

Therapists using Gottman method are encouraged to provide pulse monitors for couples to help identify a process we refer to as "flooding." This flooding experience occurs when stressful interactions with the spouse lead to a release of stress hormones causing a "flight, fight or freeze" response. Pulse monitors help the therapist identify this process early since for most people a pulse rate above 100 beats per minute signals the beginning of this process. This happens especially during conflict. Nowadays working online with computers, we can use a somewhat more advanced method: Heart rate variability (HRV), or the beat-to-beat alteration in heart rate, offers a noninvasive indicator of autonomic nervous system activity. Unlike basic pulse rate that counts the number of heart beats per minute, HRV looks much closer at the exact changes in time between successive heartbeats.

HRV can give us a window to both the Sympathetic Nervous System and the Parasympathetic Nervous System. The Sympathetic Nervous System controls our body's "fight or flight" reactions in response to internal or external stressors. The Parasympathetic Nervous System controls our body's "rest and digest" responses and is associated with recovery.

Couples benefit from an ideal balance (the "quiet-alert state") between sympathetic and parasympathetic nervous systems when both partners feel safe and secure. The Autonomic Nervous System (ANS) plays a large role in love and romance; the in-person courtship process is entirely sympathetically driven. Later stages of love and romance also depend on the parasympathetic nervous system.

The quiet-alert state allows us to be in repose with another person, relatively free of anxiety or boredom. Mutually shared parasympathetic states form the basis of long-term romantic relationships and are a hallmark of secure primary attachment relationships.

Working with computers and HRV sensors online allows us to find ways that will allow us to measure and present to the couple the balance or imbalance between these two systems.

Gottman suggests that simple heartbeat sensors that are used in face-to-face sessions can be used to detect flooding. Computer-mediated sessions allow us to use the HRV not only to detect a tension between the couple but also for various additional therapeutic tasks (see Oren et al., 2018).

Below are described steps that the therapist can carry out with the couple utilizing their psychophysiological reactions as measured by a HRV sensor. These steps can be carried out online or offline.

A   Help each member of the couple to be aware of their psychophysiological state and to find clues that will allow him/her to realize their own tension.
B   Teach each partner to find their unique way to relax and to calm down.
C   Watch how the nervous system of the spouse is activated to help each member to understand some of his partner's behaviors.
D   Each partner can watch the HRV graph of his spouse and learn how his own behavior can affect the psychophysiological status of his partner.

E   When both partners are connected each one to his computer and to his/her sensor, the therapist can see the non-verbal aspects of their interaction.

F   The couple is exposed to their psychological and physical interconnectedness in real time, thereby increasing empathy and developing sensitivity to how their actions affect their partner. The partners become aware of what it feels like to watch and be watched, and are encouraged to ask, "How can I watch more compassionately?".

G   Later, these steps can be repeated while talking about sensitive relationship content, or issues that have arisen during therapy. This allows the couple to observe the influence of these sensitive topics while learning a new language of acceptance, mutual regulation, and intersubjective awareness.

Facial Expressions as Part of Gottman Therapy

There are certain behavioral indications and facial expressions that indicate that a person might have become flooded, such as fluttering eyelids. Gottman therapists are trained to observe these indications. Using video conferencing in therapy makes it easier for the therapist to distinguish and observe these cues, because the faces show bigger and closer than in our office.

One of Gottman's unique interventions involves asking the couple to discuss a conflictual subject, while the therapist observes their facial expressions and body language. The therapist looks at the angle of their lips, the shape and position of their eyebrows, the angle of their chins, and more. This gives the therapist an indication of how close or distant the two are from one another. These observations are easier to carry out during video conferencing than face to face due to the improved view and the ability to zoom in on the subjects' face.

Using two computers one for each partner in couple therapy complicates the dynamics and is less advisable especially when discussing a conflict. There are cases especially in long distance relationships or in frequent commutes of one of the partners that two computers must be used. The advantage is that the couple can still continue couple therapy even when they are physically separated, which cannot be done face-to-face. The disadvantage is that the therapist must be aware that this is not the same data as when the partners interact in the same physical space. The observation of facial expressions in this case becomes much more difficult. The possibility of self-view in video conferencing is another interesting option or opportunity. During in-person meetings the most one can see is the tip of his/her own nose, hands, and the front of the body from the clavicle down.

This self-view or in fact "Continuous-Selfie" online, may produce various types of psychological reactions for the user (the therapist or the clients). It may evoke self-criticism – many people do not like to see themselves. Others may be narcissistically occupied in seeing themselves in various positions. Many people describe this self-view as distracting, and at times irritating, however for marital therapy, the self-view feature can be very useful.

This is a unique opportunity to learn how each one of the partners perceives himself/herself and his/her facial expression. It is interesting to note that while people are very much aware of their partner's facial expression – they are rarely aware of their own expression. An accurate awareness of one's facial expression is important in every interpersonal interaction because a considerable amount of information about one's affective state, status, attitude, cooperativeness, and competitiveness in social family and marital situations is expressed and communicated to others through facial expressions (Ekman & Friesen, 1971).

The misappraisal of facial expressions that we display to other people may have important consequences and may influence the course of the interaction. To prevent and mitigate the chances of misinterpreting our facial expressions, we need to possess a certain amount of emotional self-awareness, that is, what is expressed in our daily interactions with others.

While Gottman developed a method for the therapist to assess the couple's facial expression – now the self-view option of the Zoom, Skype, Teams, or Google Meet allows the therapist to educate and train the couple to be aware of their facial expression.

Partners' perception of the other's facial expression: although there is some universal correlation between certain facial expressions to certain emotional responses (Ekman & Friesen, 1971), it is possible that within the couple's "tradition" there are unique attitudes towards certain facial expressions. For example, it is possible that the wife interprets a certain smile of her husband as contempt, although this might be his unique way of smiling. Using the self-view option, the couple can better discuss and understand the unique meaning of each partner's smile or facial expression.

The facial expression can be also a sign of invitation to intimacy. However sometimes the other partner does not recognize the inviting gesture. The therapist might ask one of the partners to initiate some facial expression that invokes some intimate attraction. They can then discuss how much the other partner recognizes the existence of such cues.

Should we ask the couple to learn and to practice some certain facial expressions that might bring intimacy? Can people fake it (or Face it) till they make it? (Rolnick & Ehrenreich, 2019). The concept of "faking it" may seem foreign to psychologists. We usually talk about honesty, authenticity, and discovering the true self. Indeed, non-genuine facial expressions may be non-beneficial. The suggestion here is mainly to help the clients see their own facial expression (not necessarily smiles) via the video application and to be aware of the potential effect on their spouse.

Dyadic Talk and Gottman Interventions in Video Conferencing Therapy

Another emphasis of the Gottman approach is the dyadic talk. Partners must talk to each other and not to the therapist, especially when they are learning to manage a conflict. This may be easier to do in in-person sessions than in online video sessions, as during online sessions the general tendency is to look at the screen and talk to the therapist. It is important to give specific instructions so that the couple face and talk to each other and not to the therapist. Many of the treatment interventions are based on the fact that the couple has to listen and repeat what the partner is saying in a different way, therefore eye contact between the partners is very important. One of the interventions used in Gottman therapy is the Gottman Rapport exercise. This exercise helps the couple practice empathy and deepens the understanding of the other partner's position in a conflict (instead of the "harsh start up" – when a partner starts a discussion using contempt and criticism). The couple takes turns being a listener and a speaker. The goal is to feel understood by each other. The speaker has to refrain from blaming, use "I" statements and, instead talk about feelings regarding his position. The listener must tune him/herself into the partner's world and try to understand the other's perspective. At the end of the exercise the listener has to summarize and validate what he/she heard, not necessarily agree but communicate understanding and empathy to the position of the speaker. When working with couples online, the therapist can share the script of the exercise with the couple and ask the couple to practice it while the therapist gives them feedback. The work of the couple is dyadic, and the therapist is the facilitator. There are limitations in doing this work online as we do not see the whole body of each partner, even though the focus is on the couple. Some therapists turn off their video and hide their image, not to confuse the couple and make them more aware of their dyadic interaction. At the same time the therapist can observe the verbal and non-verbal cues of the couple, this would be very difficult to do in an in-person meeting.

When working online, it is easier for the couple to practice and film how they perform the intervention at home and to show it to the therapist in the following session. Given that the use of video is also part of the assessment and treatment, it is easier for the couple to accept filming their other interactions at home and to bring them back to the session. Much of the therapy that is done with the Gottman method is building skills (conflict management, friendship skills). The use of video clips that are integrated in the online sessions can be a wonderful tool to enhance the learning of these skills.

Increasing the Couple's Fondness and Admiration in Online Meetings

The first steps of the sound house are meant to improve the work of love and friendship, Gottman developed sets of activities to enhance fondness and admiration. The couple is expected to do these activities at home.

Since many couples work from distant offices till late hours, they might be too tired to do their homework. Here we can use the advantage that they work near computer screens and many of them have enough privacy to do their exercises via online communication.

One of the exercises used by Gottman is called "I appreciate," in which each partner must compliment and use a positive adjective describing a positive experience with the spouse during the week. We suggest using the web to do it in a playful way. Here is an example based on Schwanke (2020):

1   Search for a website or app that will allow you to translate phrases from one language to another one of your choice. Think about something you'd like to compliment your partner on and type that into the translator. Read it aloud or play it from the website or app.
2   Let your partner guess the compliment.
3   Switch roles, receive a compliment from your partner, and try to guess what it is.
4   Who gave the most unique or most thoughtful compliment? Try funny and unexpected compliments and switch up the languages as often as you'd like. You'll both leave the activity feeling lighter, happier, and more appreciated.
5   Try to do this once a week, every morning, or every night and make it a part of your daily routine.

The above is only one example of how we can use the computer-mediated meeting to share fondness from a distance.

We can use the computer for other exercises that the Gottmans suggest: Instead of reminding one another all the reasons why the couple chose to be together, their unique strengths as a couple and why they fell in love – using the computer the couple can share with each other pictures from their history – from the time they fell in love or spent their honeymoon.

Last but not least, Gottman suggests finding ways to be together in a playful way. The sharing screen feature of many of the video conference applications can be used to share a YouTube video of loved songs with lyrics. Singing together is a very simple way to allow a joint synchronized emotional experience.

New Internet-Based Intervention – The Coach

The Gottman Relationship Coach (www.gottmanconnect.com/relationship-coach 2021), is a series of psycho educational modules which include streaming videos demonstrating effective relationship conversations. Topics include repairing negative interactions, developing listening skills, building positive feelings, and many others. The therapist can assign these modules to the couples to enhance and reinforce changes and as a way of reinforcing the experience of the session. Couples can watch these videos of John and Julie Gottman demonstrating these skills and practice them as homework. The therapist receives information about the couple's use of the Relationship Coach Modules and can send reminders to encourage the couple to use the Builder resource between sessions.

Since the couple continues to have access to this resource after the therapy ends, it is possible to create a "post-treatment" plan with the goal of reducing relapse. Research is still needed to assess the effectiveness of the Relationship Builder for therapy and relapse prevention.

In summary, the new technological innovations of the online assessment, the recordings of the videos by the couples and the Relationship Builder modules of the interventions make Gottman couple therapy online a rich experience for both the couples and the therapist.

References

Coop Gordon, K., & Mitchell, E.A. (2020). Infidelity in the Time of COVID-19. *Family Process*, 59, 956–96610.1111/famp.12576.

Crawford, P. , & Crawford, J. O. (2021). *Cabin fever: Surviving lockdown in the coronavirus pandemic*. Emerald Group Publishing.

Ekman, P., & Friesen, W. V. (1971). Constants across cultures in the face and emotion. *Journal of Personality and Social Psychology*, *17*(2), 124–129. 10.1037/h0030377

Gordon, R. M., Wang, X., Tune, J., & Al, G. E. T. (2015). Comparing psychodynamic teaching, supervision, and psychotherapy over videoconferencing technology with Chinese students. *Psychodynamic Psychiatry*, *43*, 585–599. doi: 10.1521/pdps.2015. 43.4.585

Gottman, J., & Gottman, J. S. (2018). *The science of couples and family therapy: Behind the scenes at the "Love Lab"*. New York: W.W. Norton & Company. ISBN 978-0393712742.

Gottman, J., Levenson, R., & Woodin, E. (2001). Facial expressions during marital conflict. *Journal of Family Communication*, *1*, 37–57. doi:10.1207/S15327698JFC0101_06

Hertlein, M. K., & Earl, M. E. (2020) Internet delivered therapy in couple and family work. In Haim Weinberg and Arnon Rolnick (Eds.), *Theory and Practice in online therapy* (pp.123-136), NY : Routledge.

Kaiser, J., Hanschmidt, F., & Kersting, A. (2020). The association between therapeutic alliance and outcome in internet-based psychological interventions: A meta-analysis. *Computers in Human Behavior*, *114*, 106512. doi:10.1016/j.chb.2020.106512

Kysely, A., Bishop, B., Kane, R., Cheng, M., De Palma, M., & Rooney, R. (2020). Expectations and experiences of couples receiving therapy through videoconferencing: A qualitative study. *Frontiers in psychology*, 10, 2992.

Lewis, J., Coursol, D., & Wahl, K. H. (2004). Researching the cybercounseling process: A study of the client and counselor experience, Greensboro, NC ERIC Counseling and student services clearinghouse.

Oren, N., Gronich, D., & Rolnick, A. (2018). Stairway to togetherness: -Taking mindfulness and biofeedback into the intersubjective realm, Biofeedback, *46*(2), 30–36.

Perle, J. G., Langsam, L. C., Randel, A., Lutchman, S., Levine, A. B., Odland, A. P., et al. (2012). Attitudes toward psychological telehealth: Current and future clinical psychologists' opinions of internet-based interventions. *Journal of Clinical Psychology*, *69*, 1–14. doi: 10.1002/jclp.21912

Qu, F., Yan, W.-J., Chen, Y.-H., Li, K., Zhang, H., & Fu, X. (2017). "You Should Have Seen the Look on Your Face ... ": Self-awareness of facial expressions. *Frontiers in Psychology*, *8*, 15–21. doi:10.3389/fpsyg.2017.00832

Rolnick, A., & Ehrenreich, Y. (2019). Fake it (or face it) till you make it? Taking a deeper look. *Biofeedback*, *47*(2), 44–47. doi:10.5298/1081-5937-47.2.01

Schwanke, C. (2020). *The couple's activity book: 70 Interactive games to strengthen your relationship* (p. 40). Rockridge Press.

20 Healing Through the Screen: Using Imago Relationship Therapy Online

Kalanit Ben-Ari

'Never let a good crisis go to waste' is one of Churchill's famous quotes, which I adopted when moving all my client work online due to the Covid-19 pandemic. The lack of physical presence and its implication in therapy is well discussed in the field, from absence of the whole body, unavailable non-symbolic connection between therapist and client as a means of gestures and emotional regulation, and technology challenges to mention a few disadvantages of therapy online.

However, by deciding to let go of my preconceptions about online therapy and opening myself up with curiosity and wonder, I discovered exciting opportunities for clinical interventions when undertaking Imago therapy online, in a way which I never had before. This is not to say that one form of therapy is better or worse than the other, but to explore the different qualities that facilitating Imago therapy online offers to therapists, clients and the therapeutic alliance.

In this chapter I briefly describe the theoretical and practical implications of Imago Relationship Therapy (IRT). Following an outline about how the IRT principals are facilitated when working with couples online, I discuss how the online medium might offer a different quality of the therapeutic intervention, and how technology challenges can be used for therapeutic processes as a projection and reflection of aspects of the couple's relationship. In addition, I explore the implications of the new 'setting', and look at the blurring of boundaries between a home setting and therapy setting, as well as its implications from a neuroscience perspective. Case studies will be presented to illustrate the practicality aspect of conducting IRT online.

Imago Relationship Therapy (IRT)

Imago Relationship Therapy (IRT) is a couple relationship-focussed theory and practice, pioneered by Harville Hendrix and Helen Lakelly-Hunt in the 70s. They proposed a revolutionary paradigm shift, to move from individual-centred therapy informed by Freud and originated in the atom theory, to the 'space between' principle of the relationship paradigm, which is rooted in quantum field theory. The core principles of IRT focus on moving couples into a conscious partnership with safety, zero negativity, connectivity, and

DOI: 10.4324/9781003205029-24

joyfulness at its centre. It is the Imago assumption that we are all connected all the time: connecting is our being, and therefore it is our biggest desire and our deepest fear. It asserts that we are who we are through relationships and as we are born in relationships, and wounded in relationships we are also healed in relationships. By establishing an environment of safety within the relationship, the 'space between' is transformed from conflict into connection.

'Imago' is Latin for the English word 'image'. Imago refers to the unconscious templates (i.e., image) created in relationship with our main caretakers in childhood, that impact on the selective process of our committed romantic partnership in adulthood. This partner, who shares the same qualities as the parent we had the most difficulty with, is the person with whom there is the potential to experience the deepest hurts and at the same time our greatest transformation.

The IRT meta-theory describes four journeys of the 'self', these are: cosmic; psychological; social; and evolution. Each one of these journeys shapes unconscious romantic selection and the relationship dynamic itself. The IRT intervention takes place via a process called The Dialogue, through which couples learn to talk without judgement, listen with curiosity and openness, and connect beyond their differences. The Dialogue consists of taking turns to speak and listen, mirroring, validating, and empathising with each other. The therapist's role is to facilitate the process, and the client receiving treatment is in fact the 'space-between' the relationship, rather than either of the partners. In that sense, the Imago therapist is not the centre of the therapy process, but a facilitator of it. In the Imago process couples experience the idea of viewing conflict as growth trying to happen, and learn that all relationships move through Romantic Love into Power Struggle and have the potential to move to conscious joyful relating. Using the dialogue, within the structure of five steps for conscious partnership, they learn about their childhood wounding and how each one adapted to it, as well as the impact it has on their life and relationships. By eliminating the idea of 'right and wrong' and replacing it with a deep sense of curiosity and loving care for the partner and the relationship, transformation can emerge.

All couples come to therapy for the same reason, that is rupture in connection triggered by intolerance to differences. The sense of loss of connection replicates a more historical rupture of connection with significant others in childhood. Imago posits that everyone experiences rupture of connection in their early childhood, although people differ in the intensity and frequency of these wounds. In that sense, Imago claims that all couples want to restore safety, connection, and joyful vitality. In adult romantic relationships, the lost sense of connection starts by an unconscious process caused by anxiety, which is managed and regulated by defensive behaviours that in turn escalate the situation. Defensive behaviours can include expanding one's energy at a time of stress, which includes raising voices, seeking to talk about the issue, and needing to pursue the other on one end of the scale, and avoidance, withdrawal or shutting down when facing a conflict at the other end. Although we have a main defensive coping strategy we might, at times, flip to the other defensive strategy. Imago posits that couples fall in love with someone who is wounded in a similar way but holds a complimentary defensive strategy. Imago therapists facilitate a process of growth and healing. They do so by promoting the reclaiming of lost parts and growing into wholeness by developing safer, intentional, and relational strategies to manage differentiation. By doing so 'we help them change the energy and the elements that make up their bond, and thereby, change their relationship – and then their interior world changes' (Hendrix & Hunt, 2021).

Therapy Online

I decided to view online therapy as an opportunity to let go of my preconceptions, reflecting on Buddhist teaching that holding and resisting often brings suffering. In embracing online therapy, we do not reject in-person therapy, or try to adopt the same way of doing therapy in-person, but rather accept the different qualities that the two approaches offer.

This transformation for how I chose to view online therapy made me reflect on the meaning we give to the clinical setting. An important aspect of a therapist's office is the provision of a stable 'safe' space in which to fully be and explore. With Imago therapy taking place in the 'space between' the clinical setting can help to promote an environment of safety with one another, and of connecting and joyfulness. Unlike individual therapy where attachment needs to develop between client and the therapist for significant work to happen, couples show up to therapy with their attachment figures, i.e., their partner and therefore the focus is not on the individual but on the relationship. In online therapy, this also remains true.

When I, the therapist, have no control over the physical setting, where I create what Winnicott called a 'holding environment', what is the spiritual, mental setting I want to facilitate online for the treated couple? What is my role in the spiritual and emotional setting beyond the physical?

By letting go of the 'controlled' setting of in-person therapy and mindset of how and where therapy can take place, we also serve as a model of relational flexibility. By opening ourselves up to think about and practice therapy in new ways, we are in turn opening our couples to possibilities of change, flexibility, resilience, and growth. This is especially important at this time when we want to reduce the sense of isolation.

Another preconception of online therapy is that it is less intimate. I would like to argue that working online offers the opportunity to explore a new form of intimacy with our clients. During the Covid-19 pandemic we have been faced with mutual concerns, such as the difficulties of working from home, worry about family members, and for some the loss of income. These areas of similarity offer us the opportunity to better understand each other and can create a different kind of intimacy, a deeper understanding of the client's struggles on the one hand and a chance for our clients to feel and express concern for us on the other.

The online 'window' to both the clients' and therapist's private spaces builds another layer of intimacy to the therapeutic relationship. Seeing their space can give us a better understanding of the treated couple. For some, privacy might be an issue and occasional interruptions from children or pets can become another source of information. I have noticed several cases of clients appearing more comfortable and confident in their own space. My own experience is also consistent with those of recent studies (Kysely et al., 2020). Through sharing our intimate spaces with each other, we can be viewed as more authentic, knowable, and human.

A unique characteristic of IRT practice is the physical arrangement of the couple during a session. Each partner sits facing the other, and the therapist is placed on one side, facing the 'space between' the two. A significant technique we adopt in Imago is the use of sentence stems instead of questions. In practice this means that the therapist starts a sentence for the person who is the 'sender' (i.e., the one who speaks), then the sender repeats that sentence and completes it in their own words. For example instead of asking 'When this happened how did you feel?' the therapist might whisper to the sender 'and when this happened I felt …'. The sender then repeats the sentence and completes it in their own words. The combination of this physical positioning and verbal technique promotes a deep sense of connection and a feeling of safety between the couple, and also realigns focus from the therapist to the 'space between'. This presents a big challenge to online therapy, as couples will necessarily face the screen instead of each other, and sharing sentence stems becomes more complicated when the therapist is sat not alongside but in front and away from the couple.

It was therefore necessary for me to adapt the practice to the online sphere. I coach the couple to sit facing each other, with both of their profiles in sight on the screen. I explain the principles of the Imago session, and assert that although I will facilitate the session I am not the centre of it, neither during the session nor beyond it. In this way I can become a voice in the background. I adapt the sharing of sentence stems by naming the person whom I would like to repeat and complete what I share. For example, I might say 'Adam: And when this happened I felt …'. I found that over time, with gentle coaching, and the use of non-verbal cues such as pointing, couples quickly became competent in the process.

In some cases, the couple may not be in the same space together for a session, which might be a barrier for effective online therapy. It could be that a partner is away, and then the three of us will interact from three different locations. In this scenario, I will invite them to connect at least 15 minutes before our meeting for a small talk between them, and to create more in-timacy. I invite couples to come closer to the camera and look closely into their partner's eyes while breathing deeply together. As I do not want them to be interrupted by my screen, with their permission I will ensure my camera is off. That way I literally become a voice in the background. If faced with a highly reactive couple I will keep my camera on to support regulating their reactivity and move them to a more intentional and conscious state.

The most surprising discovery has been in finding advantages to Imago online as opposed to in-person. I have called this the blurring of home-therapy boundaries.

When the couple connects with each other at their own home with me on the screen, there is a blending of the boundaries of the session, and a merging of the therapeutic setting with home. This blurring creates a therapeutic intervention which can strengthen the couple's connection. Moreover, in the therapy room we offer couples a different 'story' and 'experience' and by undertaking therapy in their own home they can hold on to this story for longer. In contrast to Hardy et al. (2021), who argued that online therapy does not allow an appropriate distinction between therapy and home spaces, I believe that this exact blurring and stretching of the boundaries of the session is of benefit to our clients.

In the clinic the therapist controls the environmental setting. Have you ever experienced a client who says that they feel relaxed, positive, and safe, just by sitting in the space, even before the session starts? My professional research of neuroscience might offer an answer. With repeated experiences we all develop a neurological connection between the experience and the context in which the experience happened. As the neuroscientist Donald Hebb explained 'Cells that fire together wire together'. In this case, the neurological connection is between the safety and connection we facilitate (the experience) and our office room (the context/space). Yet, it is rarely the aim of therapy to be an isolated encounter with an impact limited to the office. The purpose of therapy is to learn how to process, deal with, and manage what takes place outside the clinic. Therefore, having a neurological connection between the experience and context of the clinic is great but not sufficient. Working with couples online offers the potential to develop a similar neurological connection between the experience and the context, but this time the context is the client's home. This realisation led me to a new way of facilitating the sessions. How can the couple feel the same sense of safety in the space they are in, which will stay with them beyond our time together? How can we create a neurological connection to a safe space to talk about difficult conversations within their own home?

It is my belief that online therapy does not offer a 'one size fits all' approach, and should not be recommended as the only therapeutic intervention for more complex relationship issues such as domestic violence or highly reactive and aggressive couples. In such cases home may not be perceived as a safe space for at least one of the partners and the physicality of the therapist in the room holds additional significance.

Working online is not without its challenges. Technology presents issues (Hellman & Rolnick, 2019) such as connectivity and disrupted audio. Opening up conversations about the clients' experience of therapy online offers another opportunity for therapeutic intervention. For example, does it feel close or distant? Connected or disconnected? How do they cope with technology challenges? As previously stated, in IRT the process itself is the centre of the therapy, rather than the content. Therefore having couples discuss technological challenges is, at times, a dialogue process about the 'bad object' (Klein, 1952). Whatever the technology challenges trigger, it might represent their own projected 'shadow' onto the technology. Using this therapeutically allows us to use a discussion about technological issues to represent something beyond therapy online. I can use any discomfort as a therapeutic intervention, to encourage dialogue and deepen consciousness about ourselves and relationships. This discussion can help our clients to learn to be present with discomfort, and when in pain to lean towards relationships and their partner for increasing safety, connection and healing.

We are yet to know about the long term consequences of Covid-19 on the world or therapeutic alliance. Although in-person therapy is returning, in my opinion online therapy is not going to disappear. On the contrary, many clients told me that the option of online therapy has allowed them to undertake it at all. Covid-19 opened up therapy, which is at times a rigid profession, to practice mental, emotional and cognitive flexibility as never before. It is important we keep an open mind for other possibilities for therapy, especially given recent evidence (Helps & Le Coyte Grinney, 2021; Thomas et al., 2021) from the client's perspective that there is little difference with their experience of online or in-person individual therapy. Supporting clients at their own home, via online therapy, might have an impact we are yet to understand on healing suffering and restoring connections.

To illustrate the way I facilitate the idea of blurring and merging the Imago session online I present three examples from working with couples online.

Case Studies

Couple One

The first couple is one I have previously worked with, who had a strong relationship. They reached out at the start of the pandemic because a loss of a job due to Covid-19 affected their relationship. Unfortunately, they were not in the position to afford a two-hour session as I usually recommend. I offered them flexible payment options and suggested reducing the session to an hour and a half, given they know the process and have a strong connection. However, after the first session I felt this would not be sufficient. In IRT we start sessions by stating intentions and appreciation for each other. This heartfelt dialogue not only helps to change the frequency between the couple, it allows them to feel tenderly towards each other, and focus the session. The appreciation dialogue can easily take half an hour if one chooses, and is an important foundation which sets the tone for the rest of the session. As they were familiar with the process I became aware that my facilitation was really not needed at this stage. Instead of asking them to stretch to a two-hour session I suggested they meet half an hour before our time, in the same online space we would have our session, and undertake the appreciation dialogue by themselves. At our appointed time they just needed to connect to the meeting link.

I also ended the session in a similar way. Generally, following the closure of a session I invite the couple to stand and embrace for one minute, without talking and breathing in-sync. In this instance I told the couple to stay with the hug much longer, explaining that I would just disappear from the space. This is another example of blurring the boundaries of the session and merging the therapeutic setting with home. By opening and closing the session in this more fluid way, it almost feels as if you cannot tell where the session starts and finishes, and that fluidity helped create a safe space for connection in the clients' own home.

Couple Two

The second couple, married for more than 20 years with three children, came to therapy after a crisis. They acknowledged that although the crisis was triggered by the pandemic, it was actually a result of neglecting the re-lationship for many years. Although we met online, I could still feel the tension and pain between them. The wife could not look at her husband, and he was nearly shaking from suffering. Just looking at their faces through the screen I could see the deep rupture, pain, and disconnection between them. I realised that something needed to shift before they would be able to have a safe conversation. I acknowledged the pain I saw but also their intentions to break through it. That is, that they were both feeling a great deal of suffering which we would not ignore, but we would relate to in a different way. I asked if they would be willing to try something with me. After sitting with them in silence for a moment, I asked them to identify a special 'couple song', perhaps the first dance at their wedding, or something they associated with the be-ginning of their relationship, which could serve to remind them of the sacred space between them. Looking at each other, they agreed on their song, and I invited them to find it on YouTube, as the computer was open in front of them. In a clinical setting I would never open my computer in the middle of a session, but online therapy has provided an opportunity to explore more tools like this. I invited them to stand together for a silent hug for the duration of the song. I observed and coached them to breathe together and relax.

What amazed me was that I could see even through the screen the energy move in their bodies. There was a raw physical and emotional release by both, a heart-breaking cry, emotional processing, and connection at its core. I guided them into a healing holding, which is a way to hold firmly without movement and without the need to soothe the other. This is a concept from the Imago 'holding dialogue' that I, until then, thought could only be done during in-person therapy.

The rather long song passed very quickly, after which we did some pro-cessing with words and appreciation. Given its effect I asked them to repeat the exercise with my guidance. This time we also added an eye contact ex-ercise where they were encouraged to emotionally let their partner in, and send healing energy to the other.

At the end of the session, throughout which words had not been the main focus, they sat facing each other, looking calmer and gentler. They said that the exercise changed the whole mood between them, and that they saw the person they fell in love with 20 years ago. I invited them to express what they would like to ask their partner to give them as a gift for the coming week. The wife said she wanted the same hug daily if possible, and the husband could not agree more. We clarified quantity, duration, location, presence of children, and initiations. I suggested they start doing it in the same room they met me, with the same song in the background and in time to start to explore other locations in their home. They were happy to hug at the end of the session while I disappeared from the screen. It was remarkable to me that an online session could be focussed on physical rather than verbal interventions in a way I had not thought possible.

Couple Three

The last couple I would like to present in this chapter is one whose previous session had been quite challenging and stormy. I wanted to check in to understand if and how it had impacted the rest of their week. What I learned was that although I finished the session and left the meeting they actually stayed in the same position and continued the conversation for at least another hour, in the spirit of how they talk and listen when working with me. I found it remarkable as I listened to them describing their own conversation and the healing that came out of it. Instead of forcing them to leave the office because their time is up and I need to let the next couple in, I can disappear from the call and they can stay at the same space to continue the conversation and connection. It seems that when they have done this once without me, they will be more inclined to replicate it in the future. It was then that I started to develop the idea of neurological connection by inviting couples to do their Imago dialogues or homework in the same space they meet me online. Going forward I would then encourage them to move to other areas in their homes so safety can start to be associated with their relationship throughout their space.

Conclusion

The core concepts of IRT are the fundamental of safety of the 'space between', connecting, and joy. In that sense, the significance of meeting clients and the 'space between' where they are, mentally and emotionally, has an additional meaning when facilitating Imago therapy online. Moreover, in the IRT setting, the couple face each other and the therapist facilitates the session but is not the centre of it. The effect of the therapist being on the other side of the screen is evidenced in feedback that a male client shared with me:

> "Our experience performing Imago therapy over Zoom has been great. More than could have been expected ... Perhaps X and I being together physically, vs. you being distant adds a dimension of intimacy for the treated couple ...."

Recent research demonstrates that this is not a solitary experience. Kysely et al. (2020), for example, reported that couples felt more comfortable, felt they had more control and responsibility over the space and felt less threatened by the physicality of the therapist, all of which benefited their therapeutic experience.

This supports Imago's assumption that the therapy happened in the 'space between' the couple, which hasn't changed when facilitating IRT online. Moreover, the safe place the couples create is in their own space at home, not the clinic. Promoted by online therapy, we transform healing and growth to where the clients want to experience the change – their real life outside the clinic. The case studies described in this chapter illustrate how to implement the IRT approach when working online.

References

Hardy, N. R., Maier, C. A., & Gregson, T. J. (2021). Couple teletherapy in the era of COVID-19: Experiences and recommendations. *Journal of Marital and Family Therapy*, *47*(2), 225–243.

Hellman, S., & Rolnick, A. (2019). Introduction to the online couple and family therapy section. In Weinberg, H. & Rolnick, A. (Eds.), *Theory and practice of online therapy* (pp. 103–110). Routledge.

Helps, S., & Le Coyte Grinney, M. (2021). Synchronous digital couple and family psychotherapy: A meta-narrative review. *Journal of Family Therapy*, *43*(2), 185–214.

Hendrix, H., & Hunt, H. L. (2021). *Doing imago relationship therapy in the space-between: A clinician's guide*. WW Norton & Company.

Klein, M. (1952). "Some theoretical conclusions regarding the emotional life of the infant." *Envy and gratitude and other works 1946-1963*. Hogarth Press and the Institute of Psycho-Analysis.

Kysely, A., Bishop, B., Kane, R., Cheng, M., De Palma, M., & Rooney, R. (2020). Expectations and experiences of couples receiving therapy through videoconferencing: A qualitative study. *Frontiers in Psychology*, 10, 2992.

Thomas, N., McDonald, C., de Boer, K., Brand, R. M., Nedeljkovic, M., & Seabrook, L. (2021). Review of the current empirical literature on using videoconferencing to deliver individual psychotherapies to adults with mental health problems. *Psychology and Psychotherapy: Theory, Research and Practice*, *94*(3), 854–883.

21 Online Contemporary Couples Gestalt Therapy "Two Become One" – and then there are None!

From a *Fusion* Model to a *Connection* Model of Relationships

Rita F. Resnick and Robert W. Resnick

What is contemporary Gestalt therapy and how does one work as a Gestalt Therapist with couples? Are their differences in working as a Gestalt Therapist online vs. in-person? We begin by outlining foundational Gestalt therapy, then the Resnick model of Gestalt Couples Therapy, and finally, working online as a Gestalt couple's therapist.

What Is Gestalt Therapy?

The founders of Gestalt Therapy – Frederick (Fritz) Perls, M.D. and Laura Posner Perls, Ph.D. combined old elements into new organizations (gestalts). Gestalt Therapy is arguably the first integrated and integrating (not eclectic) psychotherapy, including the current therapies of the time, (1930s) – psychoanalysis and behaviorism. Gestalt Therapy also draws from: existentialism, Gestalt perceptual psychology, biology, phenomenology, field theory and more. "There is nothing new in Gestalt therapy" (Perls, F., personal communication, 1966). What is new is the relationship among many elements.

The goal of Gestalt Therapy is to restore self-regulation, within the person's environment – by becoming aware of fixed organizing patterns of perceptually making meaning, and of responding to the world – i.e., character.

Three Pillars of Gestalt Therapy

Field Theory

It is crucial to consider the environment (context) of **which** the client emerges – history, relationships, community, and social world. Its psychological relevance came from Kurt Lewin's statement of the importance of "looking at the total situation" rather than doing a piecemeal analysis. (Lewin, 1952 p.288). "The greatest value in the Gestalt approach perhaps lies in the insight that the whole

DOI: 10.4324/9781003205029-25

determines the parts ..." (Perls et al., 1951, pg. xi). For psychotherapy, this is a huge paradigmatic shift.

Phenomenology

Phenomenology is the study of subjective experience and meaning making. It is the process by which human beings make meaning of their sensorial experience. The phenomenological *method* is about describing an experience from the point of view of the subject by carefully observing the words and actions of a particular person and staying descriptive about what you see rather than refracting meaning through an interpretive prism – thereby colonizing the client's meaning.

Dialogue

The bedrock of Gestalt Therapy is the dialogic relationship between the client and the therapist. Since the mid-1920s and heavily influenced by both Kurt Goldstein's neuroplasticity organizations and Kurt Lewin's gestalt psychology's field theory where everything is related to and effects everything else, Gestalt Therapy is essentially, definitionally, and profoundly relational. Gestalt Therapy's primarily focus of what type of relational is Martin Buber's dialogic relationship. Buber maintains there is no "I" alone, but only the "I" of "I-It" and "I" of "I-Thou." (Friedman, 2002). People alternate between these two modes of relating. The "I-It" mode is necessary for strategic living wherein the value is in the outcome. "I-Thou" fits the situation when the value is in the actual relating – and not the transactional outcome.

While *all* therapeutic approaches are (and always have been) functionally "relational" of some sort – (expert, hierarchical, directive, interpretive, horizontal, dialogic, mechanical, formulaic, protocols, etc.), Gestalt Therapy's three pillars has always been field theoretical, phenomenological and dialogic – all standing on an existential ground.

Gestalt Therapy – Foundationally Existential

Gestalt therapy is heavily influenced by existentialism. The existential themes that had the most meaning for Fritz Perls were:

1   Authenticity – Being true to oneself despite external pressures.
2   Freedom – The power to act or think as one chooses without restraint but within limits.
3   Responsibility – For our choices, the meanings we make and the actions we take.
4   Existential Anxiety – Created by being in a world that has no meaning except that which we create. Thus, existential anxiety is to a large part normalized as part of being human and not a manifestation of "pathology."

What makes Gestalt therapy so deliciously difficult to define is exactly what makes it so exquisitely creative and procreative. With the three major pillars standing on an existential ground, each Gestalt theorist or therapist organizes the various other elements within the tent of Gestalt therapy differently. Gestalt therapy is based on the meta theory that there is no single and fixed Gestalt therapy theory. Gestalt Therapy is homeo*rhetic* (returning to a trajectory) and not homeo*static* (returning to a set point).

Organismic Self-Regulation (OSR)

Gestalt Therapy's worldview sees human beings as self-regulating organisms with the need to discriminate between nourishing and toxic choices in the service of the biological imperative of survival.

Character

Character is the major interruption to self-regulation. Character is the rigidification of ways of making meaning and responding to the world. These ways were appropriate at one time – a healthy, self-regulating, creative adjustment in one situation that is now acontextual. The fur coat in Siberia in February that can save your life – can kill you in Karachi in July. *Yesterday's healthy adaptations may become today's toxic pollutants.* The new **Resnick Peacock of Character** art poster, presents many of the sources of character development

The Resnick Model of Gestalt Couples Therapy

"Two become One" and Then There are None!"

From a *fusion* model of marriage to a *connection* model of marriage.

The Resnick model of couples Therapy is based on Gestalt principles of theory and practice. The essence of what distinguishes the Resnick model of couples therapy from all other models of couples therapy is our Gestalt field theory lens which includes the anthropological/sociological "institution" of marriage as the "fusion" (confluence) of two people. This has powerful ramifications for relationships and marriage in the present as no one begins marriage with a blank slate. We all have been acculturated.

"Two Become One" – The Fusion Model of Marriage

Societal institutions, such as marriage, are analogs to individual character formation, whereby a child's survival and wellbeing is predicated on his/her/their creative adjustments to his/her/their environment. Survival is the first biological imperative of any living organism. Whatever the child does that allows him/her/them to survive and flourish in the environment, is healthy – meaning congruent with what is "due" in the situation. Similarly, the institution of marriage allowed us to survive as a species *in a former context* and now, in our current situation, raises havoc.

Each member of the couple has his/her/their own characterological style that he/she/they bring to the relationship – including introjects – "shoulds" and rules that were swallowed whole and without discrimination (introjects), as well as his/her/their attachment histories and more. The therapeutic work is to facilitate the discovery of each person's characterological style, interrupting the interruptions to self-regulation with awareness–and identifying where the difficulties lie when engaging their partner. Some introjects, hopefully, will be discarded and some will be retained and assimilated. To discard introjects without examination is as bad as swallowing introjects without examination. Sometimes, your mother was right. Maturity is doing what you want to do – even if your mother wants you to.

The patriarchal fusion model ("Two Become One") was once functional, if not the optimal way of survival for our species. This codified into the "Institution" of marriage by the same process as individual character – the unaware continuation of what was a creative adjustment in one context becoming habitual and anachronistic (in Greek, "ana" meaning wrong, "chronos" meaning time) in another.

Difference

A fusion/confluent model of relationships and marriage means little or no boundaries and therefore allows for very few differences. Confluence cannot sustain difference. Difference in western culture does not have a good reputation. Difference is associated with danger, criticism, betrayal, conflict, threats to autonomy and/or connection, etc. Ironically, difference and boundaries have *both* the function of separating *and* connecting. Without boundaries there is either confluence/fusion or disconnected separateness/isolation – each with a loss of otherness which is required for connection. As a result of differences being avoided in a fusion model, HOW (process) couples deal with differences becomes far more important than WHAT (content) the differences are. With very few exceptions, HOW couples deal with difference is the gateway issue to facilitating couples to deal with WHAT (content) the differences are in an optimal, albeit imperfect way.

Dealing with Difference

Typically, couples in a traditional confluent/fusion "Two Become One" model of marriage have three ways of dealing with difference:

1   Defer to the other (confluence) – lose yourself.
2   Withdraw from the other – lose the other.

3   Conflict – attempt to get rid of the difference by trying to make the other like you. The partner usually resists – leading to explosion and withdrawal. Difference and Conflict are not the same: *Conflict IS the attempt to get rid of difference by trying to change the other to be like you. When the other resists being changed, difference becomes conflict.*

The Resnick CONNECTION Model of Relationships and Marriage

Distilled and integrating for over 50 years, we are the only couple's therapy theorists and practitioners who fundamentally challenge the current fusion model of marriage. Although successful enough millenniums ago, it is an anathema for today's world. Ecologically, a "pollutant" is a resource out of place and so it can be for an anachronistic "institution."

In western countries, first marriages have a divorce rate (explosion/rupture) of 55%+ while second marriage divorces are 75%+ (it's easier the second time). The couples who stay together are frequently not together because they are reasonably satisfied and nourished, but because they're terrified to be alone, money, children, religion, status or because they don't want to be seen as a failure or risk social stigma. We refer to them as the "Secretly, Miserably Married" (implosion/collapse).

Couple's Therapy Issues

The Resnick model of couple's therapy, with an adjustable zoom lens, monitors at least three major areas simultaneously: 1. intrapsychic, 2. interpersonal, 3. larger field.

1   First are the individual characterological issues sourced from actual experience, introjects and attachment histories that each person brings to the table. Although these fixed ways of perceiving and reacting may not serve the person well today, they are habitual – meaning below awareness.
2   There is then the interaction between the two characterological systems – frequently creating recursive loops – often a toxic spiral.
3   The larger field context – western culture's patriarchal fusion/confluent model of relationships and marriage which makes dealing well with difference frequently impossible – "Two Become One." The fusion model of marriage has outlived its design and its "shelf life."

Gestalt Therapy in Practice

Gestalt Therapy works with clients' awareness and awareness skills rather than using the classic psychoanalytic reliance on the analyst's interpretation of the alleged unconscious conflicts. The actual dialogic relationship developing over time, adds a supportive benchmark for comparison for the client and therapist to discern possible "transferred" (characterological) organizing perceptual ge-stalts and/or habitual responses. "Transference" is character in motion.

Process

Gestalt therapy a process-based therapy. The therapist and the client notice repetitive patterns, sequences of perceptions, and corresponding behavioral responses. These habitual (procedural memory), below awareness character-ological processes interrupt healthy self-regulation in the present, and the task of therapy is to interrupt those interruptions by facilitating awareness. Therapy happens at the point of difference and awareness. ***Character in-terrupts healthy self-regulation and awareness is the solvent of character.***

Awareness

Awareness is both the goal (in the service of self-regulation) and the metho-dology of Gestalt Therapy. One of the defining characteristics of awareness is being in contact with *what* you are doing *when* you are doing it. Awareness is primarily descriptive and experiential. Accessing the relevant past as it in-terrupts healthy functioning in the present – is a "game changing" paradig-matic shift for psychotherapy, and it is possible to help clients do this online or in person.

The Dialogic Relationship

Gestalt therapy works for understanding by using the active presence of the therapist and the client in a relationship based on authentic contact – modulated with clinical judgment. Buber's dialogue includes the therapist's presence, inclusion of the client or clients, and commitment to dialogue – being open to affect the other and to be affected by the other. In the I-thou mode, this also means not trying to control the outcome. The Gestalt therapist, with clinical judgment, shares his/her/their genuine reaction to the client. Since each client and each therapist has a different phenomenological organization of the field, the engagement of these differences creates aware-ness and awareness allows for choice.

The dialogic relationship provides a rich bounty of therapeutically and personally nourishing consequences as well as 30% of the variance of therapy outcome (Wampold & Imel, 2015) – a crucible for characterological processes to emerge as a "fresh fish" in the present relationship between client and therapist.

Coming from a field theory perspective, connection to others is how human beings navigate the omnipresent basic human dilemma: *How to be connected to an other – and maintain a self* ... the ongoing dance of life. We believe that primary relationships are an attempt by many to create existential meaning. Meaning is in an ongoing relationship between me and non-me. A fusion model of marriage makes this difficult.

The Body

Body "language" refers to the nonverbal signals that function to communicate. Attention to the body leads to awareness of the client's process. The client focuses awareness (frequently using breathing and movement) on his/her/their bodily sensations. Conversely, attending to when thoughts and/or feelings awaken sensorial, kinesthetic, and proprioceptive experience can be trove of new information.

Techniques – Experiments and Others

Unfortunately, Gestalt Therapy is sometimes erroneously seen (and even sometimes poorly practiced) as if conducting experiments (or other techniques) defines Gestalt Therapy. Experiments are only one way of creating difference in the service of facilitating awareness. Importantly, experiments and all other techniques sometimes used in Gestalt Therapy such as empty chair or two chair-work, enactment, amplification, repetition, exaggeration, et al. could all disappear and never be used again – and true Gestalt Therapy can easily continue. (Resnick, R., 1984). Techniques are only the technology "du jour" to facilitate awareness, which is the durable and definitional methodology of Gestalt Therapy.

Online Therapy

If nothing else, online therapy is a challenge to re-adjust to a changed situation. Gestalt Therapy is exquisitely well suited to this challenge since fundamentally, Gestalt Therapy advocates that "wisdom" (healthy self-regulation within one's environment) is predicated on the situation (person + other + environment/history). Field theory maintains that healthy self-regulation is always relational and a function of the situation.

Online therapy is not the same as in-person therapy. There are many advantages and disadvantages of online therapy compared to in-person therapy.

Disadvantages

1   Online therapy lacks the "animal presence" of being in a shared space with another person or a couple.
2   The therapist is usually limited to the view of the client from shoulders and above with reduced visual and auditory access to the client's full body, subtle movements, flexing, breathing, perspiring and skin complexion changes, freezing, etc.

3   Sometimes a lack of safe privacy for the client as they are usually home or at work with other adults, children, noises and other distractions and threats to safety.

4   Sometimes it is harder for intimate experiences to happen screen to screen.

Advantages

1   Online sessions can provide a safe and accessible space to discuss concerns, conflicts, challenges, thoughts, and needs especially important when face-to-face is not available.

2   Online therapy is beneficial for people who live in remote, rural, or otherwise underserved areas where few or no therapists work.

3   No matter where clients are, online therapy hugely increases the pool of therapists from which clients may choose.

4   People with physical disabilities or people with mobility difficulties may find it much easier to work online than to go to an office at a designated time each week.

5   By reducing or eliminating barriers such as fear of social stigma, online therapy can reach clients who might never have sought traditional in-person therapy.

6   It can be easier for some people to reveal private information when they're sharing it online – sometimes providing more distance and accordingly, more safety.

7   The specific setting of online therapy (namely someone's home) provides some clients with a more relaxed feeling and could protect the client from the possibility of encountering someone he/she/they know in the waiting room.

8   Online therapy with couple's allows the therapist a full-face view of each of the couple at the same time – with easy mobility among one, the other, and/or the interaction.

9   The online experience is the current shared field of both the client and the therapist – a co-constructed space. It is important that the therapist explicitly acknowledges the reality of the situation, that they are online and not in the same physical space. It is very useful for the therapist to both acknowledge how that is for him/her/them, and to inquire as to how this is for the client. This acknowledgement and enquiry minimizes having an "elephant in the room" – a significant event or change that is not acknowledged.

Structure, Seating, and Screens

Usually, when a couple enters a therapist's consulting room they will find the sofa and sit down next to each other, both facing the therapist – not unlike "two birds on a wire." This supports the culturally implicit frame that the couple will both tell their stories to the therapist who will then question, clarify, suggest, support, comment, and perhaps even fix the situation. Of course, each member of the couple is frequently looking for the therapist to tell them that they are "right." In our in-person consulting rooms, we set up three chairs in an isosceles triangle (equidistant), where each person can see the other and it is observable where people are looking – and not looking – and whom they are talking to.

Example of a Working Online Advantage

Working online presents opportunities for the therapist that are not easily (or sometimes ever) available in a more traditional person to person meeting. When we meet with couples in person, as we've said, we arrange the seating in an equilateral isosceles triangle (with one therapist) or a quadrangle when we have the luxury of being co-therapists – which is largely during training workshops. This makes it "easy" to see when the person is looking at the person they are talking to and when they are not. This also avoids the tra-ditional "two birds on a wire" position, but it still does not allow the therapist to look at both people in the couple *at the same time*. Online, with a split screen of both people in the couple and the therapist's video turned off, the therapist can now see both the person speaking and the other person being spoken to – *both full face!* The couple can see each other's full face as well. Sometimes, the person speaking seems not to be aware of (and may sometimes be avoiding) how the person they are presumably speaking to, is responding non-verbally – e.g., heavenly glances, sighs of exasperation, looking away, perking up, tearing, clenching, nodding either in agreement or disagreement and more.

Frequently, we ask either the speaking partner if he/she/they noticed the impact and reaction of the listening partner, or ask the listening partner how they were affected by what their partner had just said. Further exploration as to how that impacted them (if he/ she/they noticed) or what was going on that they did not notice – inevitably leading to rich fields of each of the partner's "ground" which they carry with them. We both have had wonderful explorations open-up when attending to these phenomena. For example, sometimes the "listening" partner is not really listening at all, but is just metaphorically tapping his, her, their feet (or actually tapping but can't be seen doing that online) and waiting until his/her/their partner is finished so they can then play their familiar old tape of his/her/their point of view. Frequently, the partner reciprocates with not really listening either and poised to play their familiar old tape. We call this "a sequential monologue mas-querading as a dialogue." For actual dialogue to happen, each person must be open to both affect the other, as well as to be affected by the other.

With online and permission from all to record, it is also possible to play back some of these interactions after discussion with the couple.

Surprisingly, working with a couple online gives us even more options. By asking the couple to each have his/her/their separate device (and be in separate rooms to avoid audio feedback), we now have the additional possibility of limiting the frame to having just the split screen of the couple on view by blocking the therapist's video. This makes it clear to the couple and done transparently by the therapist saying they want the couple to look and speak to each other. Of course, when they are talking to the therapist, they can address the therapist even without a visual picture to speak to and the therapist can easily reappear visually whenever necessary. This allows the therapist a live window as to how the couple relates to each other.

Some couples even report that being on separate devices in a separate space allows them to be more direct and authentic than when touching warm shoulders sitting in front of a single screen together, looking at the therapist. The physical distance along with the visual closeness for many, offers support and safety to risk more than when sitting together. Having only the split screen of the couple being visible, clearly shows the partner and the therapist the second person's reactions to the person talking to them – e.g., looking away, rolling of eyes, intensity of focus, moving towards or away, emotionality, looking at cell phone, etc. – useful information much harder to access in an in-person format.

The Body Online

Of course, the body is one of Gestalt therapy's lenses: how one moves, how and when one breathes or holds one's breath, gestures one makes, facial expressions or lack thereof, voice tones, muscular changes, skin color changes, etc. Does being on a screen take away these bodily sensations and are sessions in danger of becoming merely cognitive? For the client to be fully seen (that is meant literally – see the whole body), it is better to work with the client in person. Online, the lower part of the body is not visible to the therapist. This may or may not be important depending upon the needs of the client and the therapist. The body also includes sensorial, kinesthetic, and proprioceptive experiences which cannot be seen directly by the therapist, regardless of whether in person or online.

One way to overcome this difficulty is to ask your client to stand up so that you can see all of him/her/them. Of course, as soon as you ask the client to do anything, the situation changes. Instead, perhaps you could ask questions of the client. Are your feet touching the ground? What is your breathing like now? For a session not to be devoid of bodily expression, the therapist must get more comfortable with his/her/their own body first. We can stand up and move and ask our clients to do the same. Hopefully, this will make us, as therapists, and our clients feel freer than if we just sit in an upright stiff position, not moving our heads and staring at our screens.

Relationships in Couples Therapy

Online also offers the therapist and the couple, new and improved ways to ensure the two people in the couple are relating *to each other* (see examples above), rather than relating just to the therapist about how they see themselves and their partner allegedly relating – without relating to their partner in situ.

The point about the therapist and his/her/their relationship to the couple is to acknowledge that now each person of the couple has their actual partner present and this relationship is privileged over either of their relationships with the therapist.

Each person's relationship to the therapist is never excluded. This is not an option in individual therapy where the dialogic relating between the client and the therapist is the "only show in town." Actually, for us, individual therapy is a kind of couple's therapy where the therapist is part of the couple.

Inclusion and I – Thou Moments

There are two parts to inclusion. The first is the process of truly getting (Buber used the word apprehending) our client's experience at a particular moment in the therapy session – to the best of our ability. The second part is conveying to the client that we do truly understand by acknowledging the impact on the therapist and his/her/their reaction to that impact. Knowing how the other is impacted lets a person know they have been received. Reacting to that impact lets them know that they have been met. These powerful moments of connection whether between the couple or even the therapist and one member of the couple, can occur in person or online.

CODA

For the Resnick's model of Couple's Therapy, the focus is on supporting a dialogic relationship between the couple. Characterological issues, how people deal with difference, and larger field issues that affect our clients (and usually ourselves as well) are crucial for the therapy. And all of us deal with the basic human dilemma: *How to be connected to an other and maintain a self …* This is the essence of couple's therapy and a central issue in individual therapy as well. Almost all therapy is about relationships – whether online or in-person. Online Couple's Therapy, although bringing some constrictions, also yields several important new options.

References

Bateson, G. (2000). *Steps to an ecology of mind*. Chicago: University of Chicago Press.

Beisser, A. (1970). The paradoxical theory of change. In J. Fagan & I. Shepherd (Eds.), *Gestalt therapy now: Theory, techniques, applications* (pp. 107–108). Palo Alto, California: Science and Behavior Books. https://archive.org/details/gestalttherapyno00faga

Buber, Martin (1970). *I and thou*. New York: Scribner & Sons.

Farber, L. (1966). *The ways of the will*. New York: Basic Books.

Friedman, M. (1976) Healing through meeting: A dialogical approach to psychotherapy and family therapy. In J. Smith (Ed.), *Psychiatry and the humanities*. (Vol. 1). New Haven: Yale University Press.

Friedman, M. S. (2002). *Martin Buber: The Life of Dialogue* (4th ed.). Routledge. 10.4324/9780203398197.

Hostrup, H. (2010). *Gestalt therapy: An introduction to the basic concepts of gestalt therapy.* Copenhagen: Hans Reitzel.

Hycner. R. (1999). Dialogical gestalt therapy: An initial proposal. *The Gestalt Journal, 8*(1) 23–49. https://www.google.com/books/edition/The_Gestalt_Journal/3M1KAQ AAIAAJ?hl=en

Lewin, K. (1952). Field theory in social science. *British Gestalt Journal, 1*(2), 69–81.

Perls, L. (1991). *Living at the boundary.* Highland, New York: Gestalt Journal Publications.

Perls, F., Hefferline, R., & Goodman, P. (1951). *Gestalt therapy: Excitement and growth in the human personality.* New York: Julian Press.

Polster. E., & Polster, M. (1973). *Gestalt therapy integrated: Contours of theory and practice.* New York: Bruner Mazel.

Resnick, R. W. (1984). Gestalt therapy east and west: Bi-coastal dialogue: Debate or debacle? *Gestalt Journal, 7*(1) 13–32. https://psycnet.apa.org/record/1985-20759-001

Resnick R. W. (2015). Gestalt therapy. (Ed) *The sage encyclopedia of theory in counseling and psychotherapy.* Thousand Oaks, California: Sage.

Resnick, R. W. (2019, Sept 19–22). *Gestalt therapy and homeorhesis: Evolution – With movement, discrimination and grace.* European Association of Gestalt Therapy. (keynote speaker, conference session) Budapest, Hungary. https://docplayer.net/158030698-Eagt-gestalt-conference-2019.html

Resnick, R. (2019). Fritz Perls: 'Narcissistic' bufoon or imperfect genius? The re-habilitation of a balanced view. In J-M. Robine, & C. Bowman (Eds.), *The psycho-pathology of awareness: An unfinished and unpublished manuscript of Frederick S. Perls* (44, pp. 65–87). [Bibliothèque de Gestalt-terapie]. St. romain la Virvée: l'Exprimerie.

Robine, J-M., & Bowman, C. (Eds.). (2019). *Psychopathology of awareness: An unfinished and unpublished manuscript,* by Frederick S. Perls, 44. [Bibliothèque de Gestalt-terapie]. St. Romain la Virvée: l'Exprimerie.

Vita, P. D., Keyes, H. A., Valantin, B. (2021). Internet-mediated gestalt therapy: Excitement and growth in an online field. *British Gestalt Journal, 1*(30), 3–10.

Wampold, B., & Imel, Z. (2015). *The great psychotherapy debate: The evidence for what makes psychotherapy work.* 2nd edition. Routledge/Taylor & Francis. https://psycnet.apa.org/record/2008-07548-000

Yontef, G. (1988). *Awareness, dialogue and process: Essays on gestalt therapy.* Highland, New York. https://books.google.com/books/about/Awareness_Dialogue_Process.html?id=NcjNkln05owC

Zinker, J. (1994). *In search of good form: Gestalt therapy with couples and families.* San Francisco: Josey-Bass. https://www.routledge.com/In-Search-of-Good-Form-Gestalt-Therapy-with-Couples-and-Families/Zinker/p/book/9780881632934

Section IV

Specific Populations

22 Online Suicide-Focused Treatment: The Telehealth Use of CAMS

Mary V. Tipton, Josh Brenner, Jennifer Crumlish, Melinda Moore, and David A. Jobes

Online Suicide-Focused Treatment: The Telehealth Use of CAMS

Suicide is among the leading causes of death for youth and adults in the United States and worldwide. The World Health Organization (WHO) estimated that 700,000 individuals died by suicide around the globe in 2019, making it the 17th leading cause of death worldwide (WHO, 2021). Rates of suicide were higher in males (12.6 deaths per 100,000 individuals) than in females (5.4 deaths per 100,000 individuals) and more than half (58%) of suicides occurred before the age of 50 (WHO, 2021). Rates of suicide are just as staggering in the United States. Suicide is the 10th leading cause of death across all age groups with about 48,000 deaths in 2019 (CDC, 2019). Suicide is the 2nd leading cause of death among 10–21-year-olds and 11th leading cause of death among individuals ages 22 and older (CDC, 2019). Out of all 202,820 adult deaths in 2019, 44,224 (22%) were from suicide (CDC, 2019). Out of all 14,945 youth deaths in 2019, 4,145 (27%) were from suicide (CDC, 2019).

Despite the statistics that indicate that suicide is a leading cause of death in the United States, the number of individuals dying by suicide is significantly lower than the numbers of individuals who experience suicidal thoughts and behaviors. About 1.4 million adults reported attempting suicide and 12,000,000 reported serious thoughts of suicide in 2019 (SAMHSA, 2020). A national survey of risky behaviors among youth found that 8.9% of high-school-aged adolescents reported at least one previous suicide attempt and about 18% reported seriously considering attempting suicide (Ivey-Stephenson et al., 2020). Despite the adoption of numerous suicide prevention efforts nationwide, such as the Zero Suicide initiative and The Joint Commission (2016) recommendation for universal suicide risk screening in medical settings, overall rates of suicide have increased over the past several decades (CDC, 2019).

Clinicians who encounter individuals at risk for suicide need empirically supported treatments to effectively decrease risk of death and psychological distress and increase hope and reasons for living. Conventional approaches to treatment include utilizing medication or inpatient hospitalization. However, these approaches do not have strong evidence to support their efficacy and

DOI: 10.4324/9781003205029-27

may increase risk of suicide following discharge (Jobes et al., 2017; Jobes & Chalker, 2019; Qin & Nordentoft, 2005). The routine practice of the routing of people who are suicidal to emergency departments (ED) became especially dubious during the COVID-19 pandemic as such referrals could put patients at additional risk of contracting the virus. Similarly, inpatient psychiatric care could also pose an increased risk of viral transmissions.

While it may not be widely known in mental health, there is strong empirical support for the use of psychotherapeutic treatments for suicide risk (Jobes et al., 2015) which include: Dialectical Behavior Therapy (DBT; Linehan et al., 1991; Linehan, 1993; Linehan et al., 2015), Cognitive Therapy for Suicide Prevention (CT-SP; Brown et al., 2005; Wenzel et al. 2009), Brief Cognitive Behavioral Therapy (BCBT; Bryan & Rudd, 2018; Rudd et al., 2015) and the Collaborative Assessment and Management of Suicidality (CAMS; Jobes, 2006; Jobes, 2012). The following chapter describes the CAMS therapeutic framework, its empirical support, and its rapid adaptation for the use via telehealth during the COVID-19 pandemic. Additional information regarding the use of each of the other aforementioned treatments within a telehealth modality is summarized in Table 22.1.

Overview of CAMS

CAMS is a suicide-focused therapeutic framework designed to specifically target patient-articulated suicidal "drivers" (problems that compel them to consider suicide) while accommodating varying theoretical orientations to treat suicidal drivers. CAMS philosophy emphasizes four pillars: empathy, collaboration, honesty, and a suicide-focus to create a strong therapeutic relationship and increase patient motivation as patient-defined suicidal drivers are identified and treated. CAMS is not a new psychotherapy, but instead functions as a framework that allows clinicians to use an integrative approach and the full range of interventions (e.g., cognitive behavioral, behavioral activation, insight-oriented, interpersonal, and psychodynamic).

CAMS utilizes a versatile assessment, treatment planning, tracking, and clinical outcome tool called the Suicide Status Form (SSF) to uncover the unique way in which the patient experiences suicidality. During the first session of CAMS, the clinician and patient review an initial SSF to collaboratively complete three sections. The first section is called the SSF Core Assessment where the patient rates and describes their psychological pain, stress, agitation, self-hate, hopelessness, and overall risk of suicide. The SSF Core Assessment is completed by the patient at the beginning of each subsequent CAMS session. In the first CAMS session, the patient also identifies their reasons for living and dying among other assessments.

There is a second section of the first session SSF that is comprised of yes/no questions about empirically supported suicide risk factors and warning signs such as current ideation, attempt history, impulsivity, substance abuse, relationship difficulties, sleep, and appetite, followed by a space for a description of the

Table 22.1 Evidence-based interventions for suicide risk & use via telehealth services

	Research Regarding Online Implementation	Suitable for Online Use?	Main Characteristics of Treatment	Main Challenges of Telehealth Use
Dialectical Behavior Therapy (DBT; Hyland et al., 2021; Landes et al., 2021; Zalewski et al., 2021; S. Rizvi, personal communication, October 19, 2021)	On-going studies across various clinical trials	Yes	Skills group; Individual therapy; Phone coaching; Team consultation	Skills group could be more difficult online; Challenges sharing materials
Cognitive Therapy for Suicide Prevention (CT-SP; G. Brown & M. Ilgen, personal communication, October 19, 2021)	On-going research of CBT-SP telehealth in Veteran Affairs	Yes	Safety Planning; Treatment of suicidal mode; Relapse prevention	Lack of clinician tech expertise and access; sharing materials; patients distracted in home settings
Brief Cognitive Behavioral Therapy (BCBT; C. Bryan, personal communication, October 19, 2021; Rojas et al., 2021)	On-going studies of BCBT-SP and Crisis Response Planning	Yes	Crisis Response Planning; Treatment of suicidal mode; Relapse prevention	Possible lack of clinician technological expertise; Difficulty sharing materials; Potential dropouts
Collaborative Assessment and Management of Suicidality (CAMS; Jobes et al., 2020; D. Jobes, personal communication, October 19, 2021)	On-going CAMS RCTs with veterans, college students, teens & young adults	Yes	SSF used for collaborative assessment and driver-focused treatment	Technology issues; use of smartphones vs. computers; patient privacy; potential dropouts

patient's experience, if applicable. The third section of the first session SSF includes the CAMS Treatment Planning section that first focuses on the development of the CAMS Stabilization Plan (see Tyndal et al., 2021) and then focuses two patient identified suicide drivers which are the issues that most compel the patient is consider suicide. The treatment plan also includes goals and objectives and the interventions that will be used to treat patient articulated suicidal drivers. A unique characteristic of the standard administration of CAMS is that we employ – with the patient's permission – side-by-side seating for certain assessment and treatment planning aspects of using CAMS. This seating arrangement is meant to underscore the collaborative nature of the intervention and ensure complete transparency about what is being assessed and treated.

There are currently five published randomized-control trials (RCTs) of CAMS across various populations including adult and college-aged individuals in outpatient and inpatient psychiatric settings. CAMS has been found to significantly reduce suicidal ideation in about 6–8 sessions (Covington et al., 2011; Jobes et al., 2017; Pistorello et al., 2020), overall symptom distress (Comtois et al., 2011; Ryberg et al., 2019) and symptoms of depression (Pistorello et al., 2020). A recent meta-analysis independently determined the efficacy of CAMS compared to other interventions for suicidal risk (Swift et al., 2021). Results showed that CAMS significantly reduces suicidal ideation, general distress, and hopelessness (while increasing hope) and that it can be considered a *"Well Supported"* intervention for suicidal risk as per the Center for Disease Control and Prevention's (CDC) Continuum of Evidence of Effectiveness criteria (Puddy & Wilkins, 2011), which is the highest designation of empirical support. Early procedures for using CAMS via telehealth have also recently been described (Jobes et al., 2020).

The COVID-19 Pandemic and Telehealth

Due to the need for social distancing to reduce the transmission of COVID-19, mental health providers had to adapt to ensure the risk of viral transmission was minimized. As a result, a surge in the necessity of conducting mental health services through "telehealth" (also called telepsychology, tele-psychotherapy, telepsychiatry, telemedicine, etc.) suddenly arose. The use of telehealth to administer mental health services is likely here to stay as some patients report finding it easier to engage in treatment from the comfort of their own homes (Severe et al., 2021). While COVID-19-driven telehealth has become pervasive, previous endorsement of using telehealth with patients who are suicidal has historically been somewhat discouraged and literature on the topic is remarkably scant.

Concerns about Working with Suicidal Risk via Telehealth

Clinical and professional concerns have long been raised about the hazards of treating patients who are suicidal (Jobes & Maltsberger, 1995) and these long-standing concerns are further now complicated by the introduction of telehealth and its use with the assessment, management, and treatment of suicidal risk. Three perceived risks were raised by 52 mental health providers in a study conducted by Gilmore and Ward-Ciesielski (2019): 1) virtual assessment issues, 2) lack of control over the patient, and 3) difficulties with hospitalizing a patient if needed. To illustrate the hesitance in endorsing the use of telehealth with patients who are suicidal, only 21.2% of the sample of the Gilmore and Ward-Ciesielski (2019) advocated for the use of Telehealth with patients who are at high risk for suicide.

While the endorsement for using telehealth with patients at risk for suicide has not been prevalent, another issue arises when patients who are acutely suicidal are typically referred to an emergency department. While it may have been routine clinical practice to refer an individual to find the nearest ED in the event of a mental health emergency, during the pandemic this practice became questionable regarding a patient's best interests as this would greatly increase the risk of contracting or spreading the virus. Given the public health recommendations, it was plainly inadvisable to suggest a patient go to an ED or have them hospitalized especially when telehealth provided a ready and safe alternative for them to receive mental health services.

Adaptations for Using CAMS via Telehealth

Because standard CAMS employs a side-by-side seating arrangement in a face-to-face visit, adjustments and adaptations for safely and effectively using CAMS via telehealth were obviously needed. We thus describe below general considerations of any remote telehealth treatment for suicidal risk and then specific adaptations for the use of CAMS.

Informed Consent

As a general matter, effective and safe telehealth work with patients who are suicidal requires thoughtful upstream thinking and extensive informed consent that anticipates the various challenges posed by telehealth. As discussed in the National Action Alliance for Suicide Prevention's (2020) Task Force document entitled "COVID Guidance: Screening for Suicide Risk during Telehealth Visits" there are important and sensible steps to take when working with suicidal risk remotely via telehealth. For example, there must be reasonable understandings about the difference between assessing and treating suicidal risk when not sharing the same physical space. Thus, arrangements should be made for a range of scenarios – for example, if Wi-Fi should freeze, either the patient or clinician disconnect from the call, or cases of emergent and imminent risk. Usually, thoughtful negotiation and the potential engagement of 3rd party contacts can ensure that care is rendered safely within telehealth even if a patient enters into an acute crisis state. Sensible general guidance around remote work with suicidal risk via telehealth has been offered by the National Action Alliance for the Prevention of Suicide (2020).

Adaptations of the Use of the CAMS SSF

While the intent and core feature of CAMS is the collaborative effort of clinician and patient completing the SSF form together, the unique difficulty of conducting CAMS via telehealth warrants an adaptation of how the clinician and patient engage with the SSF. Prior to the pandemic, CAMS in telehealth had been adopted by military behavioral health providers working with suicidal individuals in remote or underserved locations (Waltman et al., 2019). Those providers developed a process where both the clinician and patient had their own blank SSF, and during the session, took turns dictating and transcribing responses on each form, checking in with each other periodically to ensure that the clinician's and patient's form mirrored each other's as the SSF is completed in this parallel fashion. Providers noted that this process actually improved rapport as the patients often seemed particularly engaged in ensuring that the clinician was accurately transcribing the patient's responses. At the start of the pandemic, this modality was recommended to clinicians trained in CAMS who expressed an interest in continuing to provide treatment to patients who are suicidal via telehealth.

Nevertheless, it became apparent that though telehealth became more available, the ability of patients to print out their own copy of the SSF for sessions was not always feasible. To remedy this, a form-fillable PDF version of the SSF was developed and distributed so that the clinician and patient would be able to see the SSF (via screen sharing), and the clinician would become the patient's scribe, typing in the patient's responses as they moved through the CAMS assessment and treatment planning process together. This has become a more viable method for completing the SSF during telehealth sessions. Just as the clinicians using paper SSF forms would routinely check in with patients as the form was completed, it is recommended that clinicians continue to use this approach when utilizing the fillable PDF of the SSF. With the use of this form-fillable PDF, the clinician can then provide a copy to the patient to ensure the patient has a thorough and comprehensible copy of the SSF. Additionally, this process also generates a clearly legible PDF that can be easily entered into the patient's electronic medical record.

Due to COVID restrictions, three on-going CAMS RCTs needed to be converted to telehealth versions of CAMS (D. Jobes, personal communication, October 20, 2021). In the future, data will be available from these RCTs to compare potential differences in face-to-face CAMS versus CAMS provided via telehealth. In lieu of sitting next to each other, we have observed considerable success using CAMS online with both the patient and clinician appearing on the screen together using gallery mode settings. Completing the fillable SSF using the shared screen mode has worked well as the clinician transcribes assessment and treatment planning information on behalf of the clinical dyad. Moreover, the key pillars of CAMS seemed to be realized in our observations of video-recorded sessions for fidelity purposes within the RCTs. For example, both the empathic and collaborative spirit of CAMS can be seen in telehealth sessions as providers overtly endeavor to capture the patient's words and intent accurately on the fillable form and patients are invited to correct any SSF transcriptions made by the provider to ensure that the wording reflects exactly what the patient means. While we had concerns about a possible loss of empathy related to being online, thus far in our clinical trials this has not proven to be an issue. Perhaps the close-up views of the patient's and clinician's faces helps create more connection or maybe the collaborative effort of online communication helps clinicians to empathically tune-in to the patient in ways that were unexpected at the outset of online CAMS.

We also have observed that some patients actually seem to relish the opportunity to correct the clinician who earnestly endeavors to understand and validate the patient's experience. Thus far an unexpected dynamic has emerged: that of the clinician faithfully *serving* the patient to accurately record their assessment and treatment planning information, just as the patient means it. An additional unexpected benefit of the PDF SSF is a clear and legible version of the documentation that was not always ensured when hardcopies are used in standard CAMS. While these benefits are notable, there are of course some drawbacks and limits to doing this work online which include unstable internet connections, or patients not having privacy during a session (e.g., a patient in their closet whispering into his laptop to evade his intrusive mother). Moreover, telehealth CAMS is less optimal when patients use their phone versus a computer. But notwithstanding some of these issues, the use of telehealth CAMS has been largely positive.

Despite successes, it is important to address concerns raised in the survey work of Gilmore and Ward-Ciesielski (2019) related to virtual assessment, lack of control over the patient, and difficulties hospitalizing patients. Considering that every CAMS session begins with the SSF Core Assessment, any issues related to virtual assessment could be a major concern for the effectiveness of CAMS. Thus far CAMS-based assessments via telehealth have not been impacted by doing this work online – the collaborative experience of doing a thorough and empathic assessment on the fillable PDF seems intact (if not actually enhanced). The notion of "control over the patient" (who is remotely located) is frankly antithetical to a central premise of CAMS which overtly emphasizes *collaboration with* vs. *control over* the patient (Jobes et al., 2016). Across three ongoing clinical trials of CAMS that are now being conducted online, a deep sense of collaboration has been preserved. Having potential access to patient-identified third parties if needed has been helpful in certain crisis situations. Finally, another overt premise of CAMS is to endeavor to work on an *outpatient* basis (as much as possible). Within the CAMS approach to care, hospitalization is used sparingly as a last possible resort (vs. a first response). Indeed, in a recent RCT of CAMS with 62 college students – who were sometimes quite suicidal – there were zero hospitalizations initiated by study clinicians (Pistorello et al., 2020). That said, occasional hospitalizations have occurred within our on-going CAMS RCT's which have been facilitated with the supportive help of pre-identified third parties.

In summary, while there are some obvious limits to online care, there have been notable and often unexpected benefits (e.g., a case where a lethal means safety intervention was done online as the patient took their laptop into the bathroom collecting medications and turning them over to their partner for safe keeping *during* their CAMS telehealth session). While the pervasive pre-pandemic caution of working with suicidal risk remotely is understandable in hindsight, our experience to date argues that this work can be done quite safely and effectively. Moreover, a recent meta-analysis of telehealth vs. face-to-face care should give telehealth naysayers cause to check their presumptions. Fernandez et al. (2021) found in their rigorous investigation of over 100 within and between group clinical trials, that telehealth rendered care is no less efficacious than face-to-face psychotherapy (and is actually preferred by many patients).

Case Example: The EKU Clinic Use of Telehealth CAMS

For behavioral health providers in rural communities, the challenge to assess and treat suicidal individuals may be even more significant, given that rates of suicidal ideation and planning are higher among non-metropolitan, rural adults (Harp & Borders, 2019). Kentucky is one such state with significant challenges, but also has solutions to these problems. Kentucky is 96.4% rural, and most counties are considered mental health professional shortage areas (U.S. Bureau, 2016). Additionally, when behavioral health providers in Kentucky are surveyed, 43% of clinicians indicate they do not have the skills needed to engage those with suicidal intent and 48% indicated they did not have sufficient training (Covington, 2013).

To address rural mental health unique needs in Kentucky, the Eastern Kentucky University (EKU) Department of Psychology initiated a Clinical Psychology doctoral training program in 2015 with an emphasis on providing high-quality training to psychologists planning to work in rural mental health agencies and with underserved populations, with a particular emphasis on providing CAMS. From 2015 to 2019, over 60 individuals who are suicidal were successfully treated using CAMS often by doctoral student therapists who were trained in the model who were closely supervised.

COVID-19 Pandemic Challenge to the EKU Psychology Clinic

In February 2020, the EKU Psychology Clinic was serving 80 unique patients in the surrounding communities through therapy, assessment services, and group services. Of these, 20 individuals were receiving CAMS by

11 doctoral student therapists through face-to-face services. On March 17, 2020, EKU abruptly shut down in order to protect the university community from the encroaching COVID-19 pandemic, students were sent home, and all face-to-face Psychology Clinic services were discontinued. At this time, most United States universities were experiencing the same closures and were adopting telephone "check-ins" for their clinic patients who are suicidal.

Faced with the situation the EKU clinic moved quickly to adopt various telepsychology procedures and followed recommendations outlined by the American Psychological Association (APA, 2020). Eleven CAMS clinicians treating the 20 patients who were suicidal were trained in CAMS Telepsychology procedures and immediately began to deliver virtual CAMS through the Doxy.me electronic format. Throughout the pandemic, scores of suicidal college students, and community members, were successfully provided clinical care through the EKU Psychology Clinic's CAMS Telepsychology services to help save lives without any adverse incidents.

The story of the EKU Psychology Clinic's rapid transition from face-to-face suicide-focused treatment utilizing the CAMS framework to using a telehealth platform by an all-graduate student therapist team is a model for how telehealth can be applied during a pandemic and beyond. From the EKU experience, it is plain to see that mental health care has been transformed irrevocably by the pandemic compelling the field to more fully embrace telehealth. Having a workforce that is trained in suicide-focused assessment and treatment approaches is critical to addressing the problem broadly. Reliance upon a "hospitalization and medication only" approach has demonstrated failure time and time again (Jobes, 2017). Given the EKU experience, we strongly contend that training in suicide-focused assessment and treatment should begin at the graduate level at can be safely and effectively delivered both face to face and online.

The Future of Telehealth for Mental Health Services

The COVID-19 pandemic created urgency for researchers and providers to identify alternative ways of treating individuals in need of mental health services. The use of tele-mental health services was not a new practice at the onset of the pandemic (Nickelson, 1998). Although clinicians may have faced barriers to treatment including licensure across state lines and patient access to technology, many individuals who were confined to their homes were not cut off from mental health treatment. And as previously noted, the Fernandez et al. (2021) meta-analysis of video-delivered psychotherapy (VDP) has shown that it is no less efficacious than in person psychotherapy. Bottomline, conducting mental health treatment via telehealth is a clinical practice that is here to stay and ongoing and emerging clinical research will provide clinicians with best practice recommendations for providing optimal telehealth care.

Conclusion

Among the many issues addressed in this book, few can rival the life-or-death prospect that clinicians may face when working with suicidal risk remotely through telehealth. We have described a real-world pivot to providing an evidence-based suicide-focused intervention – CAMS – via telehealth early on in 2020 as the worldwide COVID-19 pandemic grew exponentially. We initially provided guidance for how to effectively provide remote care with an emphasis on informed consent and anticipating various scenarios to ensure ethical and competent care via telehealth. Within the delivery of CAMS, we initially advocated the parallel use of the SSF and have ultimately endorsed using a form-fillable PDF version of the SSF, which enables the patient to closely monitor their own assessment and suicide-focused treatment plan by using a shared screen with their provider. To date, the use of remote CAMS via telehealth has been effective in clinical practice and within ongoing randomized controlled trials of CAMS. We conclude our chapter with a systems-level case example of one clinic's real-time shift to using CAMS via telehealth at Eastern Kentucky University. It is plain to us that the pandemic has forever changed the delivery of mental health care in general including remote care for those who struggle with serious thoughts of suicide in particular.

Practical Considerations and Tips

- Patients who are suicidal can be safely and effectively screened, assessed, managed, and treated via telehealth platforms.
- While some are wary of remote work with suicidal risk, the work can be done effectively with sufficient informed consent and "upstream" thinking about how to ensure confidentiality, handling of emergent risk by having patients identify potential 3rd parties (who can be contacted), and what to do with challenges related to remote work (Wi-Fi issues or being disconnected).
- CAMS is one suicide-focused treatment approach that can be readily used within telehealth, and we have provided guidance for effectively rendering this care.
- Use of the form-fillable PDF of the CAMS SSF makes for easy medical record documentation that can be shared with the patient and sent to the patient's electronic medical record, and by its nature this extensive documentation helps decrease concerns about malpractice-related liability secondary to suicide wrongful death tort litigation.
- Even beyond the pandemic, clinicians need to get used to providing remote care via telehealth as many patients prefer it

and it has the potential to extend the reach of care to more people in need (e.g., in rural or frontier regions of a country).

- In the case of suicidal risk, remote suicide-focused care may be ethically and safely rendered to help save more lives via telehealth outpatient basis.

References

American Psychological Association. (2020). Screen your patient(s) to determine whether videoconferencing services are appropriate for them. https://www.apa.org/practice/programs/dmhi/research-information/telepsychological-services-checklist. Accessed 10/19/2020.

Brown, G. K., Ten Have, T., Henriques, G. R., Xie, S. X., Hollander, J. E., & Beck, A. T. (2005). Cognitive therapy for the prevention of suicide attempts: A randomized controlled trial. *JAMA, 294,* 563–570.

Bryan, C. J., & Rudd., M. D. (2018). *Brief cognitive-behavioral therapy for suicide prevention.* Guilford Press.

Covington, D. (March 1, 2013). Clinical Excellence in Suicide Prevention: Next Steps in Trauma-Informed Care. Presentation in Frankfort, Kentucky sponsored by the Department of Behavioral Health, Developmental and Intellectual Disabilities.

Covington, D., Hogan, M., Abreu, J., Berman, A., Breux, P., & Coffey, E. (2011). Suicide care in systems framework. National Action Alliance: Clinical Care & Intervention Task Force.

Centers for Disease Control and Prevention . Fatal injury reports, national, regional and state, 1981-2019. Available at: https://webappa.cdc.gov/sasweb/ncipc/mortrate.html, Accessed December 27, 2021

Fernandez, E., Woldgabreal, Y., Day, A., Pham, T., Gleich, B., & Aboujaoude, E. (2021). Live psychotherapy by video versus in-person: A meta-analysis of efficacy and its relationship to types and targets of treatment. *Clinical Psychology & Psychotherapy,* 28(6), 1535–1549.

Gilmore, A. K., & Ward-Ciesielski, E. F. (2019). Perceived risks and use of psychotherapy via tele-medicine for patients at risk for suicide. *Journal of Telemedicine and Telecare, 25,* 59–63. 10.1177/1357633X17735559

Harp, K., & Borders, T. F. (2019). Suicidal thoughts, plans, and attempts by non-metropolitan and metropolitan residence. *Rural & Underserved Health Research Center Publications.*

Hyland, K. A., McDonald, J. B., Verzijl, C. L., Faraci, D. C., Calixte-Civil, P. F., Gorey, C. M., & Verona, E. (2021). Telehealth for dialectical behavioral therapy: A commentary on the experience of a rapid transition to virtual delivery of DBT. *Cognitive and Behavioral Practice,* 29(2), 367–380.

Ivey-Stephenson, A. Z., Demissie, Z., Crosby, A. E., Stone, Deborah M., Gaylor, E., Wilkins, N., Lowry, R., & Brown, M. (2020). Suicidal Ideation and Behaviors Among High School Students—Youth Risk Behavior Survey, United States, 2019. *MMWR Supplements,* 69, 47–55 10.15585/mmwr.su6901a6.

Jobes, D. A. (2017). Clinical assessment and treatment of suicidal risk: A critique of contemporary care and CAMS as a possible remedy. *Practice Innovations, 2,* 207–220. 10.1037/pri0000054

Jobes, D. A. (2006). *Managing suicidal risk: A collaborative approach.* New York: Guilford Press.

Jobes, D. A. (2012). The Collaborative Assessment and Management of Suicidality (CAMS): An evolving evidence-based clinical approach to suicidal risk. *Suicide and Life-Threatening Behavior, 42,* 640–653.

Jobes, D. A., Au, J. S., & Siegelman, A. (2015). Psychological approaches to suicide treatment and prevention. *Current Treatment Options in Psychiatry, 2*(4), 363–370.

Jobes, D. A., Comtois, K. A., Brenner, L. A., Gutierrez, P. M., & O'Connor, S. S. (2016). Trials of the Collaborative Assessment and Management of Suicidality (CAMS). The international handbook of suicide prevention, 431–449.

Jobes, D. A., & Chalker, S. A. (2019). One size does not fit all: A comprehensive clinical approach to reducing suicidal ideation, attempts, and deaths. *International Journal of Environmental Research and Public Health, 16,* 1–14.

Jobes, D. A., Crumlish, J. A., & Evans, A. D. (2020). The COVID-19 pandemic and treating suicidal risk: The telepsychotherapy use of CAMS. *Journal of Psychotherapy Integration, 30*(2), 226.

Jobes, D. A., & Maltsberger, J. T. (1995). The hazards of treating suicidal patients. In M. Sussman (Ed.), *A perilous calling: The hazards of psychotherapy practice* (pp. 200–214). New York, NY: Wiley.

Landes, S. J., Pitcock, J. A., Harned, M. S., Connolly, S. L., Meyers, L. L., & Oliver, C. M. (2021). Provider perspectives on delivering dialectical behavior therapy via telehealth during COVID-19 in the Department of Veterans Affairs. *Psychological Services, 19*(3), 562.

Linehan, M. (1993). *Cognitive-behavioral treatment of borderline personality disorder.* New York: Guilford Press.

Linehan, M. M., Armstrong, H. E., Suarez, A., Allmon, D., & Heard, H. L. (1991). Cognitive-behavioral treatment of chronically parasuicidal borderline patients. *Archives of General Psychiatry, 48,* 1060–1064.

Linehan, M. M., Korslund, K. E., Harned, M. S., Gallop, R. J., Lungu, A., Neacsiu, A. D., McDavid, J., Comtois, K. A., & Murray-Gregory, A. M. (2015). Dialectical behavior therapy for high suicide risk in individuals with borderline personality disorder: A randomized clinical trial and component analysis. *JAMA Psychiatry, 72,* 475–482.

National Action Alliance for the Prevention of Suicide (2020). COVID Guidance: Screening for Suicide Risk during Telehealth Visits. https://theactionalliance.org/resource/covid-guidance-screening-suicide-risk-during-telehealth-visits

Nickelson, D. W. (1998). Telehealth and the evolving health care system: Strategic opportunities for professional psychology. *Professional Psychology: Research and Practice, 29*(6), 527.

Pistorello, J., Jobes, D. A., Gallop, R., Compton, S. N., Locey, N. S., Au, J. S., Noose, S. K., Walloch, J. C., Johnson, J., Young, M., Dickens, Y., Chatham, P., & Jeffcoat, T. (2020). A randomized controlled trial of the collaborative assessment and management of suicidality (CAMS) versus treatment as usual (TAU) for suicidal college students. *Archives of Suicide Research, 25*(4), 765–789. 10.1080/13811118.2020.1749742

Puddy, R. W., & Wilkins, N. (2011). *Understanding evidence Part 1: Best available research evidence. A guide to the continuum of evidence of effectiveness.* Centers for Disease Control and Prevention.

Qin, P., & Nordentoft, M. (2005). Suicide risk in relation to psychiatric hospitalization: Evidence based on longitudinal registers. *Archives of General Psychiatry, 62*(4), 427–432.

Rojas, S. M., Gold, S. D., Bryan, C. J., Pruitt, L. D., Felker, B. L., & Reger, M. A. (2021). Brief Cognitive-Behavioral Therapy for Suicide Prevention (BCBT-SP) via video telehealth: A case example during the COVID-19 outbreak. *Cognitive and Behavioral Practice*, 29(2), 446–453.

Rudd, M. D., Bryan, C. J., Wertenberger, E. G., et al (2015). Brief cognitive-behavioral therapy effects on post-treatment suicide attempts in a military sample: Results of a randomized clinical trial with 2-year follow-up. *American Journal of Psychiatry, 172*, 441–449. doi: 10.1176/appi.ajp.2014.14070843

Ryberg, W., Zahl, P.-H., Diep, L. M., Landrø, N.I., & Fosse, R. (2019). Managing suicidality within specialized care: A randomized controlled trial. *Journal of Affective Disorders*, 249, 112–12010.1016/j.jad.2019.02.022.

Severe, J., Tang, R., Horbatch, F., Onishchenko, R., Naini, V., & Blazek, M. C. (2021). Correction: Factors influencing patients' initial decisions regarding telepsychiatry participation during the COVID-19 pandemic: Telephone-based survey. *JMIR Formative Research, 5*(1), e27357.

Substance Abuse and Mental Health Services Administration. (2020). Suicidal thoughts and behaviors among adults (NSDUH Annual National Report). Retrieved from https://www.samhsa.gov/data/report/2019-nsduh-annual-national-report

Swift, J. K., Trusty, W. T., & Penix, E. A. (2021). The effectiveness of the Collaborative Assessment and Management of Suicidality (CAMS) compared to alternative treatment conditions: A meta-analysis. *Suicide and Life-Threatening Behavior*, 51(5), 882–896.

Tyndal, T., Zhang, I., & Jobes, D. A. (2021). The collaborative assessment and management of suicidality (CAMS) stabilization plan for working with patients with suicide risk. *Psychotherapy*. 10.1037/pst0000378

The Joint Commission . (2016). Detecting and treating suicide ideation in all settings. Retrieved from https://www.jointcommission.org/assets/1/18/SEA_56_Suicide.pdf

U.S. Bureau (2016). New Census Data Show Differences Between Urban and Rural Populations. *Retrieved from United States Census Bureau*: https://www.census.gov/newsroom/press-releases/2016/cb16–210. html.

Waltman, S. H., Landry, J. M., Pujol, L. A., & Moore, B. A. (2019). Delivering evidence-based practices via telepsychology: Illustrative case series from military treatment facilities. *Professional Psychology: Research and Practice, 51*(3), 205. 10.1037/pro0000275

Wenzel, A., Brown, G. K., Beck, A. T., editors. (2009). *Cognitive therapy for suicidal patients: Scientific and clinical applications.* Washington, DC: American Psychological Association.

World Health Organization. (2021). Suicide worldwide in 2019: Global health estimates.

World Health Organization. (2021). WHO Coronavirus (COVID-19) Dashboard. Retrieved from https://covid19.who.int/

Zalewski, M., Walton, C. J., Rizvi, S. L., White, A. W., Martin, C. G., O'Brien, J. R., & Dimeff, L. (2021). Lessons learned conducting dialectical behavior therapy via telehealth in the age of COVID-19. *Cognitive and Behavioral Practice*, 28(4), 573–587.

23 Reactivating Playfulness Online for PTSD Treatment

Mooli Lahad, Miki Doron, and Dori Rubinstein

Jack was a 51-year-old veteran with severe PTSD; nightmares, panic attacks and multiple avoidant behaviors. His anger would flare up in seconds, many a time without even knowing what ignited him. Jack had been to several PTSD treatments and was diagnosed by a psychiatrist as suffering from severe PTSD and was taking a bag full of medications. He came to us for the SEE FAR CBT treatment about 10 weeks before the COVID-19 outbreak. He was already making some progress with better sleep and less anger eruptions when due to the lockdown he stopped coming to therapy. We tried to continue the treatment over the phone, but he kept saying that playing with the cards was what helped him to revisit his trauma. Jack was one of the reasons we considered the digital option of PTSD online treatment.

This chapter will attempt to answer two critical questions regarding online PTSD treatment; A) Can and should we treat PTSD from a distance? B) Can we create an experiential playful environment via the internet. We shall examine these questions through the case of Jack whilst describing our approach. The first part of the chapter will focus on the theory and implementation behind the use of playfulness in the service of PTSD treatment.

Why Cards? Why Playfulness and Imagination?

Imagination is one of the multitudes of characteristics that make us human and unique. Without imagination, our world would be meaningless and we would be unable to interpret the sensory experience or find logic in our life's experience (Abraham & Bubic, 2015; Johnson, 2013). Imagination serves us to better plan our future and flexibly consider past experiences and past memories (Zheng et al., 2014), think outside the box (Gaither et al., 2015), stimulate and suppress emotions (Finnbogadóttir & Berntsen, 2014) and help rehabilitate learning and memory capabilities (Grilli & McFarland, 2011).

Imagination plays a central and vital role in many aspects of everyday life, involves a variety of areas in the brain, dominating all cerebral lobes and hemispheres (Fox et al., 2015). Based on our clinical, theoretical and research of trauma and recovery, we claim that as much as imagination is a source of pain and suffering during loss, trauma and in severe mental

DOI: 10.4324/9781003205029-28

conditions (e.g., depression, schizophrenia), imagination is also a source for hope, optimism and comfort in stressful situations. We argue that it can be used in the treatment of trauma adopting the known concept of Hippocrates.

By similar things a disease is produced and through the application of the like is cured.

The Possible link between Playfulness and Coping with Trauma

Two main components that can partly explain the connection between playfulness and resilience to traumatic events are positive emotions and self-regulation ability (Bonanno et al., 2011; Cohen et al., 2014). Using our imagination in a playful and social way may foster resiliency (Lahad, 2019). Without playfulness, a child cannot experience thoughts and emotions, wishes and fantasies are important. Playfulness is crucial to the development of our mentalization capacity (Bateman & Fonagy, 2004). We claim that clients (children as well as adults) who suffer from PTSD adopt a vigilant approach to prevent the painful memories from surfacing and overwhelming them and or may miss the ominous signals. Therefore they avoid playing, since play and playfulness contradict the ability to remain vigilant against the danger of the intrusive memory. This position may also be influenced by the fact that some people who suffer from PTSD also suffer from depression, therefore to them playfulness is an insufferable mental state. Thomson and Jaque (2016) found that among individuals who suffer from PTSD, creative work improves efficiency and self-management, providing meaning and satisfaction (Thomson & Jaque, 2016).

Using imagination is not new in psychotherapy. There are efficient and diverse methods of trauma-focused treatment therapy for people suffering from PTSD, mostly using imagination as a therapeutic tool, whether in-tentionally or unintentionally (Holmes, 2014; Lahad et al., 2016). Most of the therapeutic approaches in trauma refer to invasive memories and thoughts, and almost all approaches use words to process components of the traumatic experience, giving it different names: cognitive reconstruction, abreaction, de-sensitization, flooding and some even use simulated or close to reality images such as in VRT (virtual reality treatment) assuming that traumatic memory is a matter of sequentially interrupted story that once recreated either verbally or through close to reality photographic assemblage will help the client. Yet we now know that the traumatic experience is fused not only with non-verbal cognitive aspects, but also a combination of physical, sensorial, emotional and cognitive phenomena and that memory is not linear but network of facts, images, sound, smell, movement and a combination of past present and future events both reality based and wishful or horrifying ones.

Thus, retrieval of episodic and autobiographic memories serves as a common addition in different techniques for the treatment of trauma and anxiety (Cooper & Clum, 1989). Indeed some of the current treatment methods use imagination to alter traumatic memories, weaken them, and cope with them. One of the main components of CBT is exposure as a process that helps clients cope with threatening memories and situations (Choi et al., 2010). Exposure processes usually include imaginal exposure. During the exposure process the clients is asked to revisit the traumatic event, to revive the threatening memory (imaginal exposure) whilst in reality they are in the clinic, feeling safe, so that they can manage to approach the traumatic memory and emotionally process it, aiming to lessen painful and threatening reaction (desensitization) Foa & Kozak, 1986). Other forms of exposure include repeated presentation of the traumatic event in the imagination (imaginal flooding) (Keane et al., 1989; Specken et al., 2006).

However, none of these approaches use projective images that the client selects to recreate, edit and re-narrate his traumatic story, adding wishful aids to the story in the service of empowerment, not diversion of attention or denial. These missing aspects led us, Lahad and Doron (2012, 2015) to develop a therapeutic model inviting the client to gradually practice playful skills in a make-believe space, thus developing playfulness that enables change in "dead-end" or impossible situations. These are facilitated in the clinic through a fantastic reality (FR) space (Lahad & Leykin, 2012).

SEE FAR CBT

SEE FAR CBT is a protocol-based therapeutic method (Lahad & Doron, 2010,) for the treatment of PTSD and anxiety related disorders. This is a creative protocol based on empowerment by using imagination and the FR space. The model emphasizes the role of the FR and imagination in creating an alternative narrative for the traumatic event by using therapeutic cards that enable distancing and externalization of the story. As the client observes the reconstruction in cards he chose to tell the traumatic story, he becomes a spectator in his life's drama. The client also plays the role of the director as he can "remove" disturbing images, change their position, add alleviating images etc. Thus, he is able to edit an otherwise "frozen story" and "play" with its components. This model is anchored in Winnicott's, Jennings' and Landy's theories on play and also on the externalization principles of the narrative approach (Jennings, 1994; Landy, 1996; White & Epston, 1990; Winnicott, 1971) The SEE FAR CBT protocol also incorporates CBT methods and concepts for the therapeutic end of the protocol, especially components of retelling the traumatic episodes, psycho-education, real-life gradual exposure (Ellis & MacLaren, 1998; Foa et al., 2009). Additionally, the protocol includes aspects of body memory, focusing on somatic reactions of the client whilst remembering the trauma and teaching him/her how to discharge this "trapped" energy in a safe way (Clements, 2003; Levine, 1997; Van der Kolk et al., 1996).

FR (Fantastic Reality) is the link between the infinite ability of the creative imagination to create a world image, desired or required, and the actions taken to solve problems in reality within the shared space of therapy.

FR is not a condition in which clients lose touch with real reality or deny it, on the contrary, it enables a temporary experience during which the left hemisphere "relinquishes" control and command in order to transcend into the "as if" space, the space of unlimited imagination and possibilities. Processes of the right hemisphere "control" this space. They allow insights and solutions of a different kind. But "concession" is temporary, the left hemisphere stays alert, and in the return from transcendence into the FR, the control and criticism processes of this hemisphere are re-invited to examine which of the ideas that came up pictorially and in images in the FR are transferable and applicable in reality. Healing or relaxation is experienced by permitting the psyche to act like a child's, capable of creating a world out of light and shadow games. This experience is possible in a noncritical, non-judgmental, non-interpretative, non-righteous space; space that is creative, encouraging and a place where one plays. This is a space where inventing and fabricating stories are allowed, a space to daydream and to fantasize while knowing that the movement from reality to FR is in the service of the coping self and its goal is not to become detached from the circles of real life.

SEE FAR CBT has been found effective in significantly reducing post-traumatic symptoms over time (Lahad et al., 2016; Lahad et al., 2010). Another study (Lahad et al., 2016) was conducted on 25 Israeli children who live in the South of Israel in an area constantly confronted with hostilities. Children who were treated with SEE FAR CBT exhibited lower levels (40%) of PTSD than children who took part in the group CBT focused interventions (68%). Furthermore, the most significant difference was the reduction of intrusive symptoms in the SEE FAR CBT group.

We suggest that this method offers a unique aspect to PTSD patients introducing the gaining of control through the gradual utilization of playfulness and imagination and playfulness via therapeutic cards. Control is experienced in various ways: the client's choice of cards, the positioning of the cards, the ability to change their place or even remove them altogether and by choosing potential support using "If only" or " I wish I had" cards to add to the story.

If the patient experiences dissociation during the session, as the cards are laid out open to both client and therapist, the therapist has an indication where in the traumatic memory sequence the client "transcended" to dissociation. This allows the therapist to gently guide the client to return to the "concrete" external anchor (the card) that triggered the dissociation and assist the client to continue from there. The concreteness of the therapeutic cards, composed of colors, shapes, images, and hues enables a non-rational cognitive experience of the event to be present and an access to nonverbal aspects of the trauma. As the cards are "real" and are on the "outside" it also helps the client to return to the "here and now."

An empowering element lies in the potential inclusion of the "as if" positive images that the client can choose to add to his story representing wishful things or people which, if the client had had them during the incident, could have assisted him. This, without the "as if" cards changing or erasing the outcome of the incident. The new visual sequence creates a positive or more tolerable stimulation, competing in terms of the flexible brain (Doidge, 2015) with the traumatic memory pathway in the brain. We claim that beyond the sense of control, this alternative calming visual pathway directly affects the visual, sensory or experiential memory pathways of the event as well as directly acts to change perception of non-verbal and verbal levels, becoming an alternative to the traumatic memory, or at least a more flexible order of events (for more theoretical details see Lahad & Leykin, 2012). We suggest that our method that combines imagination allows "a window of flexibility" for improved health and resilience development (Lahad, 2019; McEwen, 2016). Hence SEE FAR CBT is not just another cognitive method or mind-body method for treating psycho-trauma, but an integrative approach that gives room for visual imagination as a source for healing in "impossible" situations.

Is Online Treatment for PTSD Safe?

Technology allows therapist and client to talk to each other in real time. The online session may be experienced as less threatening than a face-to-face session because of the ability to focus on the screen rather than being flooded by multiple sensory stimuli in the face-to-face session.

As early as 2007 Knaevelsrud, and Maercker, conducted a randomized control study on Internet-based treatment for PTSD found that this method reduced distress and facilitated the development of a strong therapeutic alliance and found that for PTSD symptoms (intrusions, avoidance, hyperarousal), large treatment effect was found at post-treatment and three-months follow-up. At post-treatment, a large treatment effect was also found for symptoms of depression, anxiety and mental health. After finishing the treatment, patients were asked how they experienced being treated through the Internet. 86% percent of the patients described the therapeutic contact as personal, 76% reported positive attitudes to being treated through the Internet instead of via face-to-face.

Traumatic experiences are often associated with stigmatization and intense feelings of shame and guilt. In addition, many victims report feeling alienated and estranged from the world. They refrain from social interactions and feel isolated although at the same time they often experience a great need for social support (Maercker & Müller, 2004) The Internet provides a protected environment where participants can easily control and regulate the degree of intimacy they want to share without the fear of real-life judgment, rejection, or devaluation. This way of communication lessens social risks and inhibitions and encourages the disclosure of painful experiences or shameful thoughts [Suler J., 2004, and Hoops, 2003].

Recently two studies investigated the impact of online therapy with PTSD. Lehavot et al. (2021) report on an online therapy program with female veterans and found at post hoc analyses of treatment completers and of those with baseline of significant PTSD symptoms (PCL ≥ 33) revealed that the online treatment group had greater improvement in PTSD symptom severity relative to phone monitoring with significant differences at the three-month follow-up assessment. Kirk et al. (2022) conducted an online Cognitive Behavioral Therapy, Mindfulness Meditation, and Yoga (CBT-MY) intervention. They reported that online CBT-MY program participation was associated with clinically significant symptom reductions in combination with significant PPD (peak pupil diameter) changes reflecting more normalized autonomic functioning. This evidence and the challenges of COVID-19 on therapeutic face-to-face sessions lead us to the conversion of the SEE FAR CBT to an online platform. One important aspect of PTSD treatment is availability and presence; in our opinion the protocol does not affect this aspect as the therapist is available online between sessions and client can see him or her regardless of lockdown or other obstacles preventing the session from taking place (besides maybe technological challenges).

SEE FAR CBT Online

Let's return to Jack, it is already the 5th week he is not in therapy and his condition deteriorate but SEE FAR CBT is an interactive therapy with the actual use of cards, and COVID-19 posed a challenge to our ability to continue the treatment that Jack so eagerly asking to continue. Like Jack, many other clients with PTSD reacted severely to the isolation, the lack of face-to-face communication, the impact of the lockdowns "encaging" families in very limited space making their irritability, short temper, and sensitivity to noise ever so difficult to bear. In some cases, a video conference such as zoom was a good substitute to face to face but the not seeing the client's whole body was extremely challenging, as therapist was unable to refer to it. Even more stressful for the therapist was the fact that when the client cries or shakes or vomits (known reactions to experiencing) therapist can't lay a hand or give a tissue or just sit quietly in an empathic accepting mode. In additional stressful element is the fact that if the client moves away from the camera or pushes the "end session" button unexpectedly, the therapist feels helpless. We therefore developed a pre-session protocol that includes ensuring that camera is open, agreeing that if the client wishes to terminate the session, he needs to alert the therapist, and finally, sharing the telephone number of a person the client chooses who the therapist can contact in case something happens and client "disappears" from the screen. With SE methods we were able to talk to and with the client on bodily sensation and train them to report unpleasant sensations that are not necessarily visible, to teach them the breathing methods and to create an in vivo exposure list.

Regardless, the idea to convert the SEE FAR CBT protocol into an online treatment protocol was a test to our ability to provide the method in full.

We chose an online platform (cardtherapy.online) that allowed us to emulate the physical manipulation of playing cards in the virtual realm. The platform includes 2 virtual packs of cards; 'safe place cards' and 'trauma associative cards' and allows therapist and patient to move the virtual cards, flip them, hide them, and even change the playing area (the background) behind the cards. The platform is synchronous; all actions are synchronized between therapist and client, if a client moves a card, this is presented in real-time on the therapist's screen and vice versa. The synchronicity is a key element as this allows the patient to perform all the actions independently of the therapist, an important element working with patients suffering from PTSD as we shall explain. The ability to allow our patients control during online sessions is probably not unique to working with PTSD and may be another beneficial aspect of online work.

One of the main characteristics of PTSD clients' negative cognitions is that the world is always dangerous and that they are helpless. In order to sensitively reintroduce control, we offer a choice to allow the client to find in his or her own pace a pleasant, aggreable, or safe space. As we couldn't ask the client to paint around the safe or pleasant space as we do in face-to-face sessions, we opted for a set of pre-made virtual backgrounds for the client to choose from thus adding to the sense of control. The following stage entails the client choosing the background for his safe place and then placing his 'safe place' card on the chosen background thus creating a "bigger" image of the safe space than any individual card that was put outside the "background." This act of choosing and managing the cards is central to the sense of control we wish to transmit to the client. 1. The therapist trusts you, 2. unlike the traumatic incident that was forced upon you, here you have choice and control. The therapist at this point is only an observer and supports the technical process if needed until the client is satisfied with his/her choice. The same process repeats itself later on when the client is invited to choose an unpleasant card representing a situation or place or just a sensation of unpleasantness (not connected to her trauma) of not more than 5 on a 0–10 SUD scale and place it in a manageable distance from the positive card that was created earlier. The process that ensues is pendulation or moving of the eyes between two stimuli creating a desensitization effect. This is optimized by the fact that on-line we can move the cards at a pace the client choose adding both to the sense of control and to the synchronization between client pace and therapist motion (using the mouse/cursor). Unlike the assumption of EMDR (Shapiro) that uses bilateral stimulation either by moving the therapist's finger in front of the client's eyes or using tappers to do the same on her palms, SEE FAR CBT is based on the theory of flexible brain (Doidge, 2015) and as mentioned above is based on two assumptions. The first is that the two stimuli blends and by that change the emotion and perhaps the encoded image; the second is that we provide the brain with alternative image similar to the use of cognitive restructuring in CBT as a technique for challenging underlying difficult thoughts. The screen is a very convenient space for pendulation as on the one hand it is limited in size so the client can manage it and move the two cards in a pace coordinated with the therapist or solely by the client and at the same time the screen size does not allow placing the two objects to far apart, preventing the client from avoiding looking at the "negative" card.

Next, the client is invited to choose six cards with which he will represent [for himself] the traumatic incident or episode from beginning to end. The choice of cards, their sequence, and position is in the client's control. Control and choice is further explored and experienced by the suggestion that the client can remove cards. Cards that for some reason he wishes to omit, and then see or observe what happens to the story. The empowerment is further promoted by asking the client to choose two additional cards known as the "if only" or "I wish"; that these things were with me at the time of the trauma and to weave them into the story without changing the outcome. Based on our studies therapy usually takes between 10–18 sessions of 90 minutes each leading to a considerable reduction of PTSD symptoms to manageable levels, below the clinical cut-off point. (Lahad et al., 2010).

Jack was one of the first clients to use the on-line version of SEE FAR CBT and experienced significant changes in his outbursts of anger, his ability to manage home lockdown conditions finding various in-vivo tasks to experience control.

Case Example

D. a 27-year-old woman suffered from severe PTSD with panic attacks and frequent admission to ER. Like Jack, she was in treatment a few weeks before COVID-19 and had just started the protocol. Despite the fact that avoidance was her main coping strategy, she felt that the imposed lockdown was unbearable and her symptoms increased. There were talks to hospitalize her but due to limited beds in the mental ward it was not possible. As we had just activated the online option, her therapist offered her the online SEE FAR CBT and it worked dramatically. She managed to create for herself a safe space with the cards [for her it was the image of the magician] and took a photo of it so that she can use it whenever she feels panicky and use the breathing exercise. Her mother, who was chosen as her "anchoring safe person" we could contact if something happen during therapy, "appeared" on the screen two weeks later saying how wonderful it was when her daughter had a panic attack and they were on their way to ER when she said to her mum "I will try my safe space and breathing," and they did not proceed to ER.

The availability of the therapist online made it possible to have two meetings a week during, which she completed several desensitization sessions which were very important in managing her immediate life. For example, fear of injections and fear of the night were used as the pendulation targets with her safe space reducing her fear from 8–9 (on a 0–10 scale) to 3 (Figure 23.1–23.3).

As we entered the third lockdown with the mounting numbers of infected people and rise in the death toll, the sheltered environment of being treated at home and the use of the FR enabled D. to continue therapy and work through her trauma. Her SUDs went down from usual 8 or 9 [on a 0–10 scale] to 2 and at times even to 1. Her PTSD score on the PCL-5 test scale (Weathers et al., 2013) was 68 to start with (initial research suggests that a PCL-5 cutoff

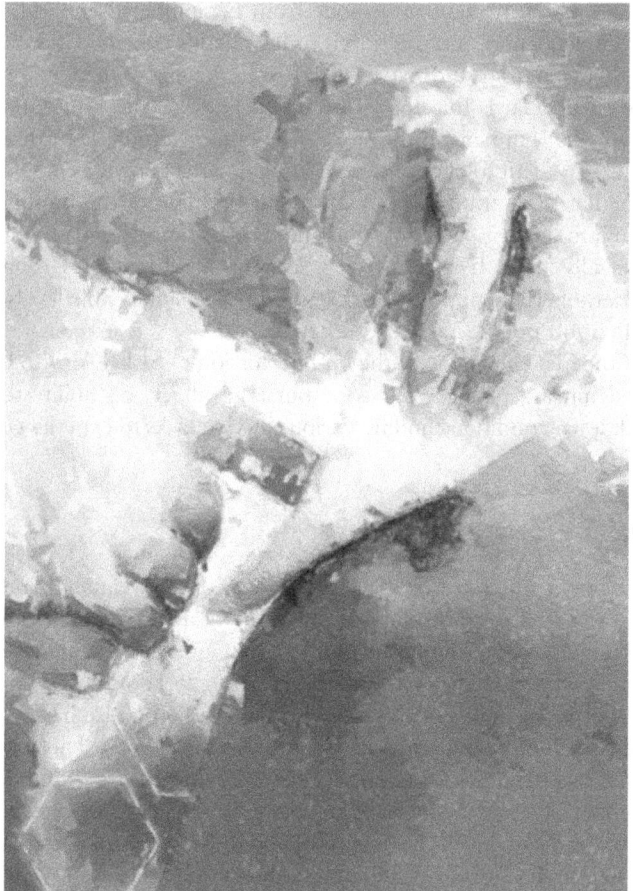

Figure 23.1 Fear of injections. From www.cardtherapy.online

score between 31 and 33 is indicative of probable PTSD) and went down to 17 which is close to non-clinical. The client's BDI depression scale (Upton, 2013) was reduced from 46 to 6 which is considered no depression. She managed to maintain a daily routine and scheduled video meetings with friends and was among the first to choose to be vaccinated. It is evident that without the opportunity to use online SEE FAR CBT, she would have been likely hospitalized in a psychiatric ward.

The fact that our method is based on playful theory was even more vivid by using the online option, as games and gaming is common online and it wasn't considered childish or belittling to the client. In fact, when she originally met the therapist in vivo she was very hesitant and somewhat resistant to the idea of "playing with cards" which did not appear when this was offered later.

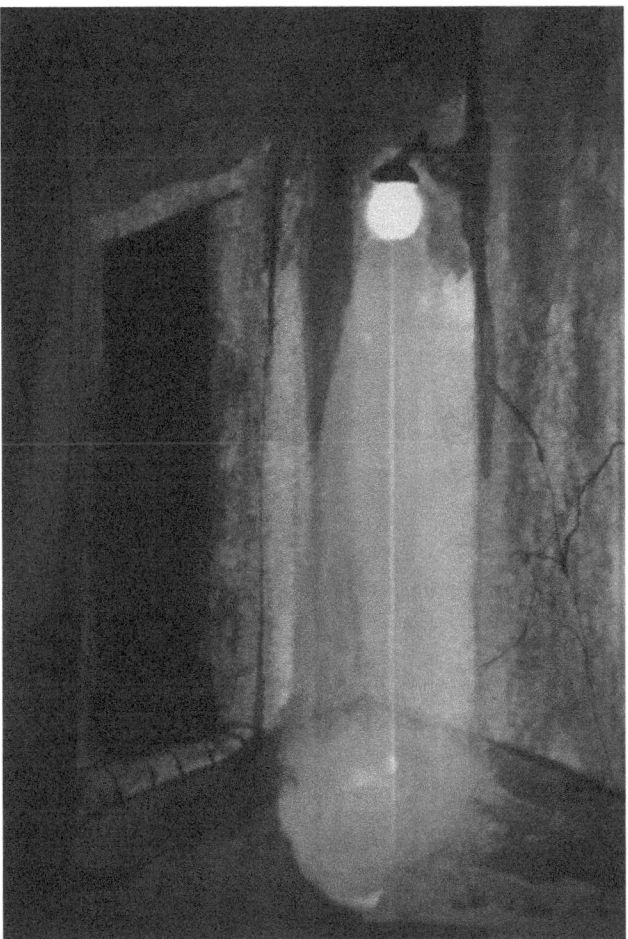

Figure 23.2 Fear of the night. From www.cardtherapy.online

As we reproduced the same cards in hardcopy, the method continues to be used now both in physical sessions and online, enabling therapy continuity if the client and therapist are unable to meet, if either have difficulty to come to the clinic or in cases the client is reluctant to leave home (at least for a while) or clients who prefer online treatment due to a variety of reasons.

Obstacles and Disadvantages

The literature on the limits of online therapy include several points to consider when dealing with a client with PTSD and depression. Keeping personal details is a major concern in psychotherapy, and online therapy adds complexity.

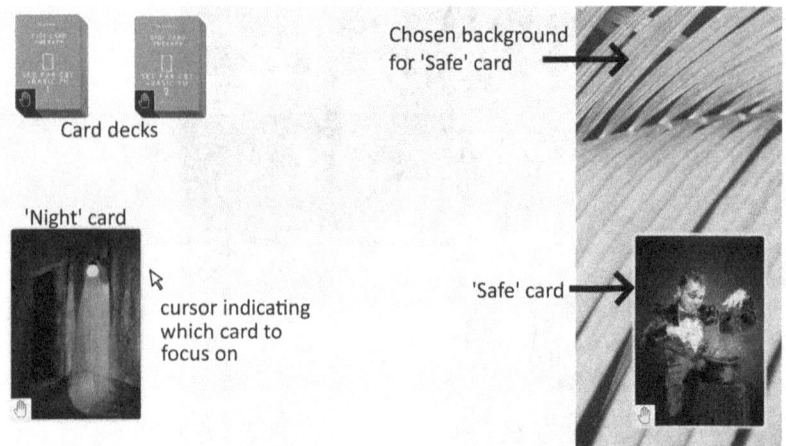

Figure 23.3 Safe place with Fear of the night. From www.cardtherapy.online

Confidentiality is difficult to handle when therapists cannot ensure the boundaries of the room with possible other family members listening to the session.

Technology issues can make therapeutic sessions difficult; the connectivity quality of the session depends on internet speed and can provoke fear and anxiety or irritability. The most common weakness is the fact that we miss part of the body language, which at times when the "terror beyond words" is vivid and the body remembers but most of it is not seen, as Van der Kolk suggests. As stated above a major concern is when a client disconnects in the middle of the session and "disappears" or even just moves away from the camera and leaves the room in an emotional state of distress. Unlike in the clinic setting, therapists can't follow the client and see that he or she is able to move on with the day. We found that a very clear contract should be made in preparation for the online session including all the possible hindrances. Even though it might affect the message to the client that we trust his abilities and that control is a basic element in this method It is extremely important to have an emergency phone number of a person the client trusts to be contacted in cases described above. This concern needs to be discussed with the client and is part of the therapeutic contract to ensure safety of the client and manageability of the process by the therapist.

Nevertheless, we found the availability of the treatment anywhere and anytime as a great benefit and we realized that training therapists with the online option is very easy. As with our face-to-face treatment, we believe that in the future we need to conduct research comparing in-vivo treatment with the on-line protocol to compare treatment outcomes.

References

Abraham, A., & Bubic, A. (2015). Semantic memory as the root of imagination. *Frontiers in Psychology*, *6*, 325. 10.3389/fpsyg.2015.00325

Bateman, A. W., & Fonagy, P. (2004). Mentalization-based treatment of BPD. *Journal of Personality Disorders*, *18*(1), 36–51.

Bonanno, G. A., Westphal, M., & Mancini, A. D. (2011). Resilience to loss and potential trauma. *Annual Review of Clinical Psychology*, *7*, 511–535.

Bryant, R. (2007). Does dissociation further our understanding of PTSD? *Journal of Anxiety Disorders*, *21*(2), 183–191.

Cohen, E., Pat-Horenczyk, R., & Haar-Shamir, D. (2014). Making room for play: An innovative intervention for toddlers and families under rocket fire. *Clinical Social Work Journal*, *42*(4), 336–345.

Chang, M. A. K., Taha, B., & Ritvo, P. G. (2021). An online cognitive behavioral therapy, mindfulness meditation, and yoga (CBT-MY) intervention for posttraumatic stress disorder: Psychometric and psychophysiology outcomes. *JMIR Mental Health*, *9*(2), e26479.

Choi, D. C., Rothbaum, B. O., Gerardi, M., & Ressler, K. J. (2010). Pharmacological enhancement of behavioral therapy: Focus on posttraumatic stress disorder. *Current Topics in Behavioral Neurosciences*, *2*, 279–299.

Clements, P. T. (2003). The body remembers: The psychophysiology of trauma and trauma treatment. *Journal of Psychosocial Nursing and Mental Health Services*, *41*(9), 56– 56.

Cooper, N. A., & Clum, G. A. (1989). Imaginal flooding as a supplementary treatment for PTSD in combat veterans: A controlled study. *Behavior Therapy*, *20*(3), 381–391.

Doidge N. (2015) *The brain's way of healing*. London: Penguin Books Limited.

Ellis, A ., & MacLaren, C. (1998).Rational emotive behavior therapy: A therapist's guide. Impact Publishers.

Finnbogadóttir, H., & Berntsen, D. (2014). Looking at life from different angles: Observer perspective during remembering and imagining distinct emotional events. *Psychology of Consciousness: Theory, Research, and Practice*, *1*(4), 387.

Foa, E. B., & Kozak, M. J. (1986). Emotional processing of fear: Exposure to corrective information. *Psychological Bulletin*, *99*(1), 20.

Foa, E. B., Keane, T. M., Friedman, M. J., & Cohen, J. A. (2009). *Effective treatments for PTSD: Practice guidelines from the International Society for Traumatic Stress Studies*. New York: The Guilford Press.

Fox, K. C., Spreng, R. N., Ellamil, M., Andrews-Hanna, J. R., & Christoff, K. (2015). The wandering brain: Meta-analysis of functional neuroimaging studies of mind-wandering and related spontaneous thought processes. *NeuroImage*, *111*, 611–621.

Gaither, S. E., Remedios, J. D., Sanchez, D. T., & Sommers, S. R. (2015). Thinking outside the box multiple identity mind-sets affect creative problem solving. *Social Psychological and Personality Science*, *6*(5), 596–603.

Gellis, A., & MacLaren, C. (1998). *Rational-emotive behavior therapy: A therapist's guide*. Atascadero, CA: Impact Publishers.

Grilli, M. D., & McFarland, C. P. (2011). Imagine that: Self-imagination improves prospective memory in memory-impaired individuals with neurological damage. *Neuropsychological Rehabilitation*, *21*(6), 847–859.

Holmes, J. (2014). *The therapeutic imagination: Using literature to deepen psychodynamic understanding and enhance empathy*. Routledge.

Hoops. S. L., Pepin. M., & Boisvert, J. M. (2003). The effectiveness of cognitive-behavioral group therapy for loneliness via inter relay chat among people with physical disabilities. *Theory Res. 40*, 136–147.10.1037/0033-3204.40.1-2.136

Jennings, S. (1994). *The handbook of dramatherapy*. London & New York: Routledge.

Johnson, M. (2013). *The body in the mind: The bodily basis of meaning, imagination, and reason.* University of Chicago Press.

Knaevelsrud, C., & Maercker, A. (2007) Internet-based treatment for PTSD reduces distress and facilitates the development of a strong therapeutic alliance: A randomized controlled clinical trial. *BMC Psychiatry, 7*, 13.

Kaplansky, N. (2009). Dissociating from death: An investigation into the resilience potential of transcendence into fantastic reality during near-death experiences. Unpublished dissertation. Anglia Ruskin University, Chelmsford, UK.

Keane, T. M., Fairbank, J. A., Caddell, J. M., & Zimering, R. T. (1989). Implosive (flooding) therapy reduces symptoms of PTSD in Vietnam combat veterans. *Behavior Therapy, 20*(2), 245–260.

Lahad, M. (2019). *The healing power of imagination: Playfulness in impossible situations.* In Jean Améry (pp. 171–197). Cham: Palgrave Macmillan.

Lahad, M., & Doron, M. (2007). *Beyond CBT, SEE FAR CBT post-traumatic stress disorder treatment protocol.* Kiryat Shmona: CSPC.

Lahad, M., & Doron, M. (2015). *SEE FAR CBT.* Kiryat Shmona: CSPC (Hebrew).

Lahad, M., & Doron, M. (2010). *Protocol for treatment of post-traumatic stress disorder. See far CBT Model: Beyond cognitive behavior therapy.* Amsterdam: IOS Press.

Lahad, M., Farhi, M., Leykin, D., & Kaplansky, N. (2010). Preliminary study of a new integrative approach in treating post-traumatic stress disorder: SEE FAR CBT. *The Arts in Psychotherapy, 37*(5), 391–399.

Lahad, M., & Leykin, D. (2012). *The healing potential of imagination in the treatment of psychotrauma: An alternative explanation for the effectiveness of the treatment of PTSD using fantastic reality {Reality}. Cognitive behavioral therapy: Applications, methods and outcomes.* New York: Nova Publishers, 71–92.

Lahad, M., Leykin, D., Farchi, M., Doron, M., Gidron, Y., Rozenblat, O., & Fajerman, Z. (2016). SEE FAR CBT therapy for children with post-traumatic stress disorder under prolonged political conflict. *Journal of Psychology and Psychotherapy Research, 3*, 1–12.

Landy, R. J. (1993). *Persona and performance.* London: Jessica Kingsley.

Landy, R. J. (1996). Drama therapy and distancing: Reflections on theory and clinical application. *The Arts in Psychotherapy, 23*(5), 367–373.

Lehavot, K., Steven, P. Millard, S. P., & Thomas, R. M. (2021). A randomized trial of an online, coach-assisted self-management PTSD intervention tailored for women veterans. *Journal of Consulting and Clinical Psychology, 89*(2), 134–141.

Levine, P. A. (1997). *Waking the tiger.* Berkeley, CA: North Atlantic.

Maercker, A., & Müller, J. (2004). Social acknowledgment as a victim or survivor: a scale to measure a recovery factor of PTSD. *Journal of Traumatic Stress, 17*, 345–351.

McEwen, B. S. (2016). In pursuit of resilience: Stress, epigenetics, and brain plasticity. *Annals of the New York Academy of Sciences, 1373*(1), 56–64.

Monahan, K. (2015). The use of humor with older adults aging in place. *Social Work in Mental Health, 13*(1), 61–69.

Specken, A. E. M., Ehlers, A., Hackmann, A., & Clark, D. M. (2006). Changes in intrusive memories associated with imaginal reliving in posttraumatic stress disorder. *Journal of Anxiety Disorders, 20*(3), 328–341.

Suler J. (2004). The online disinhibition effect. *CyberPsychology & Behavior*, 7, 321–326.

Thomson, P., & Jaque, S. (2016). Visiting the muses: Creativity, coping, and PTSD in talented dancer and athletes. *American Journal of Play*, 8(3), 363–378.

Upton, J. (2013). Beck Depression Inventory (BDI). In M. D. Gellman & J. R. Turner (Eds.), *Encyclopedia of behavioral medicine*. New York, NY: Springer.

Van der Kolk, B., Van der Hart, O., & Marmar, C. R. (1996). Dissociation and information processing in posttraumatic stress disorder. In B. Van der Kolk, A. C. McFarlane, & L. Weisaeth (Eds.), *Traumatic stress: The effects of overwhelming experience on mind, body and society* (pp. 303–327). New York: Guilford Press.

Weathers, F. W., Litz, B. T., Keane, T. M., Palmieri, P. A., Marx, B. P., & Schnurr, P. P. (2013). The PTSD Checklist for DSM-5 (PCL-5). Standard [Measurement instrument]. https://www.ptsd.va.gov/professional/assessment/documents/PCL5_Standard_form.PDF

White, M., & Epston, D. (1990). *Narrative means to therapeutic ends*. New York: W. W. Norton & Company.

Winnicott, D. W. (1971). *Playing and reality*. London: Tavistock

Zheng, H., Luo, J., & Yu, R. (2014). From memory to prospection: What are the overlapping and the distinct components between remembering and imagining?. *Frontiers in Psychology*, 5, 856. 10.3389/fpsyg.2014.00856

24 Adapting Focused Acceptance and Commitment Therapy for Individuals with Childhood-Onset Medical and Developmental Disabilities

Kristen E. Holderle and Jeffrey Iler

This chapter describes successes and challenges of providing Focused Acceptance and Commitment Therapy (FACT) via telemedicine at a multi-disciplinary clinic for individuals with childhood onset medical and developmental diagnoses. Our integrated behavioural health (IBH) team includes two psychologists, a consulting psychiatrist, mental health coordinator, and several applied behaviour analysis (ABA) providers. Broadly, we provide practice-wide depression, anxiety, and substance use screening, evaluation and short-term treatment, and medication consultation to patients (ages 16+) with childhood onset medical and/or developmental conditions within the context of a multidisciplinary team (see Holderle et al., 2021 for detailed information about services provided).

Many patients have barriers to attending therapy related to their specific medical or developmental diagnosis. Likewise, given the speciality status of our clinic, many travel from afar for care, making it impractical for them to regularly attend psychotherapy appointments. Teletherapy has allowed us to more broadly meet patient needs, especially for underserved populations.

A primary concern with telehealth is determining if patients have privacy and safety in their home setting (Abrams, 2020). Patients with intellectual and developmental disabilities (IDD) or complex medical needs often are reliant on home-health aides for activities of daily living, including connecting to appointments, and those living in group homes may not have privacy for therapy. We assess safety and privacy to ensure confidentiality can be maintained by asking patients at each session if they are in a private location where they feel comfortable talking and encouraging them to notify us if the situation changes. We encourage patients to maintain privacy and reduce distractions by wearing headphones and using a location where they can give their full attention without distraction (e.g., not while driving or travelling in a car or while in a noisy environment).

DOI: 10.4324/9781003205029-29

Implementing Focused Acceptance and Commitment Therapy (FACT) via Telemedicine

Acceptance and Commitment Therapy (ACT) is a "third-wave" cognitive-behavioural intervention. It aims to improve psychological flexibility using acceptance and mindfulness as well as commitment and behaviour change processes (Hayes et al., 1999; Hayes et al., 2013). As a transdiagnostic intervention, it is considered effective for a wide range of psychological and medical conditions (Dindo et al., 2017). The six core psychological flexibility processes include acceptance, defusion, present moment awareness, self-as-context, values, and committed actions. A primary tenet of ACT is that human suffering is ubiquitous and our attempts/desire to control suffering (i.e., experiential avoidance) are problematic. Therefore, acceptance and willingness to engage in life while suffering are important components to living a vital life.

Several studies have shown online and technology supported ACT to be acceptable for individuals with chronic illness and mental health concerns (Brown et al., 2016; Carvalho et al., 2021; Herbert et al, 2022; Thompson et al., 2021). Administration of FACT via teletherapy provides several advantages. First, it allows patients with chronic health conditions to remain in an environment where they feel safe and comfortable and limits the need to travel, which may be difficult due to physical limitations or other needs. Also, the wide-range of ACT resources available through YouTube (e.g., The Act Auntie) and on practitioner/author websites (e.g., Russ Harris) can be streamed via online methods much in the same way a patient and clinician could watch them together during a session.

A main challenge of providing ACT-based treatments via teletherapy is that the therapist and patient are not in the same environment. This can make it more difficult to assist the patient in engaging to their fullest extent in the core principles of psychological flexibility. For example, with regard to accessing the present moment, the therapist is not privy to the same environmental cues and distractions as the patient. Teletherapy also may not provide appropriate time and space for patients to emotionally prepare for the therapy session. For example, when arriving to an in person session, the built in transportation and waiting time requires planning and space that can assist a smooth transition into the psychotherapy session. Logging on for an online session can be done without the need for this additional time and space and may lead to less ability to be present due to work or household duties that remain evident in the patient's environment. One way to address this is by asking patients to reduce distractions and helping them to settle into the session with a brief grounding exercise. Finally, a key component of ACT is the therapist's ability to tune into subtle shifts in patient body language or facial expressions, which may be more difficult to do via video where views are limited. In instances where patients put their head down or go off camera this can be particularly challenging.

Focused Acceptance and Commitment Therapy (FACT; Robinson et al., 2010; Strosahl et al., 2012) condenses the six core ACT processes into three pillars: *open* (i.e., acceptance and defusion), *aware* (i.e., contact with the present moment), and *engaged* (i.e., values and committed actions). FACT was designed for work within the primary care setting and is intended for brief (<30 minute) sessions which fits well with an IBH model.

The first session of FACT includes a contextual interview to gather information about the individual's life in the following areas: *love* (living situation, relationship, family, friends, spiritual/community life), *work/school*, *play* (fun/hobbies, relaxation), and *health behaviours* (exercise, sleep, substance use, sex, medications, diet). The context of the problem also is explored including when it started (*time*), what makes it better or worse (*triggers*), and if it is better or worse over time (*trajectory*). This is followed by a contextual summary, problem identification, and plan for intervention. After creating a plan, patients are asked to rate their likelihood of following through on the plan which provides an opportunity to assess barriers and motivation (Robinson et al., 2010).

At the beginning of each follow-up session, patients are asked whether their identified problem has been better, worse, or about the same. Progress is reviewed and session focus is identified. Content is then focused on one addressing the problem using one or more of the pillars. This often involves the use of metaphors, worksheets (e.g., The Life Plan or Bullseye; Robinson et al., 2010), and in-session skills practice. The session concludes with creating a plan and assessing motivation as described above. In FACT, patients are given autonomy to decide whether to return rather than assuming regular follow-up. This is done by asking if they want to schedule follow-up or go out, try the plan, and come back as needed (Robinson et al., 2010).

FACT is easily adjusted for online therapy. Screen sharing allows for joint completion of worksheets, which can be sent to patients securely as attachments upon session completion. Videos demonstrating ACT processes and audio resources such as guided meditations can be streamed over the telehealth platform. It may be more difficult to determine patient engagement in these resources over video compared to in person.

When implementing FACT via telemedicine, we have found it useful to summarize relevant session material, resources, and plan in the patients online chart at the end of each session. This builds in a review of the material and allows the patient to refer to this information as needed.

FACT Case Example[1]

"Mary" is a 30-year-old female with cystic fibrosis (CF) referred for therapy due to increased feelings of depression, anxiety, and hopelessness. Below, we summarize her treatment utilizing FACT via teletherapy.

Session One

As an introduction, the therapist informed Mary that she is a psychologist who helps people with problems of living and outlined the session plan, which

Table 24.1 Mary's responses during the contextual interview

Love	Lives with husband, daughter (8) and son (5; non-verbal, developmental delays).
	Supportive friends
	Marital conflict around parenting
	Close with biological family and in laws who live nearby
Work	Salesperson, enjoys her job
Play	Enjoys hiking, fishing, reading
	Lately less enjoyment from these activities
Health	CF is well controlled
	Poor sleep (<5 hours)
	Minimal exercise
	Denies substance or alcohol use

included asking questions for the first 10–15 minutes then working together to formulate a plan for addressing the identified concern. We then checked in about environmental privacy and safety. Mary was located at home and nobody else was present at this time of this session.

Mary stated that she had been a "worrier" since adolescence, though this generally hadn't interfered with her life before now. In addition to her CF, which generally is well-controlled, her son has developmental delays which place strain on the family. Her self-identified coping difficulties are affecting her in multiple areas and noticed by family and friends who encouraged her to seek care.

The information learned during the contextual interview is summarized in Table 24.1.

Mary's identified problem was that she sleeps five hours a night and feels exhausted. We created a plan to go to bed an hour earlier each night. She felt very confident (7 out of 10) in her ability to implement this plan. She was given the option to schedule a follow-up or contact the provider if needed. She opted for a telemedicine follow up in 1.5 weeks.

Session Two

Session two was conducted during Mary's break at work. She connected via her phone while in her car at her workplace parking lot. While this afforded her privacy, it caused poor connectivity at times during the session, which interfered with communication at times during the session. She identified things were "better" since the first visit. She consistently reached her goal of an extra hour of sleep and noticed improvement in her mood and energy levels. She also identified feeling better after a few hours to herself during the previous week to engage in preferred activities.

During session two, Mary's identified problem was a general sense of hopelessness, often wondering "what's the point?" She reported feeling this way since she was a teenager. She also notices a tendency to get "stuck in her head" about unfinished tasks at work or home. This was evident at times during the session when Mary would become more despondent or disengaged. While Mary's full body language was not able to be seen due to the camera angle, which was primarily focused on her face, the therapist was able to notice subtle changes in facial expression (e.g., staring off, downturned mouth). When this happened, the therapist would prompt Mary to be aware of and open to her internal experiences by asking "what's happening for you right now?"

This session focused on all three pillars. We practiced a grounding exercise where Mary checked in with her physical sensations and surroundings. In some ways, this was enhanced by Mary being in her car in a parking lot as there was a lot of activity going on around her that she could tune in to, allowing her to be present in the "here and now." On the other hand, the distracted environment, which included passing cars and people, made it difficult for her to check in with herself without distraction. We identified a plan for greater present moment awareness through engaging her senses and promoting a sense of awe and wonder. This included using defusion techniques such as reminding herself "that was then, this is now" or "I'll deal with this later" when stuck in thoughts about the past or future and practicing the grounding exercises learned in today's session. She expressed confidence to implement these practices (8 of 10) and opted to schedule a follow-up in two-weeks.

Session Three

At the beginning of session three, Mary reported things were "much better." She noticed more engagement with her children and an increased sense of wonder and joy when going about her day. Because she had been more open and aware to internal experiences, she reported that she had noticed a lump in her throat that occurs when she feels anxious or overwhelmed. We discussed ways to engage her awareness, compassion, and mindfulness strategies when this occurs, including noticing the sensation without judgment or self-criticism and slowing down to consider what she needed at that moment. We also reviewed the transient nature of feelings using a weather metaphor and the therapist encouraged Mary to continue to engage her aware skills. The use of metaphors to illustrate the core-concepts of ACT is a key component treatment (Stoddard & Afari, 2014). Metaphors are usually introduced in the form of exercises using scripts, which can easily be done in an online format.

Mary reported much improvement in her quality of life since session one. She was increasingly present and enjoying time with her family and experiencing a greater overall sense of wonder and joy. Further, she felt more purposeful and less hopeless. We reviewed the open, aware, and engaged behaviours she had practiced over the last six weeks. She opted to continue implementing these without a scheduled follow-up. The therapist informed Mary she could contact her for another session at any time.

Psychiatric Consultation via Telemedicine

As many of our patients also utilize adjunctive psychiatric consultation, we briefly review the advantages to providing virtual psychiatric consultation. A majority of referrals for medication assessment in our clinic are for patients with IDD and typically involve the patient and a range of caregivers (including parents/guardians, support staff, and other clinicians). Virtual visits have made it easier to collaborate with these individuals without the need for physical arrival at the clinic or multiple out of session contacts.

Another benefit has been enhanced patient comfort. For many IDD patients, psychiatric appointments are difficult to tolerate due to their duration and the need for sustained direct communication, often with multiple individuals. The focus of visits also can be difficult, as caregiver discussion of undesirable behaviours can feel accusatory or shameful and lead to withdrawal, irritability, and emotional/behavioural dysregulation during appointments. Telehealth can help ease these by allowing the patient space to engage (or disengage as needed) in a familiar environment and allow them access to preferred coping mechanisms which may not be available in an in-person clinical setting.

The greater space allowed by telehealth can make acquiring and keeping a patient's attention more challenging. For those with IDD, this may be exacerbated by a potentially limited attention span, lack of understand of the nature of the interaction, and/or general disinterest. Although this is not always a problem, brief periods of contact may be all that is possible, and eliciting the patient's thoughts and perspective may be more challenging than it would be in an in-person setting.

Likewise, telehealth often leads to less direct observation of patient behaviour as patients may wander in and out of the visit. Clinically significant movements, expressions, etc. may or may not be visualized in this setting, leaving subjective caregiver report as the sole source of information. Although collecting this type of objective clinical information is not always possible even in person, telehealth visits often make it even more difficult.

For individuals without IDD, telehealth also has represented a reasonable alternative to in-person appointments, allowing for equivalent collection of clinical information. As with the IDD population, there are potential benefits to performing assessment in familiar and more comfortable settings, and (if necessary) allowing more individuals to participate in the assessment. Additionally, many patients have been able to more easily engage in telehealth visits compared to physically travelling to clinic.

Psychiatric Consultation Case Example

"Samantha" is a 20 y/o female with a history of a genetic abnormality and associated syndrome consisting of a seizure disorder, mitochondrial myopathy, and IDD. She was referred for a medication assessment due to a gradual worsening of longstanding anxiety around transitions. Below, we demonstrate how performing a telehealth assessment in the home setting permitted more effective information gathering and helped reduce patient distress.

For Samantha, transitions are associated with significant distress, most often emotional dysregulation (e.g., crying, screaming) and agitation (e.g., lashing out physically). Despite behavioural treatment, these symptoms gradually worsened during the coronavirus pandemic until she was unable to attend her day program. In the past, medication treatment was associated with significant improvement, yet had significant side effects.

It quickly became apparent when speaking with Samantha and her mother that Samantha had low tolerance for any discussion of her symptoms and behaviours. Even describing a typical "transition" proved distressing, restricting her mother's freedom to discuss symptoms with the clinician.

Fortunately, because she was in her home, Samantha could be safely redirected in and out of the room and could be engaged and distracted with enjoyable activities (e.g., the family's pet dog). This enabled her to remain in behavioural control for the full duration of the assessment and allowed her mother more opportunities to share important clinical information. Ultimately, the assessment was completed with minimal disruption and distress for the patient, and a plan was made to use medications in addition to behavioural treatments to better address Samantha's symptoms.

Conclusion

Providing our services via teletherapy has had a number of benefits for our patient population. These include improved access for individuals with barriers to in-person attendance, greater ease of participation for multiple parties, and increased comfort for individuals with IDD who may have difficulty transitioning to new environments

A primary challenge to telemedicine is maintaining privacy and confidentiality. We encouraged patients to use headphones, use a separate location in their house (or car), and notify us if their environment changed. Another challenge is that the provider and patient are in separate environments and subject to different stimuli, which may interfere with each party's ability to be present and focused. Likewise, while the ease and comfort of logging on from home has benefits, it may contribute to patients being less engaged in the therapeutic process or less deliberate in making emotional and physical and space required for effective behavioural health intervention.

Considering the pros and cons can help to determine whether a patient would most benefit from in-person or virtual visits. We anticipate continuing to provide a hybrid of services to meet patient needs based on their specific circumstances.

Practical Consideration and Tips

- FACT is easily converted to an online format allowing patients to engage in the open, aware, and engaged processes in much the same way they would in an in-person visit.
- It may be challenging to engage in present moment awareness when the provider and patient are in different settings.
- Providers may have greater difficulty reading patient body language or facial cues as these may not be as evident on-camera due to limitation of viewing area.
- Ensure privacy and confidentiality at each visit, encourage headphones and private location, and ask for notification if the environment changes
- Utilize secure methods to share worksheets and summarize session content
- Telemedicine allows patients to remain in a comfortable environment
- Multiple participants (e.g., caregivers) can more easily attend telemedicine sessions
- An individualized, hybrid approach may be beneficial depending on specific patient needs and circumstances

Note

1 To protect patient confidentiality, identifying information has been changed and/or removed in the case examples.

References

Abrams, Z. (2020). How well is telepsychology working? *Monitor on Psychology, 51*(5), 46.

Brown, M., Glendenning, A., Hoon, A. E., & John, A. (2016). Effectiveness of web-delivered acceptance and commitment therapy in relation to mental health and well-being: A systematic review and meta-analysis. *Journal of Medical Internet Research, 18*(8), e221. 10.2196/jmir.6200

Bush, K., Kivlahan, D. R., Mcdonell, M. B., Fihn, S. D., & Bradley, K. A. (1998). The AUDIT alcohol consumption questions (AUDIT-C): An effective brief screening test for problem drinking. Ambulatory Care Quality Improvement Project (ACQUIP). Alcohol Use Disorders Identification Test. *Archives of Internal Medicine, 158*(16), 1789–1795. 10.1001/archinte.158.16.1789.

Carvalho, S. A., Skvark, D., Barbosa, R., Tavares, T., Santos, D., & Trindade, I. A. (2021). A pilot randomised controlled trial of online acceptance and commitment therapy versus compassion focused therapy for chronic illness. *Clinical Psychology & Psychotherapy*, 10.1002/cpp.2643. Advance online publication. 10.1002/cpp.2643.

Cuthill, F. M., Espie, C., & Cooper, S. A. (2003). Development and psychometric properties of the glasgow depression scale for people with a learning disability: Individual and carer supplement versions. *The British Journal of Psychiatry, 182*(4), 347–353. 10.1192/bjp.182.4.347

Dindo, L., Van Liew, J. R., & Arch, J. J. (2017). Acceptance and commitment therapy: A transdiagnostic behavioral intervention for mental health and medical conditions. *Neurotherapeutics: The journal of the American Society for Experimental NeuroTherapeutics, 14*(3), 546–553. 10.1007/s13311-017-0521-3

Hayes, S. C., Levin, M. E., Plumb-Vilardaga, J., Villatte, J. L., & Pistorello, J. (2013). Acceptance and commitment therapy and contextual behavioral science: Examining the progress of a distinct model of behavioral and cognitive therapy. *Behavior Therapy, 44*(2), 180–198. 10.1016/j.beth.2009.08.002

Hayes, S. C., Strosahl, K., & Wilson, K. G. (1999). *Acceptance and commitment therapy: An experiential approach to behavior change.* Guilford Press.

Herbert, M. S., Dochat, C., Wooldridge, J. S., Materna, K., Blanco, B. H., Tynan, M., Lee, M. W., Gasperi, M., Camodeca, A., Harris, D., & Afari, N. (2022). Technology-supported acceptance and commitment therapy for chronic health conditions: A systematic review and meta-analysis. *Behaviour Research and Therapy, 148*, 103995.10.1016./j.brat.2021.103995.

Holderle, K. E., Poleshuck, E., Rosenberg, T., & Pulcino, T. (2021). Integrated behavioral health in primary care for adults with complex childhood onset medical and developmental diagnoses. *Journal of Clinical Psychology in Medical Settings, 29*(3), 586–595. 10.1007/s10880-021-09798-w

Kroenke, K., Spitzer, R. L., & Williams, J. B. W. (2001). The PHQ-9: Validity of a brief depression severity measure. *Journal of General Internal Medicine, 16*(9), 606–613. 10.1046/j.1525-1497.2001.016009606.x

Robinson, P. J., Gould, D. A., & Strosahl, K. D. (2010). *Real behavior change in primary care: Improving patient outcomes and increasing job satisfaction.* Oakland, CA: New Harbinger Publications.

Skinner H. A. (1982). The Drug Abuse Screening Test. *Addictive Behavior, 7*(4), 363–371.

Spitzer, R. L., Kroenke, K., Williams, J. B. W., & Löwe, B. (2006). A brief measure for assessing generalized anxiety disorder: The GAD-7. *Archives of Internal Medicine, 166*(10), 1092–1097. 10.1001/archinte.166.10.1092

Stoddard, J. A., & Afari, N. (2014). *The Big Book of ACT Metaphors: A Practitioner's Guide to Experiential Exercises and Metaphors in Acceptance and Commitment Therapy.* Oakland, CA: New Harbinger Publications.

Strosahl, K. D., Gustavsson, T., & Robinson, P. (2012). *Brief interventions for radical behavior change: Principles and practice for focused acceptance and commitment therapy.* Oakland, CA: New Harbinger Publications.

Thompson, E. M., Destree, L., Albertella, L., & Fontenelle, L. F., (2021). Internet-based acceptance and commitment therapy: A transdiagnostic systemic review and meta-analysis for mental health outcomes. *Behavior Therapy, 52*, 492–507.

25 Diving into the World of Online Play Therapy

Brian Keating

Intro

As a play therapist working in a carefully curated playroom, the restrictions put in place due to the COVID-19 pandemic brought up a lot of questions and concern for how I would continue to serve my child clients between the ages of 6 to 10. Needing to adapt my playroom to a telehealth platform, I wondered if it was even possible to ask a child to sit across a screen and continue the therapeutic arc of our play together. It was during this transitional period of uncertainty and necessity that I quickly noticed my resistance to online play therapy diminish, realizing that online play was rich with clinical value and a lot of fun.

This chapter will illustrate how I made the transition to online play therapy with specific attention given to the model of Synergetic Play Therapy (SPT). A case study is included that focuses on the challenges of the initial online sessions with a new child client and how the writer used fundamental aspects of SPT to deepen the child's work around a clinical issue.

Furthermore, the chapter may provide the reader with insight and motivation to experiment and increase his/her use of experiential aspects during their online therapy sessions.

Bringing the Playroom to the Screen

The global shift to online learning at the end of March 2020 prepared children for the experience of working with computer-based platforms, making the idea of online play therapy a workable option. In my practice, children as young as age 6 demonstrate the ability to navigate technology by logging into a device and accessing general interface commands. Play can be initiated either by choosing a game or toy from their room, or by positioning the video screen to show personal items of interest.

Children with increased technical aptitude might choose to interact via Digital Play Therapy "a modality that utilizes highly motivating, immersive activities to incorporate areas of client interest into the play therapy process to deepen relationships, gather information, implement interventions, and advance the

DOI: 10.4324/9781003205029-30

treatment plan forward." (Stone, p. 15). Through *screen sharing*, and *link sharing* play therapists could initiate additional functions of play through a telehealth platform. *Gaming consoles* such as Nintendo Switch allow the child and the therapist to play online together while addressing themes common in play therapy such as anger, frustration tolerance, turn taking, and emotional expression and regulation.

Although it is beyond the scope of this chapter to explore how children are impacted by digital media, it is important to acknowledge the experience of viewing another over video. Kirkorian (2018) studied how the interactive experiences (touching/tapping a screen) infants and toddlers participate in, are more successful than the transfer of information over television or video. She reports that these interactive experiences can be further strengthened through the attunement and presence of an adult (either on video or in person) when social cues such as eye contact, responses to behavior, and relational contact (such as the use of one's name) are used (Kirkorian, 2018). While further research is needed on the social impact of screens on young children, it is important to recognize that teleplay therapy is not passive learning or engagement, but is a social interaction that is transformed into a therapeutic interaction through the same set of clinical skills a play therapist would draw from in the playroom.

A disadvantage to being online is often the limitation of toys and items a child might have access to at home to help inspire play. Privacy, internet connectivity, and general engagement on both the part of the therapist and child are also new considerations with the online format. While training to become a Certified Synergetic Play Therapist, the study of three specific tenets of SPT became a strong asset in framing how I could support children over telehealth, helping me realize that the energy and experience of their online world was no different than being in person together.

Synergetic Play Therapy (SPT) was created by Lisa Dion, founder of the Synergetic Play Therapy Institute, and draws from a variety of play therapy modalities combining the "therapeutic powers of play with nervous system regulation, interpersonal neurobiology, physics, attachment theory, mindfulness, and therapist authenticity." (Dion, 2018). The potential benefit of combining in-person SPT with the widely practiced model of Child Centered Play Therapy (CCPT) has recently been examined, drawing attention to the focus of regulation in play (Simmons, 2020). Townsend et al. (2021), further explore the similarities and differences noting that both emphasize the need for safety in the relationship while identifying that SPT differs in that the "therapist is an active participant in the child's process and uses emotional congruence and verbal authenticity to support regulation of the child's nervous system." While the play therapist in both modalities is a witness to the child's play, in SPT the value is placed in the ability of the therapist to stay present with the child by becoming aware of, acknowledging, and attuning to the child's distress – consciously expanding their ability to move through it together by the process of co-regulation.

In joining the emotional world of the child through therapist congruence and authenticity, it is suggested that toys are simply an invitation for the child to experience co-regulation from the therapist (Dion, 2020). This framework helped bridge the gap between the playroom and the screen, relieving the pressure of having to recreate a "perfect" teleplay environment with specific toys. In essence, all a child needed to do was show up and turn on their device as I embraced the freedom and therapeutic value in following the child where they needed to go. Whether we were looking for a lizard in a home terrarium or if the child was hiding behind a closed door, angry that they had to attend the session, I began to grow confident in my ability to trust that my authentic presence could be just as healing and therapeutic as any objects in my playroom.

Through the use of the projective process, SPT asks play therapists to attune to oneself and reflect on their own thoughts, emotions and somatic sensations to consider what the child might be showing us about the challenges in their world (Dion, 2020). Regardless of which toy is being utilized, the setup provides the therapist a window into a child's experience of feelings of anxiety, fear, stress, or overwhelm (Dion, 2018). For a child who played at a distance from the video screen ignoring my observational statements or reflections, I might feel a strong lack of connection and wonder "Do I matter?" For a child who attacks the video screen with a pillow or T-Rex figure, I might question whether I feel safe or can trust the environment I am in. The setup might lead to the feeling of immense sadness and hopelessness as I watch Lego figurines be hit by a car and left behind for the remainder of the session. Could these all be feelings the child is working to communicate through his/her play?

Working with Staying Present and Self Care

Allowing oneself the space to experience the setup in a telehealth session can feel intense and even disorienting at times. Tenet 3 of SPT identifies the importance of therapist *self-regulation* in supporting both the therapist and the child in moments of hyper- or hypo-arousal (Dion, 2020). In a play therapy room, the therapist might be more free to walk around, and feel connected to their ability to regulate with the child in close physical proximity. The restriction of being limited to a video screen illustrated the importance of needing to listen to my body and my emotional experience in order to stay grounded and present. Through self-regulation, the therapist is also modeling for the child how to regulate their experience through the function of mirror neurons (Dion, 2018). This approach was something I had utilized in person and now became a helpful intervention due to being less mobile, the possibility of environmental distractions, and general screen fatigue.

Multicultural Considerations

When considering the shift to telehealth, one must consider a child and family's ability to access devices and any costs that might be associated. During the pandemic, many of the children I worked with had access to a tablet or computer due to the adjustment to online learning, but did not always have the privilege of a variety of toys or private areas to explore or play freely.

On a training call with a colleague from Namibia, I was reminded of the power of outdoor play. For the children in her country, sand, sticks, and rocks were just as fun and valuable as matchbox cars or building blocks. This reminder inspired a session where I prompted a child to move from his school tablet to a family member's cell phone allowing him to go outside and describe a picture he was drawing in the sand that ended up being a portrait of a deceased grandparent.

Case Study

Xavier is an elementary aged, white, cis-gendered male that was referred to me due to behavioral challenges and emotional outbursts at bedtime. He was living in a split family system and our sessions took place in the home of the same caregiver each week.

Our initial consultation meeting took place through the screen with his parents in the room for safety and technological support. I initiated a psychoeducational discussion about how teletherapy was different from school, how it was important for him to have privacy in our sessions moving forward, and how he could be himself over the video without feeling like it was online school.

I was feeling uncertain about how teletherapy sessions would work with Xavier. Would our next meeting be in a space that was private where he felt comfortable to be himself? Would discipline challenges at school translate to our teletherapy session feeling like an assignment he needed to complete vs. a space where he could express himself freely through play?

Our first few sessions embraced the flexibility that teletherapy offered, as well as identifying the many challenges teleplay therapists encounter. We began in a common area of his home where one of his parents could be heard and seen in the background engaging with a guest; could other people hear what we were talking about? I acknowledged this lack of privacy which led Xavier to suggest we move outside.

With his tablet, Xavier took me outside, acknowledging the technical boundaries of his wireless connection, and placed me against a curb as he rocked in front of me on his skateboard. The internet connection at times was shaky, but his ability to play via his skateboard was clear. He smiled, laughed and appeared proud when he completed a trick that he had been working on. I felt nervous on the occasions when he almost fell.

Another time when we went outside skateboarding, Xavier took a break and shared about some adults in his life. After spinning, jumping, and near-falling, he would sit down and offer snapshots of his life. At times I felt distracted by the intermittent internet connection and had a fear that the session would abruptly end. I also felt a lingering worry that I was doing something wrong and I would get in trouble for our play not being traditionally therapeutic.

When I presented my experiences with Xavier during an SPT consultation, I was encouraged to consider my feelings of fear and worry as part of the "setup." Could it be that he was "setting me up" to feel what he was feeling in his daily life? Is it possible that my fear that the session (or play) would abruptly end or that I might get in trouble for doing something wrong could also be something that he was wrestling with?

The suggestion to work with this setup was to be my authentic, true self with this child; modeling how to stay grounded and present in a hard experience. Being authentic would also mean to name what I was feeling – the emotions and the somatic sensations – as well as taking care of those feelings by regulating my nervous systems response: moving if I needed to stay alert or release energy and taking deep breaths if my heart rate was feeling escalated.

As the arc of our work continued, I held the curiosity of the setup in mind. I learned more about Xavier as our sessions moved to his bedroom. He showed me stuffed animals that had been important to him when he was younger, and I watched as he completed Lego sculptures that were half-finished on a night stand. As he continued to trust that the teletherapy sessions were different from online school (where he was expected to sit across from the screen for the entirety of a lesson) I was attuning to his experiences of distress by where he would take me with the iPad or what he would bring out to share.

During routine check-ins with his parents I was learning that he was acting out with his friends from the neighborhood. His parents noted that Xavier was a good kid who knew right from wrong, and also happened to find himself in situations that he often regretted when going to bed later in the night.

As our next session progressed I noticed there was an increase in hyper-aroused energy. Xavier was in a heightened sympathetic nervous system state where his body was much more active and he spoke faster with an increased sense of urgency. I touched into my authentic experience by identifying that things felt intense in that moment. My heart was beating faster and I needed to rock my body side-to-side to help stay focused with him. He chuckled in response and replied that he wanted to show me skateboard tricks with the iPad as a skateboard. My stomach dropped. What does that mean I thought to myself? What is happening now? I named that confusion and uncertainty as the screen across from me began to flip around, spin through the air, and then land on a pillow.

"Woah that was intense" I let out as I exhaled from a deep breath.

"Haha yeah that was fun!" Xavier replied through a smile as he plopped down on the ground. After a moment's pause, he smiled again and leaned towards the screen. "Hey, I have an idea! Do you want to go base jumping?!"

"Uh, um … like jumping out of a plane?"

"Like jumping off of a building! Except you'll jump off the side of my bunk bed!"

As Xavier was explaining this to me I realized I did not have a choice. He was already making the short climb up the ladder on the side of his bunk bed as the view on the other side of my screen became dizzying and disorienting. A pillow was quickly thrown from the bed to the floor.

"That will help give you a soft landing."

I immediately noticed my heart pounding through my chest. My stomach clenched as my belly button moved in towards my spine. I noticed I was not breathing so I took in a big breath of air through my open mouth and I spoke quickly.

"I don't know if I want to do this! I'm feeling really nervous about this! I need to catch my breath for a second because my heart is beating so fast." These words came without thought and were authentic to my experience as the iPad screen was leaned over the edge of the top bunk. Below I saw two pillows and some blankets on the ground.

Sensing my apprehension Xavier spoke. "It's okay. You'll be fine. I do this all the time. Well, actually I've never done it with the iPad, but it'll be fun."

Thoughts continued to race through my head. I wondered if the iPad might break and if I might be responsible for it in some way. I wondered how I would explain this if his parents heard the iPad hit the floor and wondered what was happening. I worried that he might not like or trust me if I did not want to do it. Then the thought of the setup came to mind and I realized what was happening: We were working through an experience of peer pressure.

Over the course of the next 20 minutes I went "base jumping" with Xavier. At first the experiences of the iPad being thrown off the bed were fast, chaotic, and perhaps borderline damaging to the device. On more than one occasion the video platform closed and he had to log back onto the call. Throughout each round I attempted to stay regulated and grounded with myself. I continued rocking side to side to discharge the energy in my arms and body, I took intentional breaths, and I named the various feelings I had.

At the top of the bed I identified my apprehension and the concerns that something could get damaged. I named my resistance and questioned if I wanted to keep "jumping off." When there was a smooth landing, Xavier would celebrate and I acknowledged the conflicting emotions.

That one was kind of fun, but I'm not sure I want to go again.

I noticed that the more I spoke about my true experience in the moment, the more he began to slow down and talk with me about his experience. He became curious about my emotions and reactions and I noticed that he began to breathe more intentionally. The rounds slowed down and he became more aware of my concerns and began to build softer landing spaces.

I am uncertain whether Xavier was specifically working through his experience of peer pressure in this teleplay therapy session; however, I can say that it was true in my experience. I was engaged with an activity that I felt apprehensive about and was unsure of how to work through it. In this experience, I worked to stay present and grounded with myself while also working to find my voice – to find a way to speak up and share my concerns and apprehension. My hope was that in being authentic to my experience of not wanting to be thrown off the bed over a video screen, I was modeling for him how to recognize his own thoughts, feelings, and actions when in an uncertain situation. By conceptualizing this as the setup, I was considering how the child might use the iPad to show me what it feels like to be him. Unlike online school, I was not limiting, restricting, or punishing his expressive play. Conversely, I was present with him in the play and staying with the intensity of his experience.

Xavier continued to meet with me online for the next few months. During that time he demonstrated an increased ability to name his emotions, and regulate himself by taking intentional breaths and moving his body. He also began to develop autonomy in his peer relationships, evidenced by sticking up for himself when situations became uncomfortable for him. Xavier began to talk about these moments more explicitly in our sessions and with his parents, acknowledging how hard it was to do something that felt right to him, even if it was not what his friends wanted.

Conclusion

Play therapists had a fast and steep learning curve when confronted with the need to adapt to telehealth. I learned that I could draw from pre-existing models of play therapy to adjust to teleplay through a screen. Alongside a variety of substitutes for physical items in the playroom, this chapter illustrated how the specific model of Synergetic Play Therapy (SPT) proved helpful in making sense of how to stay present and engaged during an online play session.

The case example illustrated how I established safety and trust by advocating for a private space and following the child's inner wisdom over multiple sessions. Similar to an in-person play therapy session, the child led and directed telehealth sessions without allowing the limitations of meeting through a video screen to reduce playfulness or session efficacy. Conceptualizing the play through the SPT lens of the setup, I was able to become aware of and attune to the child's experience of peer pressure and the request to do things he did not want to do. By giving voice to my personal experience on the other side of the screen, I helped model for the child how to stay regulated and present in ways that were congruent with his treatment plan.

Practical Tips and Considerations

- Further areas of interest include: how teleplay therapy might expose the therapist to the entire system of the child's world; ways to integrate parent-child interaction in session; ways to accommodate children under the age of 6.
- Many families have shared that telehealth sessions have become more accessible due to the lack of a commute while further expressing appreciation that telehealth can bring the playroom to them.
- A screening process specific for telehealth is recommended to determine if families are willing and able to honor the private space needed for an online play therapy session.
- The chat feature on a telehealth platform can provide privacy if siblings or family members are nearby.
- Household items such as rice, beans, or cotton balls can become the building blocks for a homemade sand tray. (Dion, 2021).
- Items can be collected from a discount store (e.g., the Dollar Store) to mail to new clients in a box that is designated only for the play therapy sessions (Dion, 2021).
- Minecraft, Roblox, and Steam are ways to play games online while traditional boardgames can be found at BoardGameArena.com
- A digital online sandtray is available online at no cost (Fried, 2021).
- "Tele-PLAY Therapy Resources and Support" Facebook group can be a resource to support play therapists in sharing digital play therapy ideas and games.
- Some children may express a dislike for the lack of physical connection and may prefer in-person interventions.
- The Synergetic Play Therapy Institute offers a variety of trainings for therapists to learn more about this specific approach to play therapy.

References

Dion, L. (2018). *Aggression in play therapy: A neurobiological approach for integrating intensity.* New York, NY: Norton.

Dion, L. (2020). *Tenets for synergetic play therapy.* Synergetic Play Therapy Institute. https://synergeticplaytherapy.com/wp-content/uploads/2021/04/SPT-Tenets-updated-6.23.20.pdf

Dion, L. (Host). (2021). *Lessons from the playroom: Episode 92: Embracing Online Play Therapy* [Audio podcast]. Synergetic Play Therapy. https://synergeticplaytherapy.com/podcasts/

Fried, K. (2021). *Online sandtray*. Oaklander Training. https://www.onlinesandtray.com

Kirkorian, H. (2018). When and how do interactive digital media help children connect what they see on and off the screen?*Child Development Perspectives, 12*, 210–214.10.1111/cdep.12290.

Simmons, J. (2020). Moving toward regulation using synergetic play therapy. *Canadian Journal of Counselling and Psychotherapy, 54*(3), 242–258. Retrieved from https://cjc-rcc.ucalgary.ca/article/ view/69443

Stone, J. (2020). *Digital play therapy: A clinician's guide to comfort and competence*. New York, NY: Routledge.

Townsend, B. J., Ishman, L., Dion, L., & Carnes-Holt, K. L. (2021). An examination of child-centered play therapy and synergetic play therapy. *Journal of Child and Adolescent Counseling, 7*(3), 193–206.

Epilogue

Arnon Rolnick, Adam Leighton, and Haim Weinberg

As we approach the end of our metaphorical journey through the chapters of this book, we would like to share our view of the main landmarks we have recognized. We will share here elements featured throughout the various chapters that illustrate new understandings regarding the transition to online therapy. Other commonalities that exist are mentioned in this book's introduction. These will be followed by a brief summary of guidelines for therapists working online.

The Main Common Elements

Creating a Shared Experience

As pointed out in the introduction, one of the main challenges of online therapy is to create a shared experience. The screen creates a barrier that interferes with this task, and our challenge is to find ways to lower this barrier and to overcome the distance created using the Internet. As said, this can be achieved by using flexibility and creativity. Along the book, different authors struggle with this difficult task, using different methods to create a shared online experience. Therapists may utilize the "here and now" of technological disruptions as a shared experience, virtually participate in base-jumping (see Keating's Chapter 25), draw on the whiteboard together, listen to music they share online or notice the impact of our self-image, to mention a few techniques described. Examining the experiential through a perspective of the physical, social, cognitive, and affective dimensions may help to identify which dimensions we may choose to emphasize and enhance during our sessions depending on the needs of the patient, therapist, and the modality.

The Therapist as a Key Factor Determining Successful Transition to Remote Therapy

The importance of the therapeutic alliance cannot be overstated. As many of the contributors discussed the impact of the therapist's outlook regarding online therapy – maybe the therapeutic alliance should be expanded to include our attitude to the digital platform itself? Our feelings as therapists towards the platform itself influence the outcome of online therapy. A lack of trust, not enough self-confidence about doing online therapy, feelings of frustration or hatred towards our video conferencing software (or even the webcam itself) can affect our online work. Just as our feelings towards our patients must be related to (each to his/her own method), thus our relationship towards this new entity cannot be ignored. Luckily, a recent survey among psychologists in the USA (Clay, 2022) found out that 96% of the therapists who responded to it said that telehealth is effective therapeutically.

Authenticity / Real Relationship

Authenticity/Real relationships as described by Gelso and Carter (1994) in their paper on the components of the psychotherapy relationship entail genuineness and realistic perceptions. They define *genuineness* as "the ability and willingness to be what one truly is in the relationship – to be authentic, open, and honest." Interestingly the theme of genuineness appears in many of the chapters as a possible advantageous outcome of the transition to online therapy. The main common denominator contributing to the genuineness we have identified is the open, shared exploration of new unknown experiences (see Galit Mor, Chapter 10). This shared experience seems to provide legitimacy for many therapists to express uncertainty and vulnerability. The humbling experience of the transition itself may indirectly contribute to the therapeutic relationship and thus to the outcome of the therapy.

Contingency Planning

As online therapy relies on technological devices and infrastructure, their functionality may critically impact the session. The therapist should minimize disruption and potential rupture by a) discussing in advance various contingencies b) prepare in advance backup means, e.g., the use of a mobile phone instead of a computer, the use of a mobile phone hotspot as a connectivity backup. c) If necessary or relevant, ensure the availability of a 3rd party to support the patient (e.g., a parent when working with children).

Additional types of contingencies that the online therapist needs to consider are patient responses to/in extreme situations. The lack of physical presence of the therapist reduces ability to respond to challenging situations; therefore, for example in certain cases the therapist may request the availability of a trusted person in the vicinity of the patient.

Working with the "Here and Now"

Most if not all modalities, utilize the content and interaction between patient and therapist during the therapy session as important content to work with. Many of the chapters describe how online therapy expands the range of content that can be related to during the session. Examples of content and events that may arise during online sessions could include the ongoing in the client's (or therapist's) background, internet connectivity issues, or feelings towards the use of technology. These background "noises" can directly contribute to the therapy session if properly discussed. Indeed, some of this noise may provide additional insight into the patient's life.

The Impact is not Limited to the Therapy Session Frame

Much has been written regarding the impact of the transition to online therapy on the session itself. An interesting aspect that we have found interwoven among the book's chapters is the impact that this transition has on therapy outside of the immediate frame of therapy. Examples include the effect on the internalization and implementation of therapy session outcomes as the patient is frequently participating in the session in his/her day-to-day environment. Another example is that the physical location of the therapy session (e.g., patients bedroom) may be the exact same location that the patient has in the past had unpleasant memories, therapy in that same location offering new experiences and possibly a new relationship to that place. Conversely, the lack of the journey to and from the therapist's clinic may have a negative impact as the patient may no longer have the opportunity for "focusing" prior to the session and the time for processing after the session, as this is often carried out during the journey home.

All Modalities can be Carried Out Online

Reviewing the chapters covering a multitude of different therapeutic modalities demonstrates that technology allows most, if not all, approaches to be carried out online. However, it is also clear that the transition requires the therapist to adjust and adapt new techniques.

Challenging Situations and Diagnoses can be Treated Online

As mentioned in the introduction, we were surprised to read convincing descriptions, based on research and the writers' experience, of treating suicidality, severe depression, patients with borderline diagnosis, and PTSD online. This contradicts our (and our colleagues') common practice. Perhaps we should reconsider this myth and acknowledge our own limitations and fears in treating these difficult cases online?

One's Image Cannot be Ignored!

A glaring visual difference between online vs face-to-face therapy is that the patient and therapist can view their own image. This is neither good nor bad, at times advantageous sometimes detrimental. However, we can confidently say that the self-view cannot be ignored. Therapists and patients may choose to remove (this is possible in many platforms) the self-view or utilize it (our preference), but in any event – therapists must be aware of its significance.

The Transition to Online Therapy Offers Opportunities

Presenting itself in many different forms, opportunity is a common theme described in the book. The transition particularly offers opportunities to examine and possibly improve our understanding of basic concepts such as setting, boundaries, rupture, or the therapeutic relationship. It requires us to ask ourselves what is important in our work, to review our own techniques and assumptions. We believe that this examination can and should contribute to psychotherapy in general, not just to online therapy.

Use of Session Recordings

This is not a new understanding or technique, simply one that potentially should be much simpler and available in online therapy. Regretfully, the commonly used platforms (at the time of writing this book) surprisingly offer little support for this feature. Although one can easily record sessions, it is not straightforward to view the same recording during the sessions. Video conferencing providers – our community needs your support on this issue!

Patient Location Is Still an Issue

Oft taken for granted, the basic conditions for providing online therapy are not always available for patients. The lack of privacy, reasonable level of background noise, or problematic internet connectivity continue to routinely prevent access to therapy. We confess to not having a simple solution to this challenge, we suggest that this may be an opportunity for a community-based solution?

The Need for Specific Training for Telepsychotherapy

Previous research before the pandemic had suggested a need for training in telehealth (Callan et al., 2017). Glueckauf et al. (2018) found that around 90% of psychologists indicated that "mental health practitioners should undergo training about the clinical, legal, and/or ethical issues related to telehealth." Most participants in their study reported the need of receiving training on technical issues around delivery of telehealth services. Furthermore, about half of psychologists reported inadequate skills in managing emergency situations when using online counseling modalities, and around 40% also reported insufficient telehealth training or education. A recent study found that an important barrier to using telepsychology was therapists' lack of self-efficacy due in part to insufficient opportunities for training (Perry et al., 2020).

In a pilot study published lately (Messina & Loffler-Stastka, 2021), the researchers found that, compared to live therapy, therapists in online therapy reported significantly less clinical skills. Another study (Sampaio, Navarro, De Sousa, Vieira & Hoffman, 2021) measured how many therapists are using online therapy before vs. during COVID-19: 39% of survey respondents used telepsychology before COVID-19, vs. 98% during COVID-19. The conclusion of the researchers was that therapists still had ethical, training, and personal concerns regarding the use of telepsychology, and gaps in therapists' knowledge on these topics were evident, indicating a strong need for increased telepsychology training for therapists in the future.

Online therapy needs specific training since it creates many obstacles and brings to the fore many challenges. These challenges can be overcome creatively, but we should learn how to do it and be trained for this shift. As said, research showed that therapists still feel unsure about their online skills and their lack of confidence affects their ability to be present and to provide better mental health care.

Training for online therapy should focus on the change of the setting and the fact that the therapist cannot create the holding environment as occurs in in-person meetings. We should learn how to share the responsibility with our clients and how to teach them to take care of the environment to guarantee their privacy. As pointed out, one of the keywords in moving online is flexibility, and training should help the therapists move away from the rigid traditional approach. Another keyword is creativity, which can help us overcome the difficulty in creating presence and the absence of body-to-body communication. Training for becoming an online therapist should be practical and focus on hands-on practice. Therapists should learn how to read facial expressions and to use this information in the session. They should learn how to use imagination while working online, self-disclose properly in order to create more presence, overcome, and repair technological and psychological ruptures, and acknowledge and take responsibility for their mistakes online.

Facing Each Other: The Long Way Psychotherapy has Gone from the Couch to the Screen

As we approach the end of the book, we can observe how psychotherapy has changed since it was formulated by Freud at the beginning of the 20th century, to the flourishing of online psychotherapy more than a hundred years later. One clear change is the movement from no face-to-face or eye contact in classical psychoanalysis to clear and noticeable facial expressions visible during online psychotherapy sessions.

Many of the methods reviewed in our book mention the clarity of facial expression during online sessions. In this section, we discuss how facial expressions and eye contact represent major changes of understating what works in psychotherapy.

In classical psychoanalysis, the couch is traditionally positioned so that the analyst can barely see the analyst's face, and there is no eye contact. The idea is that such positioning might facilitate free association. (Adler & Bachant, 1996). The free association is used by the analyst to identify repressed thoughts or feelings. According to this approach, therapy is the process of making previously unconscious thoughts and feelings conscious.

In a complete contrast, working online with videoconference software allows seeing the partner's face enlarged, thus facial expressions are very noticeable. Bailenson (2021) demonstrated that the size of the head that appears on a regular computer screen is so large that it feels like the partner on the screen is at an intimate distance from the viewer. The therapist and the patient can see their partner's face very clearly. This ability to "exchange" facial expressions between the therapist and the patient is part of the therapeutic process. We suggest that seeing each other's facial expressions allows a process of synchronization. Namely, promoting mutual emotional and social states.

Ramseyer and Tschacher (2011) mention that nonverbal synchrony has been shown to be related to the therapeutic outcome: the more synchrony between therapist and patient, the better the outcome.

Golland et al. (2019) were able to show that robust synchrony occurs via facial expression and suggested that emotional signals are constantly transmitted from person to person and might significantly shape the emotional responses of recipients. However, the shaping of the emotional responses and the synchrony itself, do not necessarily mean that the therapeutic couple continuously share identical emotions. We believe that powerful periods of synchronization occur during certain moments in therapy, and we, as therapists, should aim to increase such moments. Daniel Stern calls them "Moments of Meeting" (Lyons-Ruth et al., 1988). We suggest that creating a shared experience (as described previously in this chapter) can achieve these powerful moments.

Another way to understand certain processes in psychotherapy is the intersubjective neurobiology approach. This approach can further explain the importance of facial expression (see Chapter 6, by Hadas Mor Ofek). Porges (2021) writes about a face-heart connection in which there are mutual interactions between the vagal influences on the heart and the neural regulation of the striated muscles of the face and head. The face-heart connection enables to detect whether a partner is in a calm physiological state and safe to approach, or is in a highly mobilized and reactive physiological state during which engagement would be dangerous.

So the clear view of the faces of the therapeutic couple and the face-heart connection that enables sharing, signal safety in online psychotherapy.

While Porges refers to the safety that is communicated by facial expressions, Daniel Stern (Lyons-Ruth et al., 1988) widens the scope and discusses how non-verbal cues are the basis of "Implicit relational knowledge": Seeing the facial expression, even without being aware of their meaning, allow patients and therapist to become more connected.

Apart from facial expression, eye contact is another important aspect in creating moments of meeting. Önen Ünsalver et al. (2021 p. 1) discuss the role of eye contact in the object relations approach: "The goal of treatment is a change in the analyst's arrested or dysfunctional object relationship structure." It can be said that the essential and prominent component that establishes the therapeutic alliance is the mutual gaze between the client and the therapist. Eye contact sends a message to the receiver: "I am present with you."

Most of the authors in this book commented on the loss of such contact during online meetings. Surprisingly, Hietanenet et al. (2020) examined whether the mutual gaze effect exists when two people meet in video meetings. They compared psychophysiological responses to direct eye gaze in face-to-face meetings and in video meetings and concluded (p. 1): "Most importantly, the results suggest that the physical presence or proximity of the other person is not necessary for these psychophysiological responses to eye contact." This is a surprising result that contradicts what we intuitively think, so more research is needed.

What have We Learned about Psychotherapy from the Emergence of Online Work?

We have learned that the human species has a unique need to be in contact even from a distance. That online therapy is very much possible due to the ability to interact with each other via implicit relational knowledge communicated through non-verbal facial nuances. We have learned that psychotherapy has gone a long way: from the emphasis on the verbal or explicit components of interaction that define the traditional view of psychoanalysis; via the cognitive evolution and its focus on the explicit rational intervention, to the relational revolution and the understanding that both the implicit and explicit components of the interaction, powerfully influence the therapeutic action.

Many of the chapters of this book represent this process: even those who base their interventions on cognitive, conscious techniques understand that the nonverbal implicit process – specifically the facial expression – are crucial in explaining how online therapy works

This combination of explicit and implicit processes might explain how two physically distant people affect each other and produce a therapeutic alliance that can facilitate positive change.

Guidelines for Effective Interventions

In order to help psychotherapists to become more effective in their online interventions we summarize a set of guidelines, some of them gathered from the tips suggested by the writers of the chapters, some taken from our own experience, and others collected from different articles. Notably inclusions are

Markowitz et. al. (2021) who focused on technical difficulties in transmitting therapy online and suggested remedies for each of these difficulties and Fisher et al. (2021) who suggested several guidelines for online work focusing on ostensive cues. Ostensive cues indicate to patients that personally trustworthy and relevant information is being communicated by the therapist.

Therapist Oriented

- The virtual setting can be regarded as an entity – explore your emotions and thoughts regarding this entity.
- Ask yourself is there room for more creativity in your online sessions? Have I taken full advantage of what online therapy may contribute to the therapy? Maybe recording parts of the session could be helpful?
- Emphasize facial expressions, tone of voice and body gestures. Use your hands and show them.
- Stretch and take brief walks between sessions.
- Ask yourself if there are computer literacy skills that are holding you back?
- Allow yourself to become more active than when working in your office.

Setting

- Prior and during therapy, discuss and prepare with the patient his/her physical location for the online session. Include both physical and technical aspects as well as environmental aspects such as privacy and background noise.
- Discuss the use of self-image and how to make use of it.
- Both patient and therapist:
  - Reduce distractions – Turn off notifications such as email and messages apps. When relevant, mute mobile phones.
  - Distance yourself from the camera to show more of your body
- Examine how you may improve internet connectivity (e.g., wireless connections, Wi-Fi booster) and prepare backups for both communication (e.g., mobile phone hotspot) and the computer (e.g., mobile phone). Discuss contingencies in advance with your patients.

Session Oriented

- Examine how you may want to enhance the shared experience within sessions. It may help to examine different dimensions of experiences (physical, social, cognitive, and affective).
- Do not rush in to fill silences.
- Use Internet failures and other technical ruptures as opportunities for repair. Acknowledge and discuss them.

Relationship / Patient Oriented

- Explore your patient's emotions and thoughts regarding this entity.
- Discuss with patients how they may prepare themselves for both before and after the online sessions.
- Monitor carefully for risk of suicide or violence (Markowitz et. al. 2021)
- If prior sessions were carried face to face in order to maintain continuity, emphasize themes and topics discussed previously during the face-to-face sessions (Fisher et al., 2021).

What was Not Covered in this Book

Continuing our metaphor of this book as a journey, we are aware that the journey does not cover all grounds. We would like to include suggestions for "nearby day trips," important aspects relevant to online therapy that we have not included. A few important omissions are listed below:

- Dealing with patient's resistance to switch to online therapy. Especially with patients who have had "bad zoom experiences" (such as students in school).
- Hybrid approaches combining online sessions and other therapeutic frameworks such as online support groups and computer based learning (briefly discussed in the chapter "Looking forwards – what and how other technologies will impact online therapy").
- Additional therapeutic modalities that were not included in this book.
- Group therapy – will be covered in our next book.
- Online Supervision (this is partly covered in our previous book, Theory and Practice of Online Therapy (Weinberg & Rolnick, 2021).
- The transition back to face-to-face therapy. As this book is going to press, the present global pandemic seems to be subsiding and in many cases, online therapy sessions are transitioning to face-to-face sessions. Little has been written or researched regarding the return to face-to-face meetings.

Some of the omissions were due to the limited scope of the book, others due the editors' oversight!

Last Words

As editors of this book, we have had a unique opportunity to stand from a distance and view not only online psychotherapy, but psychotherapy in general. It has been a fascinating experience and has provided us with additional clarity and understanding. We hope you share our experience.

We thank the contributors for their important work and patience and understanding, enduring our many comments, suggestions and requests.

This work is yet another brick in the infinite construction improving our ability to allow people to live better lives.

Haim, Arnon, and Adam.

References

Adler, E., & Bachant, J. L. (1996). Free association and analytic neutrality: Basic structure of the psychoanalytic situation. *Journal of the American Psychoanalytic Association, 44*(4), 1021–1046. 10.1177/000306519604400403

Bailenson, J. N. (2021). Nonverbal overload: A theoretical argument for the causes of zoom fatigue. *Technology, Mind, and Behavior, 2*(1). 10.1037/tmb0000030

Callan, J. E., Maheu, M. M., & Bucky, S. F. (2017). Crisis in the behavioral health classroom: Enhancing knowledge, skills, and attitudes in telehealth training. In M. Maheu, K. Drude, & S. Wright (Eds.), *Career paths in telemental health* (pp. 63–80). New York, NY: Springer.

Clay, R. A. (2022). Telehealth proves its worth. *Monitor on Psychology*, January/February 2022, p. 85. https://www.apa.org/monitor/2022/01/special-telehealth-worth

Duarte, J., Martinez, C., & Tomicic, A. (2020). Episodes of meeting in psychotherapy: An empirical exploration of patients' experiences of subjective change during their psychotherapy process. *Research in psychotherapy (Milano), 23*(1), 440. 10.4081/ripppo.2020.440

Fisher, S., Guralnik, T., Fonagy, P., & Zilcha-Mano, S. (2021). Let's face it: Video conferencing psychotherapy requires the extensive use of ostensive cues. *Counselling Psychology Quarterly, 34*(3–4), 508–524.

Gelso, C. J., & Carter, J. A. (1994). Components of the psychotherapy relationship: Their interaction and unfolding during treatment. *Journal of Counseling Psychology, 41*(3), 296.

Glueckauf, R. L., Maheu, M. M., Drude, K. P., Wells, B. A., Wang, Y., Gustafson, D. J., et al. (2018). Survey of psychologists' telebehavioral health practices: Technology use, ethical issues, and training needs. *Professional Psychology: Research and Practice 49*, 205–219. 10.1037/pro0000188

Golland, Y., Mevorach, D., & Levit-Binnun, N. (2019). Affiliative zygomatic synchrony in co-present strangers. *Scientific Reports, 9*(1), 1–10.

Hietanen, J. O., Peltola, M. J., & Hietanen, J. K. (2020). Psychophysiological responses to eye contact in a live interaction and in video call. *Psychophysiology, 57*, e13587. 10.1111/psyp.13587

Lyons-Ruth, K., Bruschweiler-Stern, N., Harrison, A. M., Morgan, A. C., Nahum, J. P., Sander, L., & Tronick, E. Z. (1998). Implicit relational knowing: Its role in development and psychoanalytic treatment. *Infant Mental Health Journal: Official Publication of The World Association for Infant Mental Health, 19*(3), 282–289.

Markowitz, J. C., Milrod, B., Heckman, T. G., Bergman, M., Amsalem, D., Zalman, H., Ballas, T., & Neria, Y. (2021). Psychotherapy at a distance. *American Journal of Psychiatry, 178*, 240–246. 10.1176/appi.ajp.2020.20050557

Messina, I., & Loffler-Stastka, H. (2021). Psychotherapists' perception of their clinical skills and in-session feelings in live therapy versus online therapy during the COVID-19 pandemic: A pilot study. *Research in Psychotherapy: Psychopathology, Process, and Outcome, 24*(1), 53–59. 10.4081/ripppo.2021.514

Önen Ünsalver, B., Evrensel, A., Kaya Yertutanol, F. D., Dönmez, A., & Ceylan, M. E. (2021). The changeable positioning of the couch and repositioning to face-to-face arrangement in psychoanalysis to facilitate the experience of being seen. *Frontiers in Psychology, 12*, 718319. 10.3389/fpsyg.2021.718319

Perry, K., Gold, S., & Shearer, E. M. (2020). Identifying and addressing mental health providers' perceived barriers to clinical video telehealth utilization. *Journal of Clinical Psychology, 76*, 1125–1134. 10.1002/jclp.22770

Porges, S. W. (2021). *Polyvagal safety: Attachment, communication, self-regulation (IPNB)* (pp. 75). New York, NY: W. W. Norton & Company.

Ramseyer, F., & Tschacher, W. (2011). Nonverbal synchrony in psychotherapy: Coordinated body movement refects relationship quality and outcome. *Journal of Consulting and Clinical Psychology, 79*(3), 284–295. 10.1037/a0023419

Sampaio, M., Haro, M., De Sousa, B., Melo, W. V., & Hoffman, H. G. (2021). Therapists make the switch to telepsychology to safely continue treating their patients during the COVID-19 pandemic. Virtual reality telepsychology may be next. *Frontiers in Virtual Reality, 1*, 576421. 10.3389/frvir.2020.576421

Appendix: Looking Forwards – What and How Other Technologies will Impact Online Therapy?

Adam Leighton, Haim Weinberg, and Arnon Rolnick

The scope of our book prevents us from including many available or imminent technologies that may affect clinical online psychotherapy. In the following paragraphs, we briefly mention some notable developments and their potential impact. We examine new and evolving therapeutic frameworks and the impact through different stages in therapy (Intake/Diagnosis/Assessment, enhancing the session, therapist feedback & assessment, and between/post session).

As we demonstrate, the effect of the COVID-19 pandemic may not be limited to simply swapping our clinic for a video session.

Therapeutic Framework

The introduction of computer-assisted therapy (CAT) technologies has great potential to enhance psychotherapy. However, these technologies are frequently regarded as tools to be used separately from traditional psychotherapy. Moreover, psychotherapy tends to prefer offering one modality of therapy or another, but not incorporating a number of modalities at the same time working in synergy. Patients are often offered either self-help utilising CAT or support groups, psychotherapy with a therapist, or group based therapies but rarely a holistic approach integrating multiple approaches. DBT is a clear exception that by definition includes various modalities in parallel.

Indeed, the British initiative 'Improving Access to Psychological Therapies' led by the UK National Health Service offers a myriad of services, split into either 'low intensity' e.g., guided self-help, computerised CBT and group-based physical activity programmes or 'high intensity' such as CBT or IPT. However as the specific provider tends to be different, there are few if any combined provisions.

Developing technologies are starting to change this divergent approach. Blended care frameworks are being offered that combine support groups, interactive self-help software, immediate text-based support, and video-based therapy sessions. An interesting service offered by a US medical center is a therapeutic clinic integrating technology from smartphone apps and multiple sensors into therapy sessions. Many commercial platforms include online assessment questionnaires to assist matching client to therapist.

An area in which we are seeing innovative approaches is corporate wellness solutions or as they are known in the US, Employee Assistance Programs (EAP's). Although not within the scope of our book, the integrative blended approaches offered by many EAP service providers are worthy of mention. Companies are providing a blended approach, including online screening, triage, assessment, online therapy, and digitised self-help solutions.

We believe that these developments' impacts are twofold. Both the platforms themselves are an important offering, but furthermore, the understanding that an integrative approach is not only viable but also effective. We would like to see more providers and clinics combining different approaches and tools for their patients' best possible outcome. Therapy does not have to, and maybe should not be limited to the therapist's 50-minute slot.

Initial Stages of Therapy

Intake / Diagnosis / Assessment

The use of automated screening and triage tools is a natural step forwards. These tools are increasingly taking advantage of artificial intelligence both for the input (speech recognition) and the analysis (semantic and content). Already available are offerings for screening patients to identify, measure and monitor depression and anxiety symptoms. A UK-based provider offers online text-based CBT therapy and has integrated AI-based tools to support their therapists' diagnosis and identify patients likely to drop out. We forecast that similar tools based on voice and video will become more readily available in the near future. Lee et al. (2021) describe various technologies and use cases of AI for clinical diagnosis.

Predicting patient response to different treatments and modalities may be possible in the future utilising the ability of AI to analyse 'big data' (Lee et al., 2021). Commercial offerings are presently reaching the market predicting and identifying behaviours, such as suicidal ideation and depression. This is supported by research demonstrating the ability of using big data analysis methods with the content of social media, e.g., Lekkas et al. (2021), Roy et al. (2020), and Li et al. (2020).

Interestingly, one group of researchers found that people were more forthcoming in disclosing confidential information with a computer system than with a person (Lucas, 2014). This has interesting implications on the concept of patient intake.

In Session

Working with patients online increases the opportunities to utilise digital tools for two main reasons. The very fact that we are working with the patient in a computerised environment allows a more natural transition to the use of computer based tools. Secondly, the use of digital media during online sessions (text, sound, and image) allows access to valuable data to which AI tools can be applied both real-time and post-session.

Enhancing Sessions

Different chapters in the book relate to the use of technologies during sessions in addition to the video communication platform itself. We have learnt about the use of online games, music and videos, photographs, the use of a digital whiteboard, biofeedback instrumentation, and digital therapy cards.

There are many other technologies of different levels of maturity that can and will allow us to enhance our online sessions. These technologies may help improve our existing skills, provide additional insight, and add additional levels of experientiality. Examples of areas in which technology can enhance sessions include:

- The virtual space during video conference sessions: The popular video conferencing platforms are now offering new forms (known as immersive or together mode) of displaying participants on screen, potentially offering a feeling of a shared experience allowing the therapist and client to view the therapeutic dyad. For example, using these modes, the therapist may virtually shake hands with a patient or two members of a couple may place a soothing hand on the other's shoulder.

  These developments may also help solve issues such as the ability to understand who the therapist is looking at during couple therapy.
- Various new cameras suitable for video conferencing are becoming more affordable and available. Of particular interest are those offering the ability to move left/right (PAN), up/down (TILT), and magnification (ZOOM). These movements are usually controlled using a mouse, hand-gestures or remote control. Some can automatically track elements such as a face using AI.

  These abilities allow us to both see the patients' facial expressions and also to see their movement and preparation on the physical plane within the room. Furthermore, during couple or family therapy, the use of these cameras can also alleviate the difficulty identifying to whom the therapist is looking at.

  An interesting question is who controls the camera. For example, during a family therapy session, family members may point the camera at anyone who wants to talk at that moment or all the participants at the same time.

  The ability of a camera to track movement can remove the patient and therapists' umbilical cord connecting them to the screen, allowing them to get up from their chair, move around, and possibly play with toys in a room.

- Clinical decision support (CDS) tools – Commonplace in the traditional healthcare industry, these tools and systems aim to provide actionable clinical recommendations. Even in traditional healthcare environments, although CDS systems are becoming commonplace, user adoption is still poor due to problems of accuracy and lack of transparency (Antoniadi et al., 2021). The approach suggested by Antoniadi and his team emphasises that systems need to explain in case why it has a given that recommendation. In session CDS tools in mental health could provide insight regarding patient (and therapist) attributes, such as cognitive flexibility, mood, engagement, therapeutic alliance, and suicidal risk.

  Some of these insights are already available, for example one company provides therapists with an assessment on the therapeutic alliance based on the voices of patient and therapist during sessions.

  The data supporting CDS tools can be based on a) biomarkers, such as facial expressions, posture, breathing, eye-tracking, prosody, or direct measurement using biofeedback style instruments measuring HRV, GSR, or other signals. b) Conversation content. This data can also be directly reflected to the therapist and possibly patient during the session.

- Therapist feedback – Miller et al. (2015) describe the value (and potential dangers) of routine outcome monitoring (ROM), i.e., frequent measuring of patient related variables using different rating scales. It has been demonstrated that ROM can greatly improve effect size, and therapeutic alliance (Brattland 2019). Miller (2015, 2018) examines how deliberate practice ('measuring baseline performance, obtaining specific and on-going feedback, engaging in deliberate practice through rehearsing and evaluating a plan for improvement') (Miller et al., 2013) can offer a 'potent and reliable method for improving performance'.

  During online therapy data gathered during sessions from both patient and therapist may assist the therapist striving to apply the principles of deliberate practice. Specific therapist centric information can be generated and provided to the therapist in real time. Bickman (2020) discusses the disparity between the claimed application and actual practice of evidence-based care. Real-time (or close to real time) feedback could potentially contribute to improved application of evidence based approaches.

  An example of an available product is software for the measurement of therapist's usage of evidence-based treatment strategies. The use of such solutions undoubtedly provide therapists with an opportunity to improve performance and consequently patient outcome.

- Note taking – A fairly mundane aspect of most therapists work includes note-taking. Many different solutions are available for therapists working online to automate the note-taking process. This may allow therapists increased attention to the session itself.

- Supporting specific therapeutic techniques – for example exposure – e.g., VR, relaxation techniques, psychoeducation, and skills development.

Between Sessions

Active therapeutic approaches place great importance on the patient's work between sessions. We have described in the section 'therapeutic framework' the blended approach integrating different forms of therapy and supporting tools. Between sessions work is easily supported using various tools and technologies.

One such group of tools are interactive 'reminders' facilitating the patient's effort to implement tools and strategies learned during sessions. Various levels of sophistication are possible, starting from the most basic such as a reminder set on the patient's mobile phone, the use of interactive reminders. The most advanced level, yet to be implemented at the time of publication, would include the interaction between biomarkers measured by wearables and tailored 'reminders' set with the patient during sessions.

After Sessions

- Patient outcome measures – Brattland et al. (2018) examined the positive impact of constant monitoring of patient outcome measures at the end of each session. Working online allows simple and immediate measurement using solutions such as built in polls or dedicated solutions. The psychlops questionnaire (Ashworth et al., 2004) is a patient generated outcome measure (Roe et al., 2022) which is highly suitable for computerisation.

AI based bots may be used for brief 'interviews' at the end of therapy sessions allowing the gathering and analysis of qualitative data. Similar solutions are in common use in markets such as consumer intelligence (AI survey chatbots).

Driving Technologies

Above, we addressed the present and near-future impact of technology on online therapy. We briefly describe the driving technologies we believe underlying the above clinical applications.

- Artificial Intelligence

  - Vision recognition – eye tracking, body & facial expression analysis.
  - Voice recognition and prosody analysis.
  - Natural Language Processing (NLP).
  - Decision Intelligence.
  - Big data analysis (see examples above)
  - Virtual therapists – the provision of [limited] therapy by an AI-based agent using virtual audio and visual avatars allowing a patient to

participate in a session with a human like image. ELIZA[1] in the 22th century!

- Growing availability of wearable biometric units such as smart watches (Rolnick et al., 2021).
- Internet of things (Iot) – growing availability of non-biometric data that can provide behavioural data regarding patients' lives (e.g., opening the fridge, using cellphone).
- Metaverse and Virtual Reality (VR) – the ability to provide controlled, realistic experiences.
- Blockchain – a blockchain can be seen as a digital ledger of transactions that are linked together using cryptography, duplicated and distributed across a network of computer systems. Blockchain technology may play a key part in securely sharing personal data gathered using different devices and applications thus allowing collection of huge quantities of valuable data allowing big data analysis and providing insights as described above.

Summary

We believe that technology can and will continue to improve the quality of therapy in general and online therapy specifically. The extraordinary developments in the field of artificial intelligence will certainly enhance therapists, however we doubt that in the near future, therapy will be without 'a human in the loop'.

Note

1 ELIZA was a computer program developed in the 1960's, simulating a therapist. An example can be seen here: http://psych.fullerton.edu/mbirnbaum/psych101/eliza.htm

References

Antoniadi, A. M., Du, Y., Guendouz, Y., Wei, L., Mazo, C., Becker, B. A., & Mooney, C. (2021). Current challenges and future opportunities for XAI in machine learning-based clinical decision support systems: A systematic review. *Applied Sciences*, *11*(11), 5088.

Ashworth, M., Shepherd, M., Christey, J., Matthews, V., Wright, K., Parmentier, H., ... & Godfrey, E. (2004). A client-generated psychometric instrument: The development of 'PSYCHLOPS'. *Counselling and Psychotheraphy Research*, *4*(2), 27–31.

Bickman, L. (2020). Improving mental health services: A 50-year journey from randomized experiments to artificial intelligence and precision mental health. *Administration and Policy in Mental Health and Mental Health Services Research*, *47*(5), 795–843.

Brattland, H., Koksvik, J. M., Burkeland, O., Gråwe, R. W., Klöckner, C., Linaker, O. M., ... & Iversen, V. C. (2018). The effects of routine outcome monitoring (ROM) on therapy outcomes in the course of an implementation process: A randomized clinical trial. *Journal of Counseling Psychology*, *65*(5), 641.

Brattland, H., Koksvik, J. M., Burkeland, O., Klöckner, C. A., Lara-Cabrera, M. L., Miller, S. D., Wampold, B., Ryum, T., & Iversen, V. C. (2019). Does the working alliance mediate the effect of routine outcome monitoring (ROM) and alliance feedback on psychotherapy outcomes? A secondary analysis from a randomized clinical trial. *Journal of Counseling Psychology*, *66*(2), 234–246. 10.1037/cou0000320

Fisher, S., Guralnik, T., Fonagy, P., & Zilcha-Mano, S. (2021). Let's face it: video conferencing psychotherapy requires the extensive use of ostensive cues. *Counselling Psychology Quarterly*, *34*(3–4), 508–524. 10.1080/09515070.2020.1777535

Lee, E. E., Torous, J., De Choudhury, M., Depp, C. A., Graham, S. A., Kim, H. C., … & Jeste, D. V. (2021). Artificial intelligence for mental healthcare: Clinical applications, barriers, facilitators, and artificial wisdom. *Biological Psychiatry: Cognitive Neuroscience and Neuroimaging*.

Lekkas, D., Klein, R. J., & Jacobson, N. C. (2021). Predicting acute suicidal ideation on Instagram using ensemble machine learning models. *Internet Interventions*, *25*, 100424. 10.1016/j.invent.2021.100424

Li, S., Wang, Y., Xue, J., Zhao, N., & Zhu, T. (2020). The impact of COVID-19 epidemic declaration on psychological consequences: A study on active Weibo users. *International Journal of Environmental Research and Public Health*, *17*(6), 2032. 10.3390/ijerph17062032

Lee, E. E., Torous, J., De Choudhury, M., Depp, C. A., Graham, S. A., Kim, H.-C., Paulus, M. P., Krystal, J. H., & Jeste, D. V. (2021). Artificial Intelligence for Mental Health Care: Clinical Applications, Barriers, Facilitators, and Artificial Wisdom. *Biological Psychiatry: Cognitive Neuroscience and Neuroimaging*, 6, 856–864. 10.1016/j.bpsc.2021.02.001.

Lucas, G. M., Gratch, J., King, A., & Morency, L. P. (2014). It's only a computer: Virtual humans increase willingness to disclose. *Computers in Human Behavior*, *37*, 94–100.

Miller, S. D., Chow, D., Wampold, B. E., Hubble, M. A., Del Re, A. C., Maeschalck, C., & Bargmann, S. (2020). To be or not to be (an expert)? Revisiting the role of deliberate practice in improving performance. *High Ability Studies*, *31*(1), 5–15.

Miller, S. D., Hubble, M. A., Chow, D. L., & Seidel, J. A. (2013). The outcome of psychotherapy: Yesterday, today, and tomorrow. *Psychotherapy: Theory, Research, and Practice*, *50*, 88–97. 10.1037/a0031097

Miller, S. D., Hubble, M. A., Chow, D., & Seidel, J. (2015). Beyond measures and monitoring: Realizing the potential of feedback-informed treatment. *Psychotherapy*, *52*(4), 449–457. 10.1037/pst0000031

Miller, S. D., Hubble, M. A., & Chow, D.(2018).The question of expertise in psychotherapy. *Journal of Expertise*, 1 12-129.

National Collaborating Centre for Mental Health. (2018). *The improving access to psychological therapies manual.* UK: NCCMH.

Roe, D., Slade, M., & Jones, N. (2022). The utility of patient-reported outcome measures in mental health. *World Psychiatry*, *21*(1), 56.

Rolnick, A., Ehrenreich, Y., & Leighton, A. (2021). Psychophysiological therapy from a distance: The art of sharing. *Biofeedback*, *49*(1), 18–24.

Roy, A., Nikolitch, K., McGinn, R., Jinah, S., Klement, W., & Kaminsky, Z. A. (2020). A machine learning approach predicts future risk to suicidal ideation from social media data. *NPJ Digital Medicine*, *3*(1), 1–12. 10.1038/s41746-020-0287-6

Index